Nat...
Weight Loss

Natural Health and Weight Loss

Dr Barry Groves

with a Foreword by
Professor Joel M. Kaufman

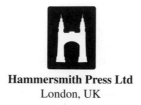

Hammersmith Press Ltd
London, UK

First published in 2007 by Hammersmith Press Limited
496 Fulham Palace Road, London SW6 6JD, UK
www.hammersmithpress.co.uk

Whilst the advice and information in this book are believed to be true and accurate at the date of going to press, neither the author nor the publisher can accept any legal responsibility or liability for any errors or omissions that may be made. In particular (but without limiting the generality of the preceding disclaimer) every effort has been made to check drug and supplement dosages; however, it is still possible that errors may have been missed. Furthermore, dosage schedules are constantly being revised and new side effects recognized. For these reasons readers are strongly urged to consult printed instructions before taking any drugs or supplements recommended in this book.

British Library Cataloguing in Publication Data: A CIP record of this book is available from the British Library.

ISBN 978-1-905140-15-2

Commissioning editor: Georgina Bentliff
Edited by Carolyn Holleyman
Designed by Julie Bennett
Typeset by Phoenix Photosetting, Chatham, Kent
Production by Helen Whitehorn, Pathmedia
Printed and bound by TJ International Ltd, Padstow, Cornwall, UK
Cover image: Woman Meditating by the Sea © Angelo Cavalli/Befa/CORBIS
Illustration on page 313: Still Life with Eggs by Jennifer A. Mills

Table of Contents

Table of Contents

Preface

My story

This is where it all started for me: if I and my wife, Monica, hadn't been overweight, I probably would not have written this book – or any other.

When we were married in April 1957 I weighed 11½ stones (161 lb or 73 kg) and Monica weighed ten stones (140 lb or 62 kg). These were quite normal weights as we were five feet nine inches (1.75 m) and five feet six inches (1.67 m) tall respectively.

Monica was a good cook, and used to cooking for her parents and sister as well as herself.

We hadn't got much money so Monica made her own bread; she also made cakes and biscuits. It wasn't long before we started to put weight on.

Over the next five years our weights yo-yoed as we tried low-calorie dieting, sweaty clothes, 'inert fillers' and played tennis and badminton, swam, and walked everywhere. We lost weight, put it on again; lost weight, put it on again, and so on. I'm sure you know what I mean.

Nothing worked in the long term. Monica weighed 12 stone (168 lb or 74 kg) at her peak and my weight went up to 13½ stone (189 lb or 84 kg).

In 1960 we started to cut down on the carbohydrates (carbs). In those days it was the thing to do, but it only worked up to a point. Just cutting calories didn't work; we got hungry. Replacing the carbs with protein was not only expensive, we didn't feel right eating that way – it was as though something was missing, and we still struggled with our weight.

In 1962, I was posted by the Royal Air Force to Singapore. We hadn't been there long when I discovered a doctor who guided me to the other half of the equation: 'When you cut down on carbs, you must replace them with fat,' he said.

He had to be joking, right? We knew that fat contained far more calories than carbs or protein. It seemed ridiculous to suggest we eat fat. But, having tried everything else, we decided to give it a go.

It worked! By 1963 Monica's weight was 8 st 10 lb (122 lb or 54 kg), a loss of over 40 lb; mine was the 11 st 7 lb it had been when we married. That started me thinking. If what looked like a high-calorie diet was good for weight loss, why were we told to eat a low-calorie diet? I wanted to know.

At the time, being in the RAF, I couldn't do much research. Monica and I ate our fried egg and bacon breakfasts, fat meat followed by fruit and cream dinners – and our weights stayed down. The fatter cuts of meat were also cheaper because they weren't so popular and that suited us just fine. But the best part was that we had no difficulty living this way at all, and our weights continued to stay down.

In 1971 I started to give a talk about our experience entitled 'The Fat of the Land' to clubs like Women's Institute, Young Farmers, and anyone else who would listen. By the late 1970s, however, we started to hear that the sort of diet we ate, which was high in animal fats, was bad for us: it caused heart disease, they said.

With my previous experience, I wondered how much truth there was in this. I therefore determined to leave the RAF as soon as I could, and research diet to find out. In 1982 I did just that, and have been doing full-time research into nutrition and health in general ever since. This book is based on what I have learned.

As I'm sure you have discovered, the difficult part of weight control isn't actually losing weight, it's keeping it off – for life. Monica has now had 45 years of eating fried breakfasts, fat meat, extra-large eggs, full-fat cheese, and fruit and cream and so on, as well as vegetables and fruit. Her weight has been around 9 st (126 lb or 54 kg) and mine has been around 11 st 7 lb (161 lb or 73 kg) for as long as we can remember.

It is a diet that works – for life!

Barry Groves 2007

Foreword

Much more than a re-write of his 1999 book on diet (*Eat Fat Get Thin*), Barry Groves' new book is far more complete and even better referenced. The low-carbohydrate theme is expounded consistently and to good effect. Groves has not lost his talent for exceptionally readable prose, and his ability to explain nutritional concepts clearly to non-specialists is fully intact.

The progression of abdominal obesity to syndrome X to hypoglycæmia to adult diabetes is well known now. The cause of it all is shown to be excessive consumption of carbohydrates in food choices. The seriousness of the condition is that it leads to atherosclerosis, including in the coronary arteries, as well as to all the other complications of diabetes.

Unlike many credentialed 'experts', Groves is not fooled by the supposed holiness of whole grains. He writes that starches in these grains, as well as most sugars, are converted to glucose when digested. Too high glucose levels lead to too high insulin levels. One effect of the latter is body fat formation.

Groves is not seduced by 'low-carb' synthetic foods. He notes that their protein content may be inferior to that of animal protein; that their sweeteners may reinforce a long-term craving for sweets, which we would do well to lose; and that such foods are very expensive. He advocates real food, pointing out that 'slimming foods' are a profitable industry. He also counsels avoiding diabetic foods, as the premise for them is faulty; and they are also expensive.

Groves is one of the few who praise the British contribution to world cuisine – the wonderful breakfast of bacon and eggs, noting its lasting quality throughout the day compared with rapidly digested carbs, however trendy, such as a croissant or baguette.

He notes that 'healthy eating' in the UK is not healthy, that a calorie in is not always a calorie absorbed, making calorie-counting useless, and that the Glycæmic Index is of limited use, since it varies so much with the duration of cooking and for other reasons that he explains.

A simple theme is pursued throughout the book – eat no more than 50-60 grams of carbohydrate per day. Replace the carbohydrate not eaten with fat, not with protein. Leave the fat on meat. Try to have some organ meats. Lose the nonsense that saturated fats are dangerous in any way. Half the fat in human breast milk is saturated!

Get set for an entertaining yet accurate read. This is the best non-technical book on diet I have ever seen.

Joel M. Kauffman, PhD
Berwyn, PA, USA
2007

Introduction

One must attend in medical practice not primarily to plausible theories
but to experience combined with reason.

Hippocrates

Firstly, thank you for buying this book. I hope you will ultimately thank me for
writing it. It's possible that you have a weight or health problem; or maybe a delayed
flight in a far-flung airport drove you to buy the only English book left on the book
stall. Your dieting journey has perhaps taken you along the disappointing route of
low-calorie, low-fat, high-fibre 'healthy eating' – but with no satisfactory results for
you. For many it's a life of counting calories and cutting fat off, of eating bland, dry
food, inert fillers, and meal replacements, and taking lots of exercise when you have
better things to do. And the result a year later? After a brief weight loss,
disappointment and even wider hips.

I, too, have been on that journey, until I managed to solve the dieting conundrum
over 40 years ago. Yes, I have not had a weight problem since 1962.

In the 1950s and 1960s the solution to being overweight was to cut back on sugar
and starchy foods such as bread and potatoes. My wife, Monica, and I started to do
that in 1960. It worked, but only up to a point. The essential ingredient missing until
1962 was the other half of the equation: eat more fat. After we added that in 1962 it
was easy. I shrank from a fat 189 lb and rising body-weight to a 160 lb normal

weight in less than a year – and I have maintained that weight to this day. Monica also lost her excess weight. We didn't starve; we were never hungry; we didn't deprive ourselves; our meals were, and still are, all enjoyable.

In those days the only fast food was fish and chips, with none of the temptations of Kentucky Fried Chicken (KFC) and McDonald's. The food we ate then, and still do today, was fresh, unprocessed and mainly locally produced.

We were told then, as now, that eating fat makes you fat. It doesn't – and I speak with nearly half a century of experience. But don't just take my word for it; there is an overwhelming body of clinical and population study evidence to disprove that idea, but no-one bothers to read how other races and tribes live very healthily on their 'unhealthy' diet. Clinical trials, conducted under controlled hospital conditions, which show that eating fat actually makes weight loss easier are also ignored. The historical evidence for the effectiveness of the way I eat has been gathering dust in medical libraries since the mid-1800s. We are brainwashed into believing all we hear, especially by ill-informed TV pundits and 'celebrities'. The constant propaganda churned out by the media is rarely medically or scientifically based; it is driven by profit motives and ignorance.

So, with a picture of a pretty girl who has probably never had a weight problem, the cover of the women's magazine stacked on the newsagent's shelf exhorts you to 'Fit in that bikini: lose 20 pounds in two weeks with our easy weight loss plan'. It's not alone: there is a whole row of similar magazines and newspapers, all with variations on the same message. There are new ones every week, and new diet fads seem to appear with similar regularity, not to mention advertisements and programmes for women (mainly) on TV and radio.

We are constantly inundated with a new 'magic' formula that (we are assured) is tried and tested, and guaranteed to work miracles. Everyone, including many doctors, are agreed that if we want to 'melt' the fat off our bodies, all we have to do is reduce our calorie intake and do a bit more exercise. Do that, they all say, and your fat will disappear so fast you are in danger of leaving a greasy streak behind you.

But, if that works, and if it is so easy to do, why are there so many fat people about today? The answer, of course, is because this plausible theory is totally wrong! Calorie control doesn't work in the long term. You're being 'had' every day.

The 10 September 1994 edition of the *British Medical Journal* published two papers about obesity. One expressed grave reservations about the effectiveness of present dietary treatments for obesity[1] while the other asked: Should we treat obesity?[2] Being overweight has affected a small proportion of the population for centuries, but clinical obesity was relatively rare until the late twentieth century. Indeed obesity remained at a fairly stable low level until about 1980. Then the numbers of overweight people began to increase dramatically. By 1992 one in every ten people in Britain was obese; a mere five years later that figure had almost doubled. In the USA it is even worse: by 1991 one in three adults was overweight. That was an increase of 8% of the population over just one decade despite the fact that, as a commentary in the 16 July 1994 edition of the *Lancet* pointed out, Americans spend a massive $33 billion a year on 'slimming', as well as taking more exercise, and eating fewer calories and less fat than they did ten years ago. There is now a pandemic of increasing weight, and the diseases that accompany this condition, across the industrialised world.

It may be hard to believe, but this has occurred in the face of increasing knowledge, awareness, and education about obesity, nutrition and exercise. It has happened despite the fact that calorie intake had gone down by 20% over the past ten years and exercise clubs have mushroomed. More people are cutting calories now than ever before in their history yet more of them are becoming overweight. Why should this be?

'Civilised' man is the world's only fat animal

The fact is that obesity does not afflict any other animal species. Wherever you look around the world, you will not find an overweight animal in the wild. Animals in their natural habitat are either hunters or hunted. If they were overweight, either they would have difficulty catching their prey, or they would be easier for the carnivores to catch. An overweight animal would not survive for long. It is true that there are animals which carry a large amount of fat: whales, for example, who have it as insulation against the cold Arctic waters; or bears who store fat as a food reserve for hibernation in the winter. But this is natural; they are not overweight. Whether it is a herd of cows, a hive of bees, a pride of lions, or any other animal species, all the animals in a species are essentially the same size and none is obese. Obesity is also noticeably absent in primitive human cultures.

The only animal to get overweight is 'civilised' man – and his pets – and that fact is highly significant. The reason cannot be genetic or hereditary, as some argue. If it were, obesity would have plagued us for generations, and it cannot be simply that we eat too much, although many of us do. If an abundance of food were the cause, other animals with an ample food supply would also get fat, yet they don't. If that were the reason, cutting calories would work, yet it doesn't, except in the short term.

Fat facts

The prevailing wisdom over the past several years has been that fat makes you fat, and that if you simply stop eating fat, you'll lose weight without even trying. I'm sorry, it doesn't work – but you have probably discovered that for yourself.

In a supplement to the *American Journal of Clinical Nutrition* in 1998 entitled 'Is dietary fat a major determinant of body fat?',[3] Professor Walter Willett of Harvard University School of Medicine wrote of a study which confirmed what many of us have realised for years – that if there is a weight loss associated with changing to a low-fat dietary regime, it is statistically small and the results are highly short-lived – when he found:

> '. . .fat consumption within the range of 18–40% of energy appears to have little if any effect on body fatness.'

So cutting fats doesn't work. Dr Willett continued:

> 'Moreover, . . . a substantial decline in the percentage of energy from fat consumed during the past two decades has corresponded with a massive increase in obesity.'

This has become blindingly obvious. Could cutting fat be the *cause* of obesity? Dr Willett concluded:

> 'Diets high in fat do not appear to be the primary cause of the high prevalence of excess body fat in our society, and reductions in fat will not be a solution.'

He's quite right, but there is more: as fat in the diet is a significant contributor to being satisfied with a meal, low-fat diets often leave dieters very hungry. In other words, those who tell you that, to maintain a normal weight you must cut down on fats, want you to live your life being hungry most of the time, and you simply can't do it. Your body is not designed to operate in this way and it rebels. No other animal on this planet counts the percentage of fat calories (or any other calories) in its diet, and there is no reason we should either.

When a calorie isn't a calorie

The first orthodox Golden Rule for treating overweight is: **Calories in minus calories out equals weight change**. As you will see later, although this hypothesis looks plausible on the surface and has what looks like umpteen good, solid, rigorous, clinical studies appearing to support it, it is actually quite wrong.

However, if we assume it is correct, that brings up the first big problem; how do we answer the apparently simple question: *How many calories are there in this food item?*

Despite supermarkets' desire for uniformity, natural food products can vary widely from item to item. An early season fruit, for example, may be much lower in sugar than one from the peak of the season; a green banana is mostly starch, while an overripe one is mostly sugar.

And that is only the first problem. The second is even harder to answer: *How much energy do you use when you do something?* If you walk a mile you will use less energy than someone else who walks the same distance, but weighs more. If you walk quicker your energy usage will differ from someone who walks more slowly.

Dr Willett's study talked about how, when people changed to a low-fat diet in a metabolic ward experiment for a couple of weeks they lost some weight. However, a few weeks later, when the subjects had returned home, the regulatory systems in their bodies ensured that the weight they lost was replaced. Therefore, it doesn't work. The problem with this approach is that you cannot know how much energy to take in. Neither can you know how much you are using.

The second Golden Rule of orthodoxy is: **'A calorie is a calorie'** – no matter where it comes from. This means that if you eat X number of calories more than you use up, you will put on Y amount of weight, wherever those calories come from. However, as will be demonstrated later in this book, studies looking at diets with equal calorie content but different constituents have proved conclusively that this is not the case. Dieters on fat-based diets in clinical trials have always lost much more weight than dieters on carb-based diets, even when both types of diet had exactly the same number of calories.

So 'a calorie is a calorie is a calorie' is not so meaningful after all: a carbohydrate calorie is obviously much more fattening than a fat calorie. So do calories count? Of course they do – but some don't count as much as others.

There is an emerging scientific consensus that the old ideas that overweight people are lazy gluttons are as absurd and insulting as the overweight have always thought they were.

Carbs are worst

Over the last few years, things have started to change. There is now little argument that an excess of dietary carbs is the prime cause of overweight and obesity (and, incidentally, many other diseases). This is widely recognised. In fact, there is so much evidence against carbs in the literature that anyone who tells people to eat more of the stuff must have an ulterior motive. We will come to that in a moment.

But there is no way that we as a species can cut down too much on carbs unless we either eat more of something else or starve. Scientists, therefore, started to study whether some carbs might be less harmful than others. They found that this was the case, and the Glycaemic Index (GI) was developed. Carbs that didn't raise glucose as much were called 'low-GI', while those that did were labelled 'high-GI'. This principle now forms the basis for many of the diet books around today.

Unfortunately, what started out looking like an exciting breakthrough isn't the be-all and end-all it is claimed to be.

Low-GI is only half of the answer . . .

When I wrote *Eat Fat, Get Thin!* in 1999, it was one of the first popular weight loss diet books to talk about the Glycaemic Index. At that time GI looked like a useful aid, not only for weight loss, but also for health in general. However, in the six years since I wrote that, I have been dismayed by the way that the GI has been misrepresented in popular diet books where it has now been hijacked by the discredited 'healthy eating' dictocrats in an attempt to reinforce their low-calorie message.

GI is concerned only with the amount that *carbs* raise blood glucose levels. As proteins and fats don't raise glucose levels, they aren't included in the GI.

This is unfortunate as it allowed many popular diet book authors who had previously exhorted their readers to cut calories and eat low-fat diets, merely to modify their message to talk about 'good carbs' and 'bad carbs' – and then continue to preach exactly the same low-calorie advice that is a major cause of the obesity epidemic we see today. Foods that have a GI of zero – and, thus, are the lowest GI of all – are stigmatised if they don't fit with preconceived low-calorie ideologies.

One current low-GI diet book, for example, states clearly that the authors believe that saturated fats are not unhealthy.[4] But the authors have deliberately left out red meat and restricted dairy products and eggs because, they say, they want 'no contentious elements whatsoever'.

In other words, the GI in this book is deliberately misrepresented and the readers misinformed because, in fact, the 'saturated' fats on red meat are firstly mainly *un*saturated and secondly, *not* unhealthy as, indeed, the authors acknowledge. They and dairy products such as butter, cream and cheeses also contain a fatty acid called *conjugated linoleic acid* which a mountain of evidence proves is a powerful anti-cancer agent as well as a very useful aid to weight loss. And the most saturated fat of all in nature, coconut oil, is probably the healthiest oil of them all as well as being the best for weight loss. So, in bowing to convention, this book deprives its readers of some very important medical evidence.

I refuse to toe that party line – which tends to make me unpopular with my peers – but it does give you, the reader, the only source of reliable evidence on which to base your dietary decisions.

GI is discussed in Chapter 11 of this book but, as it stands now, GI is over-sold and over-hyped. Presented honestly, GI can be a useful tool – and this book does present GI honestly.

. . . The other half of the answer is insulin

The amount of glucose put in the blood by carbs is only half the story. Excess glucose in the bloodstream is harmful. Our bodies know this and so they produce insulin to get that excess out. They do this by storing the excess as body fat. In this sense, insulin is a fattening hormone. If you eat lots of carbs, the high levels of insulin that result not only stop you losing weight, they also increase the risk of other serious diseases such as heart disease and cancer. So it is not only glucose that must be considered, but insulin as well, and in this respect, once again many books mislead dangerously.

While proteins don't raise glucose levels, they do raise blood insulin. For this reason, it's no good looking at carbs alone. We have to consider the whole picture. This book does just that and, in so doing, it goes beyond current low-GI books.

The overweight are a ready source of income

And so back to the ulterior motive: the slimming industry really doesn't want you to know these facts, and neither do some popular diet book publishers. They all rely on you for a very comfortable living, so you are kept in the dark unless (1) you know where to look for the right information and (2) you know what is truth and what is not. So let's look at how you are exploited.

Jules Hirsch, of Rockefeller University, New York, observed in the 1994 Herman Award Lecture to the American Society for Clinical Nutrition:[5]

> 'The public must understand that all current methods, from thigh creams to stomach staples, are like gropes in the dark, and as such, are either totally ineffectual or are no more than counterforces to an incompletely understood regulatory disorder. There are no cures at this time.'

Although the first sentence of this statement is correct, Hirsch was wrong in the second, as this book will show. However, Dr Hirsch put his finger on a major stumbling block when he continued:

> 'The ambiguities inherent in [the] problem . . . [have] led to the growth of a flourishing industry for weight control. The basic tenets of this industry are that there are commercially available programs that can safely lower body weight more easily than those of competitors and unlike their competitors, once the weight is lost, it will remain that way for ever. On this basis an endless set of new products, new diets and drug interventions play legal tag with governmental regulatory agencies while reaping profit from a public desperate for answers.'

Bingo! Hirsch hit the nail squarely on its head: the many commercial interests that rely on overweight people to make a living – and that includes most nutritionists and diet or lifestyle gurus – compound today's weight epidemic.

Walk into any large newsagent's shop today and count the number of slimming magazines. Then add the number of slimming articles in women's magazines, plus also the slimming clubs and manufacturers of slimming products: foods, counselling, exercise equipment and clothes. 'Slimming' is an enormous money-maker. You may not have realised it, but the first concern of slimming businesses is not to help people to slim. They are like any other business, working to make a profit, to increase their market share and, above all, to stay in business. If they published a dietary regime which really did slim you as easily and permanently as they all say they will, would you need to buy the next edition or pay the next club fee? Of course not: if they did that, it would be tantamount to committing commercial suicide. So they don't.

Over the past 20 years or so a number of diet books, videos and regimes have been marketed with miraculous claims for their effects. They claim that a dieter can lose more weight than is safe, yet be safe. One has only to read the medical journals to discover how untrue those claims are. These diets tend to have three things in common: they all restrict fat intake, they all restrict calories, and they all don't work. Yes, you will lose some weight but in over 97% of cases it all goes back on again – and usually a bit more besides. So you try another diet, buy another book or join another club and, of course, spend more money.

Over 90% of the British population has tried dieting at some time or other, and at any one time a third of the adult population is trying to lose weight. As the British spend £850 million on top of the Americans' $33 billion (£25 billion), a prosperous slimming industry can look forward with confidence to a never-ending income as products and articles that promise unattainable goals persuade women (mostly) to attempt the impossible.

The magazines know that many women are so desperate to lose weight that, although they constantly fail, they will try any and every new diet that comes along. Whatever it is, they want to be the first to try it. It is not a new phenomenon: as long ago as 29 March 1957, a 108 kg (17-stone) woman appeared on the British ITV programme *State Your Case for £100*. She said that she wanted the money so that she could attend what she called a 'slimming farm'. She did not get the money. No doubt if she'd had £100 (about two months' wages for the average man in 1957) at the time she would have spent it all on slimming. The mere fact that she appeared on the programme at all in front of millions of viewers demonstrated the strength of her need. So diet after diet is published – all destined to fail, but fail in such a way that they make you need the next one. It becomes an addiction that is created and nurtured by the slimming and food industries for profit. For example, did you know that Weight-Watchers, probably the best-known slimming organisation, is a wholly owned subsidiary of Heinz Foods?

In November 1998 a British Channel 4 television series featured a similar weight loss club, Slimming World. The programme showed club members who had shed the most weight being given awards by Margaret Miles Bramwell, Slimming World's founder and Managing Director – and she was obese! Talking on the programme was Pat Sheppard, one of Slimming World's most popular 'co-ordinators'. She was also obese. Pat Sheppard admitted that she believed that if she had never dieted, she would never have had a weight problem – yet she runs a club for dieters that pushes the same message that made her fat. Let's face it, if the people running such clubs and who are, one assumes, experienced and knowledgeable, can't control their weight, what hope is there for their less knowledgeable club members?

Even in specialist hospital obesity clinics, you may not be much better off (although there is the advantage that, as part of the NHS, attendance at one won't cost you anything). An audit of treatments and outcomes was carried out by workers at the Medical Unit, St Bartholomew's Hospital, London, in 1998. They found that only a third of patients lost more than 5% of their body weight during their treatment phase; 43% lost between nothing and 4%; and 25% actually gained weight. Twenty-four per cent of patients reported depressive symptoms and required psychiatric or psychological care or antidepressive drugs.

'Healthy eating' is not the answer

And forget about 'healthy eating'. While the government spends millions on promoting a 'healthy' diet and exercise for weight loss, the truth is that what they are promoting as healthy today is not healthy! The so-called 'healthy diet' is being increasingly questioned by the medical world for the simple reason that, since the low-fat, carbohydrate-based 'healthy eating' recommendations were published in the 1980s, many studies have shown that it is part of the problem not the answer to it.

It is no coincidence that obesity and a whole host of other diseases have 'taken off' since healthy eating was introduced. It is an example of cause and effect.

The idea that a fatty diet leads to heart disease has never been proven – and it isn't for want of trying! Recent studies discussed later in the book have demonstrated that the reverse is true: that high-fat, low-carb diets are far healthier and that the recommendations to base meals on starchy foods and 'eat five portions of fruit and vegetables a day' are not supported by the evidence. These recommendations have increased the numbers of people becoming overweight and contracting other serious diseases such as type-2 diabetes – as well as heart disease, the very disease against which the recommendations were aimed.

And you don't need to eat 'five portions of fruit and vegetables a day' after all. The evidence presented in this book shows that, while two portions a day may be of benefit, you won't gain anything by eating more. The simple fact is that, like practically all other health advice, the '5-a-day' mantra which is parroted increasingly is, as Professor Sir Charles George, medical director of the British Heart Foundation, admitted in 2003, nothing more than unsupported dogma (see Chapter 14).

You will get quite sufficient fruit and vegetables with the way of eating outlined in this book.

Low-carb is best for you

My family and I, after having been overweight, have lived on the low-carb diet described here and maintained a normal weight now for well over 40 years. I have championed this way of eating (it's not a diet), researched, lectured and written about the health benefits of low-carb diets for over 30 years. Even the medical profession is now coming round to this way of thinking: for example, Dr Sylvan Lee Weinberg, a former President of the American College of Cardiology, a former President of the American College of Chest Physicians and current editor of the *American Heart Hospital Journal,* asserted in a paper published in the 4 March 2004 edition of the *Journal of the American College of Cardiology* that it was no longer acceptable to promote on faith alone the current low-fat, high carbohydrate approach to coronary health.[6]

Introduction

Dr Weinberg's critique follows the history of the 'diet-heart' hypothesis for the last century. This hypothesis has historically suggested that diets high in fat intake increase the risk of coronary artery disease, but Dr Weinberg called for a balanced re-evaluation of that belief as he suggested that the current crises of obesity, type 2 diabetes, heart disease and the metabolic syndrome reached epidemic proportions due, in part, to those recommendations which began in earnest in 1984.

Dr Weinberg concludes that 'This diet can no longer be defended . . . by rejecting clinical experience and a growing medical literature suggesting that the much-maligned low-carbohydrate, high-protein diet may have a salutary effect on the epidemics in question' simply because it conforms to current traditional dietary recommendations. You will not be surprised to learn that, while low-carb diets have come in for a great deal of criticism in the media over the past few years, this review by Weinberg in support of them received very little media attention either here in Britain or even in the USA.

Ten days later, Professor Julian Peto, a British cancer specialist also called for children to be put on low-carb diets. He said that he believed the rising numbers of overweight children would prove a bigger threat than cancer – and cancer now affects almost one person in two in this country. That's three times as many cases as when 'healthy eating' was introduced! Professor Peto also received only slight coverage in the news media.

There are certainly vested interests at work to cover up the huge body of evidence supporting the benefits of a low-carb, high-fat diet. I imagine that, in such a litigious society as the USA, and increasingly in the UK, the nutritionists and dieticians, who really should have a better knowledge of their professed subject, dare not admit that they have been wrong and done so much harm, for fear of being sued by the millions of people harmed by their advice. However, the cracks are beginning to show and it only needs a trigger to cause this precarious house of cards to collapse. Weinberg's paper could be that trigger.

No more dieting

So, what should you be eating to reduce and maintain a normal weight? There are so many apparently conflicting theories about diet. You not only need reliable information; to be of use, that information must be filtered through the lens of understanding, interpreted through experience. Without a knowledgeable guide, information – particularly in the medical field – can quickly create a great deal more confusion than it dispels.

Thus, this book looks at our evolution to see what foods we are adapted to eat. It discusses the reasons why we alone, as a species, get fat, and it explores the history of slimming over the past 140 years. It presents an eating plan that has been shown to be effective, safe and based on hard evidence. It may seem a revolutionary regime but it is not a new one. For more than a century it has been proven to be safe and effective, both in population studies and in clinical trials – and that evidence is presented in Part Two. This dietary regime is both natural and healthy but more than that:

- it does not restrict calorie intake;
- it is easy to maintain;
- and, above all, it works – for life.

That it works should come as no surprise as this regime, unlike any other on offer today, is based on the natural diet for our species.

This is not a 'diet' – and it's not difficult

'Diet' implies limits, restrictions, lots of counting and thick, complicated books. All of these are unnecessary: nobody has to tell a lion what, when and how much to eat; and no primitive human carries calorie charts around. Weight control combined with good nutrition needn't be dreary or difficult.

However, that does not mean you won't have to change the way you live. I'm afraid you will – and for the rest of your life. There is no point in 'going on a diet' only to end it and put the weight back on again. That's what got you into the situation where you felt you had to buy this book in the first place. If you are going to stay with one way of eating for life, any satisfactory weight-reducing diet must be healthy, economical and palatable: you have to enjoy it and eat the foods that you like.

So this is not a 'diet' in the way dieters usually interpret the word. It is only a diet in the sense that everything you eat constitutes your diet. The way of eating presented here is actually the correct way to eat: eating naturally; eating to enjoy food, with you in control of your food rather than having the food controlling you.

Introduction

It is easy today to lose weight – all you need to do is starve. The problem is keeping the weight lost from going back on again. This is where this book is unlike all the others: you really can stay on this 'diet' for the rest of your life. The only difficulty that I find is getting people to believe it can work!

If you are overweight, there is doubt that you will have to change the way you eat, but eating this way you will no longer have to count calories consciously. Given the right foods, your body will do that for you automatically, the way it was designed to do naturally.

Eat real food

One question I am asked more than any other by people starting to eat low-carb diets is: 'Where can I buy low-carb foods?'. They have been misled into thinking that this is just another 'diet' that needs special 'diet foods'. It isn't! You don't need to eat anything 'special' when eating this way; you will no longer be 'on a diet' and you don't need to eat low-carb diet products such as those now increasingly being sold for the 'low-carb' market. These are designed for one purpose only: to keep you dependent on them so that the manufacturers can continue to make a good living out of you. And it was probably such highly processed food that made you overweight in the first place, so avoid the highly processed bars, shakes and smoothies heavily advertised and promoted for the 'low-carb' market. A properly constituted low-carb diet is one that is based on real foods.

Fats and health

Natural Health and Weight Loss advocates a diet that does not cut out fats. Until a couple of decades or so ago this would not necessarily have been thought odd. However, dietary fat has had such a bad press for so long that to advocate such a diet today could make the average dietician shudder. But evidence published in the medical journals shows that the opposite is true. Fats are essential for health. Make no mistake, cut them out and you will shorten your life. And, as you will learn, fat actually helps you to slim.

Dieting and health are big business. Without fat people, the slimming industry would crumble; without ill health we would not need doctors. They all have vested interests. As a consequence, they have subjected you to only one side of the debate. One thing I can promise: *Natural Health and Weight Loss* gives you a rare opportunity to read the other side of the slimming and health arguments and the evidence on which they are based. *Natural Health and Weight Loss* presents the evidence that the experts have presented. It is a matter of record. The final judgement rests with you.

The proof of the pudding

You know the old saying: 'The proof of the pudding is in the eating'. It couldn't be better illustrated than in the subject of diet, weight loss and health. Try a properly constituted, low-carb diet and prove its benefits for yourself, not just for weight loss but also for health generally.

Your choice, therefore, is either to eat the diet we are designed to eat and be a normal weight and healthy without much effort, or resign yourself to hunger, deprivation and self-denial as a lifestyle.

How to use this book

Part One sets out in simple terms what you need to do to begin your new, lighter, healthier life. It lets you get straight on with natural weight loss without having to read lots of information first.

Part Two tells why and how it works. It looks at the evidence supporting the *Natural Health and Weight Loss* way of eating. Most of what you have been told about both 'healthy eating' and GI is not evidence-based and is quite misleading. And there is a lot of evidence of the harm that 'healthy' advice has done. But the fat-cholesterol-heart disease dogma is now so ingrained in our psyche that this fact has been lost. For this reason, I have written Part Two in some detail. I have also included references to back up all statements and details of how you can access the studies to check them for yourself.

At the back of the book you will find additional information including a glossary, height/weight tables and comprehensive tables of the carbohydrate content and Glycaemic Index of foods, and sample recipes.

References

1.   Wooley SC, Garner DM. Dietary treatments for obesity are ineffective. *BMJ* 1994; 309: 655.

Introduction

2. Garrow JS. Should obesity be treated? *BMJ* 1994; 309: 654.
3. Willett W. Is dietary fat a major determinant of body fat? *Am J Clin Nutr* 1998; 67 (3 Suppl): 556S–562S.
4. Clark C, Clark M. *The Healthy Low GI Low Carb Diet.* Vermilion, London, 2005, p.3.
5. Hirsch J. Herman award lecture, 1994: Establishing a biologic basis for obesity. *Am J Clin Nutr* 1994; 60: 613.
6. Weinberg SL. The Diet-Heart Hypothesis: a critique. *J Am Coll Cardiol* 2004; 43: 731–733.

Part One

Natural Health and Weight Loss
in practice

Chapter One

Let's get started

If you do what you've always done, you'll get what you've always gotten.

Peter Bender

Start now

If you have been overweight for any length of time, and tried many diets, you will probably want to get started on this one as quickly as possible. For that reason, this chapter sets out in brief the basics of the way of life I hope you are going to follow for the rest of your life. The reasons why it works and why it is so much healthier, together with the medical evidence supporting this way of living, are all in the following chapters. You can read these later at your leisure but, for the moment, bear with me.

If you are overweight and don't want to be, be under no illusions: you are going to have to make some changes to the way you eat – permanently. However, if you think that means eating very little and being hungry for the rest of your life, think again. That's what made you overweight in the first place and I am not about to ask you to repeat it.

The best way to get down to a normal weight – and then maintain it for the rest of your life – is not to 'eat less' but to 'eat properly'. And that means eating the foods your body needs, and eating as much as your body tells you it wants. In other words, you must not go hungry.

It is as well to be aware of what you are trying to achieve before starting this way of life. What you are embarking on is a way of eating that doesn't count calories. You may be eating 1500, 2000 or 3000 calories a day. But don't bother counting them; they are irrelevant. You must, however, restrict your intake of sweet and starchy foods. For weight loss, you may find that merely cutting down on these foods is sufficient, or you may have to make a more conscious effort to avoid eating too much of them, but either way let your appetite be your guide. You can eat as much protein and fat as your body tells you it needs. Historically people have preferred these combined in the proportions of one part fat to between three and six parts lean.

How to lose weight

If you are overweight, what is it that you actually want to lose? That's not as silly a question as you might think. You don't want to lose weight – you can do that by having a leg amputated; what you really want to lose is fat.

The point is that, *to lose fat, your body must use that fat* as a fuel; there is no other way. And the only way your body will use its stored fat as a fuel is if you force it to. That means depriving it of its present supply of fuel – the blood sugar, glucose – so that it has no choice in the matter.

There are two ways to cut your body's glucose supply:

- you either starve, which is what low-calorie, low-fat dieting is, or
- you reduce the starches and sugars from which glucose is made and make it up with a source of a different fuel – fat.

This latter approach has two advantages over the traditional calorie-controlled approach: it means that you no longer have to go hungry and, by feeding your body on fats, it will stop trying to find glucose and change over naturally to using its own stored fat. This is by far the easiest way.

The rules

If you are to live this way for the rest of your life, then you must enjoy what you eat. For this reason, I want to let you choose the foods that you like rather than preach to you and tell you what you must and mustn't have. Nothing is forbidden, but there are a few rules that it is wise to follow:

1. Reduce your intake of carbohydrates, particularly refined carbohydrates . . . but don't reduce them too much.
2. Eat a high-protein breakfast.
3 Eat real food.
4. Replace the loss of calories from carbohydrates mainly with calories from fat, not protein.
5. Leave the fat on meat.
6. If you are overweight, don't try to lose more than 1 kilo (2 lb) a week.
7. If you are not overweight, don't try to slim.
8. Exercise only if you want to.

These rules are considered in more detail below.

Reduce your intake of carbohydrates

You can eat as much as you want of any meat, fish, poultry, cheese, cream, butter, eggs – indeed anything that is high in proteins and fats and low in carbohydrates.

You can eat as much as you like of green leafy vegetables such as cabbage, Brussels sprouts, cauliflower, broccoli, lettuce, celery, and so on. You can also eat root vegetables that have a low Glycaemic Index (GI).

Although it is advisable to cut out altogether if possible carbohydrate foods such as sugar and breakfast cereals, it is not necessary to stop eating fruit and vegetables, merely to cut down on the sweeter and starchier ones. It is necessary only to reduce the amount of them you eat so that your total carbohydrate intake is no more than about 50–60 grams a day (but see Rule 2). This is equivalent to about 5 slices of bread or a small mountain of green leafy vegetables (see Appendix E).

The foods that you should be most wary of are:

- Sugar, sweets and candies.
- Bread, biscuits, pasta, breakfast cereals and rice.
- Rice cakes, sweet pies, puddings and other sweet desserts.
- Jams, jellies, honey and syrups.
- Sweet, fizzy drinks, even the low calorie ones (see Chapter 3).
- Beer and sweet wines.

- Fruits that are tinned or cooked in syrup.
- Dried fruits.
- High GI root vegetables such as parsnips and swedes.

You do not have to go through life never tasting these again. They are listed here because they are the foods with the highest carbohydrate content. Appendix E has a list of common foods, their carbohydrate content and their GI.

Some people have difficulty giving up certain foods. Bread seems to prove a particular problem, but you do not have to give up eating bread altogether (although it is a good idea to give it up if you can). Just cut down to a maximum of two slices a day, or substitute a starch-reduced bread, but beware of regular and low-carb breads that are made with soya (see Chapter 3).

So, instead of sandwiches for lunch, why not eat a chunk of cheese and an apple if you plan to have a larger meal in the evening, or take a bowl of cold meat, egg and cheese with salad instead. If you like fruit juice at breakfast, drink grapefruit juice in preference to orange juice and reduce the amount by watering it down. Breakfast could be, for example, grapefruit juice, fried egg and bacon, one slice of thickly buttered toast or fried bread, and cocoa, tea or coffee with cream rather than milk (try to manage without sugar). This will give you a good start for the day, and easily keep you going until lunchtime, even though it comprises only about 18 grams of carbohydrate. Compare this with a small bowl of cornflakes and a 150 mL (a quarter of a pint) of skimmed milk; together these contain about 30 grams of carbohydrate, which is half your daily carbohydrate allowance and you will be hungry again by mid-morning.

Don't reduce carbs too much

The object of eating this way is to reduce glucose and insulin levels in the blood by changing your body from using glucose from dietary carbs as an energy source to using fats. To make the changeover, it is necessary to reduce your carb intake, while increasing fat intake. However, there are two possible problems at the start which must be addressed.

Writers of low-carb diet books and articles realise, quite rightly, that women want to lose weight fast. For this reason several recommend cutting carbs to very low levels at the start. If you reduce carbs to around 20 grams a day or less, you can achieve a dramatic loss of weight. At first sight, from a psychological point of view, this seems a good idea as it gives many dieters who have failed in the past a feeling of success. Unfortunately, this feeling frequently doesn't last, and when the weight loss 'stalls' as it almost always does, this can engender a feeling of 'here we go again, another diet that doesn't work', with a consequent loss of self-esteem and self-confidence, and depression. And, as it is very hard to motivate yourself under these conditions, you are likely to give up before you have really started.

And there is another concern – an important one. If you change your body from using one fuel (glucose) to another (fats) too quickly, it can put your body under stress. This is because your body's whole endocrine system – the hormones that govern your metabolism and keep it on track – have to readjust to the changeover, and this takes time. This is why people on diets that cut carbs too much at the start often complain of nausea, headaches, fatigue, sleeplessness, and so on. So the benefits of this way of eating are best when circulating glucose levels are gradually reduced in conjunction with elevations of ketone bodies derived from dietary and body fats.[1,2] The emphasis here is on the term 'gradual', as ketone bodies cannot be used for energy following an acute low blood-sugar condition.[3] It can also have more serious consequences if your health is already compromised. The 50 to 60 gram carb minimum advocated in this book is deliberately chosen to avoid these symptoms.

It is much better, not only for your self-esteem and success with this way of eating, but also for your health, to make the changeover more gradual and to lose weight, if you need to, slowly but surely. So try not to be in too much of a hurry.

If you know that you have a serious health problem already – and I include diabetes in this category – then be even more cautious: halve your current carb intake for a couple of weeks, then reduce to 100 grams, then reduce again to the recommended 50 to 60 grams. You will do yourself no harm by eating only 50 grams of carbs a day – or even less – for the rest of your life, but do take it easy during the changeover period. You will reap the benefits later. However, if you have kidney disease, seek medical advice first. Eating high levels of animal proteins may put an excessive 'strain' on your kidneys.

Eat a high-protein breakfast (see Chapter 2)

It is essential that you start the day in such a way that your energy levels are sufficiently high that you will not want to snack between meals, and your brain has a constant, unvarying supply of energy. A good, old-fashioned, cooked breakfast – eggs and bacon – is ideal, followed by, say, an apple or orange. Ring the changes with eggs and kidneys, eggs and liver or liver and bacon. (Yes, I'm serious. Calves liver, if properly cooked, can be particularly delicious.) Add tomatoes or mushrooms. If you can't face, or haven't time for, a fried breakfast, you could have cold meats, continental sausage, cheese, hard-boiled eggs, or fish instead. You can also think of breakfast as just another meal and have steak and salad if you like. But whatever you do, *never* make do with cereals or toast and marmalade.

Eat real food (see Chapter 3)

In 2001 I joined a low-carb forum on the Internet to help people having difficulty as a result of one of the low-carb dietary regimes aimed at weight loss that had been published. This one was American and recommended meal replacements and special 'low-carb' products. It's perhaps not surprising that the most frequently asked question by far was: 'Where can I buy low-carb foods?' The answer, of course, is simple: at any supermarket, butcher's shop, dairy, grocer's or farmers' market, because it is not necessary to buy anything 'special' with this way of eating. All you have to do is eat real, unprocessed food in as natural a state as possible.

Some authors give the impression that pills, nutritional supplements, meal replacements or special diet foods are required. In some cases that's because they sell them or have a financial reason for advertising them, but these simply aren't needed. In fact, I believe they defeat the whole object of this way of life, which should be as natural as possible. You should not look for low-carb bars, which contain processed protein powders, artificial sweeteners and harmful fats. You don't need protein smoothies – made with cheap ingredients because the manufacturer is looking for a hefty profit. These are not healthy – what is the point in swapping one disease for another?

All the foods you need, to provide your body with all the nutrients it needs, and you with the pleasure you need, can be found in the meat, cheese, dairy, fish, and fruit and vegetable departments of any supermarket. You may have to add butter and other fats as meat today is bred so lean as to be tough and tasteless. But even this is far healthier than the junk that is beginning to be sold for the 'low-carb' market. And don't be afraid of eggs; they have a nearly perfect balance of nutrients, and are excellent dietary sources of protein, vitamins, minerals and trace elements, and essential fatty acids. Again, buy normal, natural eggs, not 'special' eggs with added omega-3 fatty acids.

In fact, if a diet tells you that you need supplements of one sort or another, you know it is not nutritionally balanced.

Replace the carbs mainly with fat, not protein (see Chapter 15)

The propaganda against dietary fat has been powerful and relentless during the past 20 years. You may still be very frightened about adding more fat to your diet, particularly if your doctor has told you that you have a high cholesterol level. Don't be. You will inevitably increase the amount of protein in your diet to some extent but you should not overdo it. For you to be healthy, *your main source of energy with this way of eating must be fat.* A high-protein diet in which both carbs *and* fat are restricted is probably the least healthy diet of all because your body will continue to use glucose – which we don't want – but it will make that glucose from the protein. While your body can do this in an emergency, it certainly isn't healthy to use protein as a source of energy long term. It is also inefficient and expensive.

Leave the fat on meat

One big difficulty these days is that, after two decades of 'healthy eating' dogma, it isn't easy to buy really healthy food. This means that getting sufficient of the right fats into your diet is made more difficult than it was half a century ago. So:

- Buy the fattiest meat you can find.
- Don't cut the fat off meat.
- Don't remove the skin from chicken and other poultry.
- Use duck or goose in preference to chicken and turkey. They are fatter birds, taste better and provide lots of lovely, tasty fat for cooking.
- Use full-cream milk in preference to semi-skimmed or skimmed; or better still, as most of the milk is water, why not just buy cream? It's cheaper in the long run. And you can get your calcium and protein better from cheese. The best cheeses for calcium are the hard Italian cheeses such as Parmesan, Swiss cheeses and Cheddar.
- Eat your fruit with cream if you wish; put butter rather than gravy on cooked vegetables; and use an olive oil dressing on salads.

Chapter One

If you are overweight, don't try to lose more than 1 kilo (2 lb) a week

It is dangerous – and usually counterproductive – to lose weight too quickly, particularly if you are only moderately overweight. Be patient; with this way of eating you may not lose weight as quickly as on some other plans, nor should you try to. If it took you 10 or 20 years to put the weight on, it is unrealistic to think you can lose it all safely in as many weeks. Large weight losses are always followed by a 'stall' when you don't lose weight for weeks at a time. This is demoralising and the reason why most people stop any diet and start another one – usually with the same result.

You may find that you do lose quite a lot in the first week or so. This is normal on any new diet as your stocks of glycogen (one form in which our bodies store energy) and its associated water are used up before your body changes to using fats as an energy source. But after that, weight loss should be slow and steady. One kilogram (2 lb) a week may well be less than you are used to losing on a low-calorie diet, but don't give up. Your weight will come down, safely and comfortably. On the other hand, you will not go hungry. It is the easiest of 'diets'.

If you are not overweight, don't try to lose weight (see Chapter 17)

If you are within the acceptable weight range for your height, you may not lose any weight on this regime, as it will not let your weight fall below your natural weight. This is another reason why it is so much healthier than low-calorie diets that rely on starvation to achieve results.

However, even if you are within the acceptable weight range for your height, there is no reason why you should not adopt the principles of this way of eating as a precautionary measure. This will ensure that you never do become overweight. It will also protect you from many other modern diseases that are listed in Appendix A.

Get the ratios right

For the best of health and for weight maintenance research has shown[4] that you should try for the following ratios of the three macronutrients:

Carbs: 10–15% of calories.
Protein: 15–25% of calories.
Fat: 60–70% of calories.

The day's meals

I don't want to dictate what you must eat. That is for you to decide based on the information given here, in conjunction with your own preferences and other aspects of your life style. The Recipes section (page 313) will give you some ideas, but below is a broad pattern your meals for the day might follow. The examples are from a typical daily menu for my family. While I have said 'Don't weigh your food' I have used weights here in order to be able to give you exact nutrient values by way of example.

Eat food

You don't eat 'nutrients', you eat 'food'. When you look at these examples remember, if you look to the carbs and use fat wherever you can, your body will take care of the amounts without your having to count anything. Once you get used to this way of eating, it will soon become second nature.

Breakfast

Select from:

- Fried bacon, eggs, kidneys, omelettes.
- Cold meats, ham and continental sausage (British-type sausages, unfortunately, usually have a high proportion of cereal filler and are high in carbohydrates. If you have British sausages, do not have bread as well).
- Kippers (smoked herring), bloaters (pickled herring), or haddock either lightly fried or stewed in milk and butter.
- Tea, cocoa or coffee with milk or cream, with a little sugar if you must.
- Starch-reduced bread (if you can find one that doesn't contain soya) with butter, but not jam or marmalade.

If you prefer not to fry, try scrambling eggs in lots of butter. You will be amazed at how much butter scrambled eggs will absorb. Just three eggs scrambled in 20 grams of butter for breakfast could keep you going until well into the afternoon.

If you have insufficient time to cook in the morning, prepare cold meats, hard-boiled eggs, cheese, etc, the night before. Or cook a meal the previous evening while making dinner, and re-heat it in the morning. After such a breakfast you will not get hungry and you shouldn't need to eat anything until lunchtime, but you should drink at least three cups of liquid.

Example: *This is to illustrate what the meal might include. I've used weights because there is so much variation in food sizes.*

73 g very large egg
75 g streaky bacon
Lard for frying
75 g apple
70 g single cream (in cocoa)
18 g 100% cocoa powder
1 pint water (for cocoa)
Carbs = 13.5 g; Protein = 40.3 g; Fat = 68 g; Total calories: 787.2.

Lunch

For lunch you may eat:

- Any meat with its fat left on.
- Any offal: liver, kidneys, etc.
- Any fish, poached, grilled or fried (not in batter); oily fish are best.
- Cold meats.
- Omelettes.
- Cheese.
- Eggs, cooked any way.

Eat these with salad or vegetables with as much butter or olive oil as you like. Follow with:

- An apple or other small fruit, with or without cream; cheese.
- Coffee, cocoa or tea with cream or milk but no sugar.

If you normally eat sandwiches at lunchtime, there are some alternative ideas for take-out meals without bread in the Recipes section. The easiest meals consist of meat, eggs, cheese or fish with salad or pickles. Many department stores sell covered compartmentalized plastic containers that are ideal for this. You could also have fruit and cream in one of the compartments. If you need to have, or prefer, sandwiches, the almond and parmesan pancake recipe on page 328 makes a good flour-free substitute for bread.

Example

115 g pork loin
31 g onion
50 g lard for frying the above (and poured over the meal)
60 g carrot
80 g butternut squash
56 g cheddar cheese
Carbs = 14.9 g; Protein = 39g; Fats = 70 g; Total calories: 846.

Evening meal

The evening meal or dinner follows the same rules as breakfast and lunch. If you like an alcoholic drink with your meal, bear in mind its carbohydrate content and treat it as any other food. Dry (as opposed to sweet) drinks are recommended.

Having said that, it is better to make dinner the smallest meal of the day if you can. My wife and I usually eat only about 100–140 g of a full-fat cheese such as Brie or cream cheese, and fruit either on its own or with cream. We also usually drink unsweetened cocoa made with 100% cocoa powder, water and cream.

Example

140 g Brie
274 g apple/pear
8 g 100% cocoa powder
35 g single cream
Carbs = 43.9 g; Protein = 32.5 g; Fats = 44.9 g; Total calories: 709.7.

DAY'S TOTALS

Weight: Carbs = 72.3 g; Protein = 111.8 g; Fats = 182.9 g
Percentage calories: Carbs = 12.1%; Protein = 18.8%; Fats = 69.1%
Calories: Carbs = 289.2; Protein = 447.2; Fats = 1646.1; Total = 2382.5 calories.

As you can see, this way of eating is not low-calorie.

Snacks

There is a tendency with 'diet' books these days to recommend 'grazing': that is, eating little and often all day. This is generally to 'ward off the hunger pangs' or 'to keep blood sugar levels up' because they recommend diets that are so energy deficient the authors know you will be hungry if you don't. However, it's not a good idea to graze or snack in this way. If you graze, it is easy to be unaware of what and how much food you are eating. It also doesn't allow your body to use its stored fat – which is what you are trying to lose; and it doesn't allow the insulin system to rest.

A 'three-meals-a-day' regime creates a freedom from what many find is a relentless slavery to overeating in case they become hypoglycaemic (have low blood sugar). To go without hunger because your meals have satisfied you, and for your body to trust that it will be well fed until the next meal, is a freedom you will learn to cherish. It also allows your stomach to rest, as nature intended.

So, with three meals a day like those above, you should not feel the need to snack. But if you do occasionally feel the need to nibble something, have a piece of cheese, some nuts or a hard-boiled egg.

Make sure you drink enough

Many people drink far less than they should. As a general rule, I recommend that you drink around 2 litres (3½ pints) of liquid a day; more on a hot day or if you are engaged in any pursuit that makes you sweat a lot. Don't wait until you are thirsty, this means that you are already dehydrated to some extent, and spread your water intake out over the day; don't drink more than about half a pint with a meal as this may dilute your stomach acid.

Please note that when you are thirsty, this is your body telling you it needs water – not food. It's very easy to 'eat' too much by drinking a drink that contains calories, usually in the form of sugar in soft drinks and fruit juices.

Relax

What I mean by 'relax' is: if you are overweight, don't get all uptight about rates of weight loss. I do realize that this may not be easy; you will want to lose weight, to look good on the beach, to be able to buy clothes more easily, and so on. This is natural. But do try not to do it too quickly and try not to be anxious if it doesn't happen as quickly as you would like. You are much more likely to achieve your goals if you are relaxed. If you are stressed, this increases the levels of stress hormones in your blood, which increase blood glucose levels, and that, in turn, makes weight loss more difficult.

The same happens if you are constantly rushing about under pressure at work. Try to take it easy, particularly during meals and for the first hour afterwards. Working lunches are devastating.

Exercise only if you want to (see Chapter 16)

Exercise increases fitness by promoting suppleness, strength and stamina. It also has its place in a healthy lifestyle by improving your cardiovascular system, and it has a social function. However, as a means of losing weight it is a dead loss. If you are overweight to the point of obesity, bear in mind the fact that you are already 'exercising' merely because you are carrying a large amount of weight every time you walk about. I remember when I was building my house what it felt like to lug a heavy bag of cement around. At that time these were hundredweight bags – 112 lb, or 8 stone, or 51 kg. That was a form of exercise I wouldn't want to make a habit of doing. So, do please exercise if you like – but only do the exercise and sport you enjoy.

Making the transition

If this way of eating is foreign to you, it can take some getting used to. You may have to battle with your mind as it will probably go against all you have come to believe in; you will have seen all the adverse publicity that the 'Atkins diet' received; friends may tell you that this way of eating will undermine your health. However, the evidence from published research, detailed in this book, which shows that this way of eating is in reality much healthier than what many people call 'healthy eating', refutes all of these criticisms.

It is certainly true that there are problems with the Atkins approach. This is mainly for three reasons:

1. The induction period at the start produces stresses on the body and adverse side effects that I mentioned earlier.
2. It also causes a much too rapid weight loss. In this situation, the first initial flush of success comes to an abrupt halt a few weeks in, when your body says: 'Whoa, that's enough', and weight loss 'stalls'. My wife, Monica, has a saying that 'rapid weight loss is no weight loss'. It's all too true, as you may find when your weight plateaus and starts to increase again.
3. Many low-carb plans also rely on, and promote, meal replacements, diet supplements and vitamin and mineral pills. These are quite unnecessary, particularly in Britain. The Atkins diet also relies heavily on soya as a source of protein, but soya is not a healthy food and it can actually stop you losing weight (see Chapter 3).

The start

It's a good idea not to plunge straight into this way of eating. You will have developed menus and ways that you are used to, but will have to modify them. You won't want to give up all the things you like to eat and all the ways you have habitually prepared them. It's too much to do all at once. It's a good idea to take stock of your usual way of eating, and see how you can adapt it to the new regime so that it fits in, as much as possible, with what you like doing now.

Then plan a strategy to reduce the carb proportion of your diet while increasing the fat and protein proportions to make up. One way is to continue eating the sweet, starchy foods you like, but reduce the amount. Halving the amount is a good guide, so you would have two slices of bread instead of four, for example, but spread the butter on them thicker. Or if you have a glass of fruit juice, only half fill the glass with juice and top up with water. Try to spread the amount of carbs evenly over the day's meals.

You may have difficulty cutting down on certain foods: bread, for example. If you find that your two slices of bread is creeping up, becoming three or four, don't feel guilty. As I mentioned, you must enjoy your food, and you won't if you are worried about it. In this case, you might find it easier to cut it out altogether, but if you do, don't have it in the house. If you haven't got it, you can't eat it. One of my clients told me she couldn't see the point in eating one sandwich, she had to eat the loaf, so she stopped altogether. After about six weeks, she found that she no longer felt a need for bread at all. In fact, she told me that she wasn't even tempted to eat bread when she was out with other people who were eating it.

The changeover period is when most of your problems will occur. It takes time for your body to adjust; it is particularly difficult for people whose belief that this way of eating may be harmful is ingrained. Those who were taught this from an early age will have the greatest difficulty coming to terms with it. Older people may remember what they ate before 'healthy eating' and, with a bit of luck, will also remember how much better they felt then.

Lazy bowel

Another problem you may encounter at the beginning is constipation. Eating lots of fibre has meant that your bowel has become 'lazy' and the muscles will have been weakened. The changeover to a diet which contains less fibre means that your bowel muscles will have to work again – and they might take a short while to recover their fitness. If this is the case, you should find that drinking more water will help. If not, then either add fibre by eating more uncooked vegetables such as a green salad, until your bowel's muscle tone improves.

Note that these difficulties, if they occur at all, will only be temporary. You will find that, within a few weeks, they will no longer bother you. But you may have to be patient for a while.

When your target weight is reached

When you have reached a weight that is acceptable to you, you may increase the amount of carbohydrate in your diet or indulge yourself with chocolate once a week, but avoid the popular British chocolates. Not only do these chocolates contain so little cocoa that they don't deserve the name 'chocolate', they have an extremely high sugar content (sugar is invariably the first named ingredient). The dark continental chocolates with at least 70% cocoa solids are better. Better still – as well as cheaper – are some supermarkets' own brands, which usually contain 72% cocoa solids. However, watch the scales occasionally and if your weight starts to creep up, just reduce your intake of the carbohydrates again.

A *healthy balanced diet*

If you just want to maintain a normal weight, keeping carbs down to about 60 g a day and increasing fats to compensate is sufficient. However, for optimum health, the ratio of carbs to fats to proteins is more important. It is determined, like everything else, by our evolution and our body's needs.

Carbs

Although I have given a figure of 60 grams for carbs, this is really only a starting figure. It was chosen to avoid the problems caused by a too drastic change of energy source during the few weeks after changeover period. It is also the maximum amount that a diabetic should have. After your body has become accustomed to not getting the level of carbs it had previously, you can eat more or less as you like. Sixty grams will provide 240 calories; that is 12% of a 2000-calorie diet.

Protein and fat

To maintain your body and provide it with the amino acids it needs for cell regeneration and repair, and the enzymes that control almost all body functions, your consumption should be at least 1 to 1.5 grams of good quality protein for each kilogram of lean body weight. This means in practice eating some 50 to 100 grams of protein, but this has to be balanced to the evolutionary intakes our bodies are genetically programmed to eat. People who live on a wholly meat diet generally prefer to eat between three and six parts lean to one part fat. As the lean is only about 23% protein (the rest being mostly water), whereas the fat on meat is about 90%, that gives a ratio in terms of weight of 100–200 grams of protein to each 140 grams of fat.

Not everyone eats the same amount; a smaller person will eat less than a tall one and a child will eat a different amount from an adult. Thus laying down specific amounts can be misleading. Taking all this into consideration, let me put it another way, and suggest that you aim for the ratio of between three and six parts lean to one part fat mentioned above.

You should also include organ meats like liver and kidneys as these contain the widest range of the vitamins, minerals and trace elements your body needs.

Diet for diabetics (see Chapter 5)

If you are diabetic, whether type-1 or -2, the primary aim of any dietary treatment must be to normalise your blood glucose levels and, thus reduce your need for insulin. As it is carbs that have the greatest effect on blood glucose and insulin, it is not surprising that the way of eating advocated in this book is ideal for diabetics.

Merely lowering your carb intake will automatically lower the amount of insulin your body needs, but there are other considerations. For example, you will be told by your diabetes counsellor that all you need to do is eat 'low-glycaemic' foods, and that fruit is low glycaemic. What she won't tell you is that fruit is actually worse for your health as it increases the complications of diabetes far more than starches (see Chapter 5).

So for a diabetic, the Glycaemic Index, a scale which measures the speed with which foods increase glucose levels in the bloodstream, can be misleading. You must understand that *all* carbs regardless of how quickly they raise glucose, are still going to produce that glucose and your body has to deal with it.

Before you start, particularly if you are a type-1 diabetic, it is important that you read Chapter 5 for more detail to avoid the pitfalls of changing to what will eventually be a much healthier way of life.

Conclusion

This dietary regime may be new to you and a radical departure from the type of dietary philosophy you're used to, but it is one that has proven itself for nearly one and a half centuries. It is completely safe and may be followed for life. No other diet is as healthy or offers so much. In fact it offers so many filling foods to satisfy you that the small sacrifice you make by reducing your intake of such foods as sweets, bread and pasta is really no sacrifice at all. You need never be hungry again. And this diet really does work; it could dispel the slimming magazines' myths and put them out of business.

I know of many people successfully losing weight and maintaining their new weight with this way of eating. A typical example is A.N., an overweight civil airline pilot. His wife, also overweight, came to see me and started on this way of eating in mid-1997. Her husband decided he would join her although he thought that having to eat the set meals his airline supplied it would be difficult to do. It was not; he found he merely had to eat more of some things and leave others. After a couple of months his weight, as well as his wife's, had dropped significantly. He told me: 'I can't believe this is working; I enjoy it too much'.

The only difficulty I have is getting people to believe that it can work. Cross that hurdle and your weight problems are over – for life.

That, then, is the theory in brief, and it works remarkably well in practice. There are five important advantages to eating this way:

1. You can live with this way of eating for the rest of your life without ever again being hungry. There is no stressful 'yo-yo' effect. Instead of starving the weight off, it gets the body to burn fat more efficiently.
2. It is very easy to live with and maintain socially. As all you have to do is reduce your intake of carbohydrates; you can eat whatever you are offered without having to disclose that you are 'on a diet'. You simply need to take a little more meat and a little less pudding.
3. With this way of eating, your weight cannot fall below its natural level. This is important; being overweight may be undesirable, but being underweight is potentially far more dangerous. Serious risks of sudden death are associated with extreme leanness.
4. It is a much healthier way of eating. This way of eating supplies all the essential nutrients. On top of that, you will also be amazed at how much better you feel, and your lack of a need to see your doctor.
5. It is a natural way of eating.

References

1. Greene AE, Todorova MT, Seyfried TN. Perspectives on the metabolic management of epilepsy through dietary reduction of glucose and elevation of ketone bodies. *J Neurochem* 2003; 86: 529–537.
2. Seyfried TN, Sanderson TM, El-Abbadi MM, et al. Role of glucose and ketone bodies in the metabolic control of experimental brain cancer. *Br J Cancer* 2003; 89: 1375–1382.
3. Fanelli C, Di Vincenzo A, Modarelli F, et al. Post-hypoglycaemic hyperketonaemia does not contribute to brain metabolism during insulin-induced hypoglycaemia in humans. *Diabetologia* 1993; 36: 1191–1197.
4. Kwaśniewski J. *Jak Nie Chorować*. Wydawnictwo WGP, Warsaw, 2005, pp.92–119.

Chapter Two

Breakfast: The most important meal of the day

The foundation course

The time to start any new diet or way of eating is tomorrow! So, with that in mind, the obvious starting meal is breakfast.

French cuisine is admired the world over; the Chinese, in the West, are renowned for takeaways; the Italians for their pastas and pizzas; the Japanese for raw fish. Although in gastronomic terms, England tends to be thought of only in terms of fish and chips, the fact is that the English have given the world what is without doubt the finest and most important meal of all: breakfast.

In the face of a traditional cooked English breakfast, French croissants and Swiss muesli pale into nutritional insignificance; only the German cold meats, cheese and hard-boiled eggs, come close. For breakfast – a good breakfast, that is – makes all the difference: not only does it determine how well you will perform and how well you will feel throughout the day; it also plays a crucial role in determining whether or not you will be healthy.

Whether you are trying to lose weight or not, it is better to take meals spread out over the day, rather than have one large one. The pattern that has been suggested for centuries is: 'Breakfast like a king, lunch like a lord and dine like a pauper.' In other words, the biggest meal should be at the start of the day, when energy for work is required, instead of the more usual practice of having it in the evening when all you are going to do is sit and watch television and then go to bed. It makes a great deal of sense.

Several lines of research have suggested that both children and adults get fatter and perform less well if they do not have breakfast.

The average working woman and man needs some 2100 and 2800 calories a day respectively. If you are engaged in heavy physical work, you require more. If you are to spread out your calorie intake over three meals a day sensibly, therefore, you really should be thinking in terms of eating a breakfast comprising around 800 or 1000 calories. And you can't do that on muesli and skimmed milk.

Blood sugar deficiency

Although I have a fried breakfast every day now, I didn't always do so. I like cornflakes. So even after I had started to eat this way, I had cornflakes with Jersey milk for breakfast every Sunday as a treat. At about 10 o'clock on a Sunday I would get the car out to wash it and start work. I noticed, however, that after I was about halfway through, I started to get what I called 'weak and wobbly'. So I would come in, have something to eat and sit until the feeling passed. I must be dense because it was years before I realised that this *only* happened when I had breakfast cereal; I never had these 'weak and wobbly' episodes after a fried breakfast.

Our bodies need over 40 different nutrients to function properly. Fresh fat meat supplies them all; refined sugar, on the other hand supplies only one.

Normally we eat such a wide variety of foods that deficiency of one essential nutrient seems impossible, but there is one deficiency that can happen and when it does, even for a few hours, it can ruin your whole day: that is a deficiency of the blood sugar, glucose.

All body cells and the brain need energy to function. This energy comes from the oxidation of glucose or glucose and fat. Only when blood glucose levels are adequate can the cells that need it obtain the amount of energy they need.

Breakfast is the most important meal of the day because it determines what your energy levels will be, not just for the immediate period after it has been eaten, but throughout the day. That, in turn, determines how you will feel and act, and how efficiently you will operate. But just eating something is simply not good enough: for breakfast, quality is much more important than quantity. Eating too much of the wrong foods is as bad as, and in some cases worse than, not eating enough of the right ones.

If you have not eaten for 12 hours, your blood sugar level will be between 3.8 mmol/L (millimol per litre) and 6.1 mmol/L, with an average at about 4.5 mmol/L. This figure is known as the fasting blood sugar level. It depends on what and how much food was eaten at the last meal.

At the level of 5 mmol/L or above, energy is readily available, but as energy is used and your blood sugar level falls, energy becomes scarcer and you start to become tired. Below about 4 mmol/L you will feel hungry and your tiredness will become fatigue. If your blood sugar level continues to fall, you become progressively exhausted, develop headaches, weakness and tremors in your limbs, palpitations of the heart, and nausea. It requires only a small reduction in blood sugar levels for your brain's energy supply to fall to a level where thinking is confused and slowed. As this process continues, you become depressed and uncooperative, irritable and aggressive. This is a natural reaction to starvation, programmed into all of us by our evolution: it is our body's signal to us to go out and kill something to eat.

In contrast, if your food intake ensures that your blood glucose is maintained at a level above fasting, you will feel on top of the world with plenty of 'go', be quick and alert, and have no feelings of depression or hunger.

Results of early breakfast studies

Many studies have been conducted into the effects of various foods and mealtimes on blood glucose levels. They have all demonstrated the importance of the breakfast meal.

- In one study conducted at Harvard University in 1943, glucose levels were measured for six hours after breakfasts that were high in carbohydrate, protein or fat.[1]
- In the light of breakfasts today, the high-carbohydrate breakfast, which consisted of orange juice, bacon, toast and jam, a packaged cereal with milk and sugar, and coffee with milk and sugar, might seem quite good. It wasn't. After this meal the subjects' glucose levels rose rapidly, but fell just as quickly to a very low level, causing inefficiency and feelings of hunger and fatigue.

- The high-fat breakfast consisted only of a packaged cereal with whipping cream. This time blood glucose levels rose only slightly and then returned to the fasting level throughout the period.
- The high-protein breakfast contained skimmed milk, lean minced beef and cottage cheese. This time blood glucose levels rose to 6.6 mmol/L and stayed at that level throughout the whole six hours.

Unfortunately, in this series of tests, although it did show that a high-carbohydrate meal, which resembled what many today would consider a 'normal' breakfast, was the worst, neither of the others was representative of breakfasts in the real world.

Six years later another American test addressed this flaw.[2] This time the subjects ate a variety of commonly eaten American breakfasts. To assess their relative influence, blood sugar levels were measured before breakfast and then at hourly intervals for three hours afterwards.

The findings, looked at today, are quite remarkable as breakfasts that gave the worst results are those that are now the most popular:

1. Black coffee alone was the first breakfast to be tested. This caused a drop in blood sugar levels, and feelings of hunger, fatigue, lassitude, irritability, nervousness, exhaustion and headaches that became progressively worse.
2. Two doughnuts and coffee with milk and sugar caused a rapid rise in blood sugar, but it fell again within one hour to a low level, giving similar symptoms to the coffee-only breakfast.
3. A glass of orange juice, two strips of bacon, toast, jam and coffee with cream and sugar, the typical American breakfast, was the next meal tested. Again, blood sugar rose rapidly but fell to a level below the pre-breakfast level within an hour, remaining low until lunchtime.
4. As (3), with breakfast cereal added. The result was the same: a rapid rise followed quickly by a fall to abnormally low levels.
5. As (4), except that the cereal was replaced by oatmeal served with milk and sugar. Again there was a rapid rise in blood sugar followed by a fall which, this time, was more rapid and to an even lower level.
6. The same again but with two eggs added. This time, blood sugar levels rose and stayed up all morning, as did efficiency and a feeling of wellbeing. A similar breakfast replacing the eggs by fortified full-cream milk was also beneficial.

The effects on the subjects of these various breakfasts were then studied after they had eaten lunch. Those who had eaten the most protein at breakfast retained a high blood sugar level all afternoon. Where blood sugar levels had been low in the morning, after the largely carbohydrate breakfasts, however, levels after lunch rose only for a matter of minutes, falling to a low level that lasted all afternoon.

Both these studies showed that the amount of protein eaten at breakfast time was highly relevant.

Several similar studies have since been conducted. Where the foods eaten were realistic, the results were remarkably consistent: efficiency and feeling of wellbeing experienced after meals was directly related to the amount of protein eaten.

Twenty-two grams of protein seemed to be the minimum for a breakfast to be effective. This kept blood glucose levels up for the three hours. Fifty-five grams of protein was required to keep the levels high for six hours. To put these figures in perspective, an egg contains between 6 and 7 grams of protein; an average rasher of bacon is about the same. Two eggs and two rashers of bacon, therefore, give you more than your 22-gram requirement. The best breakfasts of all were those that also included fat and a little carbohydrate. This was true of all meals.

Weight control

Breakfast is also important for weight loss. In 1989 there was an important meeting of the Forum on Food and Health that discussed a number of aspects of the various common breakfast meals[3] of the contributors. Dr F. Belleisle of Paris told of a study of French schoolchildren which showed that fat children ate breakfasts that contained, on average, 75 fewer calories and ate significantly more in the evening than their slimmer peers. 'Statistically,' he stated, 'the energy value of breakfast was inversely related to corpulence.' In other words, the less you eat for breakfast, the more weight you put on.

In 2002 another study also showed that overweight children were less likely to have eaten breakfast.[4] And in the following year yet another study showed that people who skipped breakfast were four and a half times as likely to be overweight.[5]

Stress

However, whatever the breakfast, most recent studies show that eating something is better than eating nothing for a range of health issues. Scientists at the Cancer

Research UK Health Behaviour Unit, University College London, investigated associations between stress and dietary practices in teenagers from a wide range of socioeconomic and ethnic backgrounds.[6] They found that those who were stressed were less likely to have eaten breakfast and were also more likely to have other unhealthy eating patterns.

Breakfast for brain power . . .

If you are to perform at your best and be bright and alert, breakfast is a must. Missing breakfast has consequences as far as both mental and physical work are concerned. Energy intake at breakfast affects the performance of creativity tests, memory recall and voluntary physical endurance in children before lunch, and food craving during the whole day.

In 1995, Dr Ernesto Pollitt, Professor of Human Development in the Program in International Nutrition at the University of California's School of Medicine, conducted a review of papers published in refereed journals since 1978 on the differences in children's abilities after breakfast compared with fasting.[7] He concluded, on the whole, that children performed better after having breakfast, but there were some notable exceptions. In some, breakfast made no difference to performance and in one study children did better when they did *not* have breakfast. It is significant that in all the cases where breakfast was ineffective, those breakfasts were almost entirely carbohydrate based: cornflakes, semi-skimmed milk, sugar, wholemeal toast with margarine and marmalade.

Doctors at the Massachusetts General Hospital, Division of Pediatric Gastroenterology and Nutrition and at Harvard Medical School, wanted to know whether a recently introduced, universal, free school breakfast programme aimed at children who were at nutritional risk would help their academic abilities and psychosocial functioning.[8] After six months, students who improved their nutritional status with the school breakfasts provided showed not only the expected decreases in hunger, but significant improvements in attendance, and improvements in mathematics and behaviour.

A French study of teenage boys and girls set up to assess the adequacy of breakfast energy supply and energy expenditure in adolescents during a school day with either no exercise or with a two-hour physical education lesson in the morning confirmed the American results.[9] With no physical education (PE) lesson, it needed nearly a quarter of the day's energy at breakfast to do it, so a simple bowl of cereal wouldn't do.

. . . and physical work

That French study above also demonstrated that a level of energy intake at breakfast of only a quarter of the day's total energy was not enough if the two-hour PE lesson was involved. The study stressed the need for a heavier breakfast for children and adolescents on the days with PE in the morning.

Similarly, Canadian scientists conducting a study of hill walkers to examine the effects of breakfasts with different energy intakes – either 616 calories or 3019 calories – also found that energy intake was important for a range of responses that were relevant to the walkers' safety.[10] The group who'd eaten the smaller breakfasts showed significantly slower one- and two-finger reaction times, were not able to balance as well, and were compromised in their ability to maintain body temperature, when compared with the bigger-breakfast group. The researchers say that this 'impaired performance (particularly with respect to balance) and thermoregulation during the [lower energy intake] condition may increase susceptibility to both fatigue and injury during the pursuit of recreational activity outdoors'.

Exceptions

By the 1970s, the practice of having any breakfast was declining, and cooked meals were being replaced by more cereal-based meals. As fat became 'unhealthy', full-cream milk on those cereals was replaced with semi-skimmed or skimmed milks. After the end of the 1970s, therefore, trials aimed at testing the effects of breakfast on mood, cognitive response, problem solving and obesity also increasingly used only carbohydrate-based foods. Results from these have tended to question the previous findings by purporting to show that high-carbohydrate breakfasts are best.

If these studies are taken alone, without knowledge of the previous studies' results, this seems to be the case. For example, workers at the Institute of Food Research and the University of Reading conducted a study of 16 people given low-fat/high-carbohydrate, medium-fat/medium-carbohydrate, high-fat/low-carbohydrate breakfasts or no breakfast at all.[11] This study found that not having breakfast did not have any marked detrimental effects. This suggests that breakfast is not so important after all, and that seems to refute the findings of the previous studies. However, this is not surprising when you discover that all the breakfasts were made up of varying amounts of white bread, margarine, jam, a sweetened milk drink, extra thick double cream, maltodextrin (a commercially produced sweetener made from cereals) and water. These meals are all seriously protein deficient. Had breakfasts contained protein, the results would undoubtedly have been very different.

Another study, conducted by Professor Andy Smith of the University of Bristol, sent completely the wrong message to readers of *The Times* on 5 April 1997. This reported a study of 600 people's breakfast habits and concluded that those who regularly ate cereal first thing in the morning had a more positive mood than those who ate other foods or had no breakfast. It also reported that elderly cereal eaters were found to have higher IQs. But Professor Smith, speaking to the British Psychological Society, admitted that not only did his study not look at the type of cereal eaten to see if one was any better than others; the study also provided no information about cooked breakfasts because the diets of non-cereal eaters were not recorded. In other words, this study looked only at cereals to reach its conclusion that cereals were better. 'Better' is a comparative word. How can cereals be 'better' if they were not compared to other foods?

Three other good reasons for having breakfast

- **Gallstones.** The avoidance of gallstones is the first good reason not to miss breakfast. A study of French women with gallstones found that they had fasted on average for two hours longer overnight than women without the disease.[12]
- **Constipation.** The second reason is that breakfast, for most people, is followed by a trip to the lavatory. This is caused by the 'gastrocolic reflex', which works best in the morning. Although a cup of coffee can set off this reflex action, the strongest stimulus is dietary fat. Anyone who is constipated would do well to cultivate the fried breakfast habit.
- **Cancer.** And the last reason is because, according to a study at the Aichi Cancer Center Research Institute, Nagoya, Japan, a Western-style breakfast and salty food reduces the risk of oral cancer.[13]

Conclusion

There is no doubt that breakfast is the most important meal of the day. Many people have their major meal at the end of the day, sleep badly as a result and then have no appetite for breakfast. You must change this regime. Even if it takes some time to get used to it, do persevere. I urge you to make time for breakfast – the time it takes will soon be made up later as you will work more efficiently. A good meal of eggs, meat, cheese or fish will give you an amazing amount of energy throughout the whole day. If you are used to feeling weak and hungry by mid-morning, you will be astonished by the difference a good breakfast makes. If you truly haven't time to cook in the morning or cannot face a cooked breakfast, why not try a real Continental breakfast? Keep some hard-boiled eggs in the fridge and have one or two for breakfast with cold meat and/or cheese, a piece of fruit or salad and a drink. Never 'make do' with a slice of toast and a cup of coffee.

References

1. Thorn GW, Quinby JT, Clinton M Jr. A comparison of the metabolic effects of isocaloric meals of varying compositions with special reference to the prevention of postprandial hypoglycemic symptoms. *Ann Int Med* 1943; XVIII: 913.
2. Orent-Keiles E, Hallman L F. *The Breakfast Meal in Relation to Blood Sugar Values*. US Department of Agriculture Circular 1949; No. 827.
3. Heaton KW. Breakfast – do we need it? Report of a meeting of the Forum on Food and Health, 16 June 1989. *J R Soc Med* 1989; 82: 770.
4. Boutelle K, Neumark-Sztainer D, Story M, Resnick M. Weight control behaviors among obese, overweight, and non-overweight adolescents. *J Pediatr Psychol* 2002; 27: 531–540.
5. Ma Y, Bertone ER, Stanek EJ 3rd, et al. Association between eating patterns and obesity in a free-living US adult population. *Am J Epidemiol* 2003; 158: 85–92.
6. Cartwright M, Wardle J, Steggles N, et al. Stress and dietary practices in adolescents. *Health Psychol* 2003; 22: 362–369.
7. Pollitt E. Does breakfast make a difference in school? *J Am Diet Assoc* 1995; 95: 1134.
8. Kleinman RE, Hall S, Green H, et al. Diet, breakfast, and academic performance in children. *Ann Nutr Metab* 2002; 46, Suppl 1: 24–30.
9. Vermorel M, Bitar A, Vernet J, et al. The extent to which breakfast covers the morning energy expenditure of adolescents with varying levels of physical activity. *Eur J Clin Nutr* 2003; 57: 310–315.
10. Ainslie PN, Campbell IT, Frayn KN, et al. Physiological, metabolic, and performance implications of a prolonged hill walk: influence of energy intake. *J Appl Physiol* 2003; 94: 1075–1083.
11. Lloyd HM, Rogers PJ, Hedderley DI, Walker AF. Acute effects on mood and cognitive performance of breakfasts differing in fat and carbohydrate content. *Appetite* 1996; 27: 151.

12. Heaton KW. Breakfast – do we need it? Report of a meeting of the Forum on Food and Health, 16 June 1989. *J R Soc Med* 1989; 82: 770–771.
13. Takezaki T, Hirose K, Inoue M, et al. Tobacco, alcohol and dietary factors associated with the risk of oral cancer among Japanese. *Jpn J Cancer Res* 1996; 87: 555–562.

Chapter Three

Eat real food

Food is an important part of a balanced diet.

Fran Lebowitz

Introduction

The overweight and obese have always provided a very lucrative and ready market for food companies to exploit with expensive, nutrient-poor, highly processed, 'slimming foods' and diet products. Some of these, the liquid powders you made into a drink, were made largely from skimmed milk powder, with added chemicals and artificial flavours. The ingredients were very cheap for the manufacturers to buy (skimmed milk powder is almost given away), but were very expensive for the dieter to buy. Others included inert fillers which contained little or no food at all.

I had hoped that when the new low-carb way of eating caught on, these rip-off merchants would be unable to sell their products and go into liquidation. How naïve I was! It merely gave them yet another market to exploit.

The question I am asked most often is: 'Where can I buy low-carb foods?' The answer of course is simple: you can buy all the foods you need in any high street at the supermarket, butcher's shop, dairy and farm shop because it is not necessary to buy anything special with this way of eating.

Nevertheless, shopping for natural, fresh and healthy food was undermined when low-carb books promoted low-carb products such as meal replacements and dietary supplements. Readers were misled into believing that they needed these special products to be successful, but because most books were from the USA, these products were not at first available in the UK. As low-carb diets increased in popularity the products were shipped to Britain and British food producers adopted a 'me too please' attitude and likewise jumped on the low-carb bandwagon.

No joy with soy

Vegetarians have long used soya products as a replacement for meat, and it is not just vegetarian foods such as tofu that use soya. Soya is a cheap bean that has a relatively low carb content while being high in protein, and it is now being increasingly used in all manner of foodstuffs from meat sausages and fish fingers to salad creams and breakfast cereals. It is also used in almost all breads. Bovine spongiform encephalopathy (BSE) and other health scares related to meat have also led to rocketing sales of soya-related products in Britain. Since we are trying to reduce our intake of carbs, and at the same time seem to be relying more and more on convenience foods, we tend to look for foods that combine these two elements; soya looks promising.

Read the recipes in any American book on weight loss and see the number that incorporate soya in one form or another, in breakfast cereals, soya breads, convenience foods, smoothies, protein shakes, low-carb meal replacements, meat substitutes, and so on. Those who find giving up or cutting down on bread difficult also look for low-carb breads. Again, one that incorporates soya flour seems to provide the answer.

Soya also has a reputation of being 'healthy'. Each year, research on the health effects of soya and soybean components seems to increase exponentially with suggestions that soya has potential benefits that may be more extensive than previously thought, not only for low-carb dieting for weight loss but also in the fields of cancer, heart disease and osteoporosis.

Another incentive, at least for the manufacturers, is that the USA, where many of the 'low-carb' meal replacements come from, has 72 million acres under soya. With that much to sell, soya is relatively cheap. Not surprisingly, all these low-carb junk foods from the USA contain lots of soya and many of the British ones do as well.

However, soya has a dark side which needs to be considered very carefully because, far from being the perfect food it appears at first sight, modern soya products contain antinutrients and toxins that not only reduce the absorption of vitamins and minerals, but they also have other adverse effects including reduction in thyroid activity, which affect our metabolism.

A *brief history of soya*

Soya is a legume, a bean, which hails from Southeast Asia. You may be surprised to learn that, originally, the Chinese did not eat it, but merely used it to fix nitrogen in the soil.[1]

The Chinese did not eat the soya beans for a very good reason: soya beans contain large quantities of natural toxins which made the beans uncomfortable and unsafe to eat. These include:

- **Protease inhibitors** that block the action of trypsin and other enzymes needed for protein digestion. These inhibitors are not completely deactivated during ordinary cooking. They produce serious gastric distress and reduce protein digestion to cause chronic deficiencies in amino acid uptake. In test animals, diets high in trypsin inhibitors cause enlargement and pathological conditions of the pancreas, including cancer.[2]
- **Phytic acid** which inhibits the absorption from the gut of several important minerals, particularly calcium, iron and zinc.
- **Phytoestrogens and isoflavones** which mimic the female sex hormone, oestrogen. These are heavily promoted as an alternative to hormone replacement therapy (HRT) for menopausal women – but imagine what female hormones might do to men or growing children.
- **Goitrogens** which inhibit thyroid activity.

Fermentation and precipitation

Fermentation of soya destroys or neutralises the various toxins, making soya safe to eat. It was only after this discovery, during the Chou dynasty (1134–246 BC), that soya started to be eaten – but always in fermented form. The first fermented soya foods were products like tempeh, natto, miso and soya sauce. The use of fermented and precipitated soya products soon spread to other parts of the Orient, such as Japan and Indonesia.

Some soya products – notably tofu and bean curd – are precipitated rather than fermented. In this process, enzyme inhibitors concentrate in the soaking liquid rather than in the curd. Growth depressants are reduced in quantity in these products but not completely eliminated. Today, unfortunately, many of the products sold in supermarkets which contain soya, contain unfermented soya flour and soya milk. Eating these is not without risk.

Soya and the thyroid gland

The thyroid gland produces hormones that have a profound effect on our bodies' metabolism – the rate at which our bodies use energy.[3] This in turn has implications for the cause and treatment of overweight and obesity. It also affects such seemingly unrelated things as blood cholesterol levels.

In the condition known as *hypothyroidism* – underactive thyroid – the thyroid gland does not produce enough thyroid hormone, thyroxin. As this condition progresses, the thyroid may increase in size in an attempt to make more thyroxin. This produces an unsightly swelling in the neck called a *goitre*. The most important cause of goitre is a lack of iodine and goitres are endemic in parts of the world that are deficient in iodine. However, these are rare in the West, where other causes of hypothyroidism and goitre are more prevalent, such as *goitrogens* which suppress thyroid function. One such is fluoride, which will be discussed later in this chapter. Soya also contains goitrogens.

In 1991, Japanese researchers reported that consumption of as little as 30 grams – about two tablespoons – of soya beans per day for just one month caused a significant increase in thyroid-stimulating hormone (TSH), the hormone which instructs the thyroid to produce more thyroxin.[4] This caused goitre and hypothyroidism to appear in some of their trial participants and many complained of constipation, fatigue and lethargy, even though they had an adequate intake of iodine. In 1997, researchers from the United States Food and Drug Administration's National Center for Toxicological Research made the embarrassing discovery that the goitrogenic components of soya were the very same isoflavones that were promoted to help women through the menopause.[5]

When the thyroid gland does not produce sufficient thyroxin, this slows down the body's metabolism – the rate at which it uses energy. For this reason, including soya in the forms of flour, powder or milk in your diet could cause weight gain or stop your weight loss.

Phytoestogens

Soya contains *phytoestrogens*: isoflavones such as *genistein* and *diadzen* which are similar to natural oestrogen. These are used by many women to stave off the effects of the menopause, despite a British Government assessment which failed to find much evidence of benefit and warned against potential adverse effects.[6] A new soya-enriched loaf from Allied Bakeries was targeted at menopausal women seeking relief from hot flushes in the 1990s. It was so successful that sales in 1997 were running at a quarter of a million loaves per week.[7] Today you will be hard pressed to find any bread that doesn't contain soya flour.

Twenty-five grams of soya protein isolate contains 50–70 mg of isoflavones. Yet it took only 45 mg of isoflavones in premenopausal women to exert significant biological effects, including a reduction in hormones needed for adequate thyroid function. These effects continued for three months after they stopped eating the soya.[8]

In 1992 the Swiss health service estimated that 100 grams of soya protein provided the oestrogenic equivalent of the contraceptive pill.[9] With that in mind, what of its effects on children and men?

Soya consumption has been linked to numerous disorders, including infertility, increased cancer and infantile leukaemia, and studies dating back to the 1950s showed that genistein in soya caused disrupted hormone production in animals.[10]

Laboratory studies also suggest that isoflavones inhibit synthesis of oestradiol and other steroid hormones.[11] Several species of animals including mice, cheetah, quail, pigs, rats, sturgeon and sheep displayed reproductive problems, infertility, thyroid disease and liver disease due to dietary isoflavones.[12]

Isoflavones in infancy are probably the greatest cause for concern, as they are likely to affect the way a child develops. In 1998, investigators reported that circulating concentrations of isoflavones in infants fed soya-based baby formula were 13,000 to 22,000 times higher than plasma oestradiol concentrations in infants fed baby formula made with cow's milk.[13] An infant exclusively fed on soya formula receives the oestrogenic equivalent (based on body weight) of at least five birth control pills per day.[14] By contrast, almost no phytoestrogens have been detected in dairy-based infant formula or in human milk, even when the mother consumes soya products.

Did you know that the age of puberty has been coming down significantly for a number of decades? Girls, for example, used to reach puberty in their teens. In general that age has dropped to around ten to eleven years old. However, a more alarming number of girls are entering puberty at a worryingly earlier age. An American study found that one girl in every hundred had started to develop breasts or pubic hair before the age of three; by the age of eight, almost one in six white girls and one in two African-American girls had one or both of these characteristics.[15]

The effect of the female hormone on boys is potentially far more serious. During the first few months of life, boys have testosterone levels that may be as high as those of an adult male. Although this is long before puberty, it is the period when a boy is programmed to express male characteristics after puberty. These include not only in the development of his sexual organs and other masculine physical traits, but also sets patterns in the brain which are characteristic of male behaviour. Little experimentation seems to have been done on human babies for obvious reasons. However, a deficiency of male hormones in monkeys has been shown to impair the development of spatial perception, which is normally more acute in men than in women, as well as learning ability, and of visual discrimination tasks such as are required for reading.[16] Learning disabilities, especially in male children, have reached epidemic proportions. It is possible that feeding soya to infants could be responsible for this situation.

It should also be obvious that the early hormonal environment might also influence future patterns of sexual orientation.

Dr Daniel Doerge of the Division of Biochemical Toxicology at the National Center for Toxicological Research, who is one of America's top soya researchers, and Daniel Sheehan, who at that time were the Food and Drug Administration's (FDA) two key experts on soy, protested the health claims approved by the FDA on soya products, in an official letter of protest to the FDA dated 18 February 1999, saying:

'there is abundant evidence that some of the isoflavones found in soy, including genistein and equol, a metabolite of daidzen, demonstrate toxicity in estrogen sensitive tissues and in the thyroid. This is true for a number of species, including humans. Additionally, isoflavones are inhibitors of the thyroid peroxidase which makes T_3 and T_4. Inhibition can be expected to generate thyroid abnormalities, including goiter and autoimmune thyroiditis. There exists a significant body of animal data that demonstrates goitrogenic and even carcinogenic effects of soy products. Moreover, there are significant reports of goitrogenic effects from soy consumption in human infants and adults.'

In 2002, Doerge published the results of follow-up research.[17] In this new research, Doerge looked at the goitrogenic and oestrogenic effects of soya in greater depth. Research had already shown that soya consumption was linked to increased risk of goitre. When iodine is deficient, the antithyroid effects of soya are intensified. Soya's ability to affect the thyroid, he found, therefore, depends on the relationship between iodine status and thyroid function. In animal studies, rats given genistein-fortified diets showed an increase in thyroid antibodies, while other measures of thyroid function apparently remained normal. These findings led Dr Doerge to conclude that additional factors appeared necessary for soya to cause overt thyroid toxicity. These factors included:

- iodine deficiency
- consumption of other soya components
- other goitrogens in the diet
- other physiological problems in synthesizing thyroid hormones.

According to Dr Doerge, more needs to be known. He concluded: 'Although safety testing of natural products, including soy products, is not required, the possibility that widely consumed soy products may cause harm in the human population via either or both estrogenic and goitrogenic activities is of concern. Rigorous, high-quality experimental and human research into soy toxicity is the best way to address these concerns.'

Phytic acid and mineral status

Lastly, many nutritionists condemn low-carb diets because, they say, they are unbalanced, leading to deficiencies in some nutrients. With a properly constituted diet that is simply not true, but with a dietary regime in which soya features, deficiencies could become a problem because soya is high in phytic acid, a chemical that inhibits the absorption of a range of minerals. Scientists are in general agreement that diets high in phytates contribute to widespread mineral deficiencies in third world countries.

Soya beans have one of the highest phytate levels of any grain or legume that has been studied.[18] With wheat and other grains, long slow cooking and fermentation will neutralise the phytate they contain, but the phytates in soya are highly resistant to these techniques.[19] Only a very long period of fermentation will significantly reduce the phytate content of soya, and in most of the foods which contain soya today this simply doesn't happen, as it adds to the cost of production. When precipitated soya products like tofu are consumed with meat, the mineral-blocking effects of the phytates are reduced, but that is all.[20]

Vegetarians who consume tofu and bean curd as a substitute for meat and dairy products risk severe mineral deficiencies. The results of calcium, magnesium, zinc and iron deficiency are well known.

The mineral most affected by soya is zinc. Soya-based infant formula is particularly harmful because zinc is needed for proper development and functioning of the brain and nervous system. It also plays a role in protein synthesis and collagen formation; it is involved in the blood sugar control mechanism and thus protects against diabetes; it is needed for a healthy reproductive system. Zinc is a key component in numerous vital enzymes and plays a vital role in the immune system.

Soya and cancer

The food industry touts soy products for their cancer-preventing properties. This is because the *isoflavone aglycones*, contained in fermented soya do have an anti-cancer effect. However, in non-fermented soya products such as tofu and soya milk, as well as the raw beans, the flour used in bread, and protein powders used for the low-carb market, these isoflavones are present in an altered form as *beta glycoside conjugates*, which do *not* have an anti-cancer effect.[21] Indeed, some researchers believe the rapid increase in liver and pancreatic cancer in Africa is because of the introduction of soya products there.[22]

Summary

Soya processors have worked hard to get soya's antinutrients out of the finished product, particularly out of the soya protein isolate which is the key ingredient in most soya foods that imitate meat, dairy products and the protein powders used in commercial low-carb meal replacements so beloved of American low-carb diet gurus. It is true that much of the trypsin inhibitors can be removed through high-temperature processing. However, not all are removed, and there may be as much as a fivefold difference between the trypsin inhibitor content of one soya protein isolate and another.[23]

There is one last problem: the high-temperature processing needed to neutralise these toxins has the unfortunate side-effect of so denaturing the other proteins in soya that they are rendered largely useless.[24]

All in all, it makes sense to avoid products containing unfermented soya.

Fluoride

To finish I want to look briefly at one other 'nutrient' that should be avoided at all costs: fluoride. Fluorides are promoted to help teeth, but they are powerful enzyme disruptors with the power to affect every cell in our bodies.

Up to the middle of the last century, fluoridated water was used to treat people who had an overactive thyroid.[25] It was a very effective treatment, but for any person with normal thyroid function, ingestion or absorption of fluoride produces hypothyroidism – underactive thyroid. So here is another chemical that makes weight gain more likely and weight loss more difficult.

Do you live in a fluoridated area?

Fluorides are not just found in toothpaste; the stuff may also be in your water supply. You can call your water company to find out. If you do live in a fluoridated area, then you should think seriously about complaining to your water company and area health authority, because you have a legal right not to be medicated without your consent. Your only other options are either to move to an unfluoridated area or buy an expensive Reverse Osmosis water filter or water distillation equipment.

If you continue to drink fluoridated water, or bath in it, or wash your clothes in it, and you have difficulty losing weight when you know you are eating properly, it could be your health authority's fault.[26]

Artificial sweeteners

There is some debate about the role of the artificial sweeteners as used by dieters. Saccharine and aspartame contain no calories so, on the face of it, they appear to be an ideal substitute for those people with a sweet tooth who cannot give up sugar. But there are two problems with them:

1. A great deal has been said in the media about artificial sweeteners hampering weight loss. The suggestion is that the pancreas may start to produce insulin for

the purpose of reducing blood glucose levels before those levels are elevated, merely in response to a sweet stimulus. Thus eating a calorie-free sweetener can trigger the production of insulin. However, as no glucose enters the bloodstream, glucose already there is removed for storage as fat, blood glucose levels are driven down and the result is hunger and increased food intake.

2. Whether or not the above is correct, it is true that eating foods containing artificial or any other kind of sweeteners maintains the taste for over-sweetened foods. It is much better to reduce your use of *all* sweeteners gradually until the natural sweetness of foods tastes right for you. The sweetness to aim for is the natural sweetness found in fruit.

Artificial ingredients

Lastly, there is a great difference between the fresh foods you buy in butcher's and greengrocer's shops and the pre-packaged, processed foods supermarkets are full of. It's no secret that processed foods are liberally laced with colourings and preservatives so that foods look more attractive and have a longer shelf life. They are also usually made from the cheapest materials available. But there are two other aspects:

1. First is that heating, which is the most common form of processing, tends to denature many foods. If you buy these foods and cook them at home, they are heated twice, which harms them even more.

2. Second is that real flavours tend to be more expensive than artificial ones, because the real flavours have to come from real food. So, if, for example, you buy strawberries and some plain yogurt and mix them, you have an entirely natural and healthy dessert. If you buy strawberry-flavoured yogurt, however, you are likely to end up with a very different product. In Britain it is impossible to discover what these flavourings are made of – it seems that it is a trade secret. Fortunately, this is not the case in the USA so by asking there, we can discover their formulae. The widely used strawberry flavour, MF129, is made up from a 1000 gram mixture of the following:

> Corps Praline (trade name of Firmench and Co) (17.25 g)
> Alcohol, 95% (362.05 g); agitate and heat until dissolved, then add:
> Propylene glycol (530.00 g)

Glacial acetic acid (10.00 g)
Aldehyde C$_{16}$ (30.25 g)
Benzyl acetate (22.75 g)
Vanillin (11.25 g)
Methyl cinnamate (4.25 g)
Methyl anthranilate (2.25 g)
Methyl heptine carbonate (0.20 g)
Methyl salicylate (2.25 g)
Ionine, beta (2.25 g)
Aldehyde C$_{14}$ (2.25 g)
Diacetyl (2.25 g)
Anethol (0.75 g)

Additives in processed foods

Even though additives have to be listed on product labels, those labels may tell only half the story, for enzymes used in the processing of the product do not have to be listed. They are used to tenderise meat, to clean milk contaminated with antibiotics, to make modified starches and in the baking and brewing industries. Some of these enzymes are made from plant or animal tissue, but most are made by microbial fermentation. Naturally the industry says that they are safe but there have been a number of reports of allergic reactions to them in workers in the industry.

Conclusion

Although I have focused on weight loss, I can't see any point in swapping one disease for another. For that reason, this book is really concerned with promoting a much healthier lifestyle altogether. As all highly processed and packaged foods are usually chemical laden, nutrient poor and not fresh, I don't recommend you buy them. Stick to the real thing and buy fresh or frozen foods except, perhaps, in an emergency when nothing else is available. Although, having said that, I can't imagine any time when a 'low-carb' bar will be available, where some form of real food isn't.

The soya ridden, low-carb bars and shakes should be avoided at all costs. This is a particularly important consideration for children.

References

1. Katz SH. Food and biocultural evolution: A model for the investigation of modern nutritional problems. In *Nutritional Anthropology*. Alan R. Liss, New York, 1987, p.50.

2. Rackis JJ, et al. The USDA trypsin inhibitor study. I: Background, objectives and procedural details. In *Qualification of Plant Foods in Human Nutrition*, vol. 35, 1985.

3. Nyrnes A, Jorde R, Sundsfjord J. Serum TSH is positively associated with BMI. *Int J Obesity* 2006; 30: 100–105.

4. Ishizuki Y, et al. The effects on the thyroid gland of soybeans administered experimentally in healthy subjects. *Nippon Naibunpi Gakkai Zasshi* 1991; 767: 622–629.

5. Divi RL, et al. Anti-thyroid isoflavones from the soybean. *Biochem Pharm* 1997; 54: 1087–1096.

6. *IEH Assessment on Phytoestrogens in the Human Diet*. Final Report to the Ministry of Agriculture, Fisheries and Food, UK, November 1997, p.11.

7. Bakery says new loaf can help reduce hot flushes, Reuters, 15 September 1997.

8. Cassidy A, et al. Biological effects of a diet of soy protein rich in isoflavones on the menstrual cycle of premenopausal women. *Am J Clin Nutr* 1994; 60: 333–340.

9. Bulletin de L'Office Fédéral de la Santé Publique, No. 28, 20 July 1992.

10. Matrone G, et al. Effect of genistin on growth and development of the male mouse. *J Nutr* 1956; 235–240.

11. a. Keung WM. Dietary oestrogenic isoflavones are potent inhibitors of B-hydroxysteroid dehydrogenase of *P. testosteronii. Biochem Biophys Res Comm* 1995; 215: 1137–1144;
    b. Makela SI, et al. Estrogen-specific 12 B-hydroxysteroid oxidoreductase type 1 (E.C. 1.1.1.62) as a possible target for the action of phytoestrogens. *PSEBM* 1995; 208: 51–59.

12. a. Setchell KDR, et al. Dietary oestrogens – a probable cause of infertility and liver disease in captive cheetahs. *Gastroenterology* 1987; 93: 225–233;
    b. Leopald AS. Phytoestrogens: Adverse effects on reproduction in California Quail. *Science* 1976; 191: 98–100;
    c. Drane HM, et al. Oestrogenic activity of soya-bean products. *Food Cosmet Technol* 1980; 18: 425–427;
    d. Kimura S, et al. Development of malignant goiter by defatted soybean with iodine-free diet in rats. *Gann* 1976; 67: 763–765;
    e. Pelissero C, et al. Oestrogenic effect of dietary soybean meal on vitellogenesis in cultured Siberian sturgeon *Acipenser baeri. Gen Comp End* 1991; 83: 447–457;
    f. Braden AW, et al. The oestrogenic activity and metabolism of certain isoflavones in sheep. *Aust J Agric Res*1967; 18: 335–348.

13. Setchell KD, et al. Isoflavone content of infant formulas and the metabolic fate of these early phytoestrogens in early life. *Am J Clin Nutr* 1998; Supplement: 1453S–1461S.

14. Irvine C, et al. The potential adverse effects of soybean phytoestrogens in infant feeding. *NZ Med J* 1995; May 24: 318.

15. Herman-Giddens ME, et al. Secondary sexual characteristics and menses in young girls seen in office practice: A study from the Pediatric Research in Office Settings Network. *Pediatrics* 1997; 99: 505–512.

16. Hagger C, Bachevalier J. Visual habit formation in 3-month-old monkeys (*Macaca mulatta*): Reversal of sex difference following neonatal manipulations of androgen. *Behav Brain Res* 1991; 45: 57–63.

17. Doerge, DR. Goitrogenic and estrogenic activity of soy isoflavones. *Environ Health Perspect* 2002; 110 Suppl 3: 349–353.

18. El Tiney AH. Proximate composition and mineral and phytate contents of legumes grown in Sudan. *J Food Compos Anal* 1989; 2: 6778.

19. Ologhobo AD, et al. Distribution of phosphorus and phytate in some Nigerian varieties of legumes and some effects of processing. *J Food Sci* 1984; 49: 199–201.

20. a. Sandstrom B, et al. Effect of protein level and protein source on zinc absorption in humans. *J Nutr* 1989; 119(1): 48–53;

    b. Tait S, et al. The availability of minerals in food, with particular reference to iron. *J Res Soc Health* 1983; 103: 74–77.

21. Coward L, et al. Genistein, daidzen and their betaglycoside conjugates: Antitumor isoflavones in soybean food from American and Asian diets. *J Agric Food Chem* 1993; 41: 1961–1967.

22. Katz SH. Op cit.

23. Rackis JJ, et al. Op cit.

24. Wallace GM. Studies on the processing and properties of soymilk. *J Sci Food Agric* 1971; 22: 526–535.

25. Gorlitzer von Mundy. Einfluss von Fluor und Jod auf den Stoffwechsel, insbesondere auf die Schilddrüse. *Münch Med Wochenschrift* 1963; 105: 234–247.

26. Groves BA. Fluoride: Drinking Ourselves to Death? Newleaf, Dublin, 2001.

Chapter Four

Tips for successful dieting

A friend asked me 'Do you think you will spend the rest of your life without ever eating potato again?' I thought about it, and said, 'Have you ever had a potato dish that was worth you weighing 21 stone? No, I didn't think so.'

R.B.

Today, children's education is sadly lacking in most of the skills needed to live a healthy life. When my generation went to school, we were taught how to cook and how to manage and provide foods for a family. If anything is taught at all these days, it seems to be restricted to how to get a packet out of the fridge and put it in a microwave. This simply is not good enough, if only because it puts the population at the mercy of food-producing companies whose only real motivation is profit. For this reason, they will use the cheapest ingredients available; they will also include artificial flavours and flavour enhancers as cheap ingredients usually means 'bland'. And, as shelf life is an important consideration, these foods will also include preservatives. None of these additives is desirable in a truly healthy diet.

The most important tip

There is one tip that must come before all others in this book. That is: Don't think of this plan as just another 'diet'. It's a way of life. But if you are going live this way for the rest of your life, you must enjoy what you eat. For this reason, while you should stay within the general guidelines, pick foods that you like.

Tips to keep the cost down

Many people think that cutting down on carbs and replacing them with foods high in protein and fat is expensive. Indeed it can be, but it can also be as cheap, if not cheaper than the way you are eating now – especially if you deduct the price of slimming clubs, exercise gear, magazines and personal trainers. The tips in this chapter are all common sense really, but it is as well to reinforce that. It is also invaluable for anyone used to eating only fast food. Let's face it, processed food has to be an expensive option because processing and packaging has to be paid for. So:

Get back to basics

Rather than paying someone else to cook, pack, advertise and then ship inferior food to you, it's much cheaper and certainly more nutritious to buy basic ingredients and make your own meals.

Don't buy special 'low-carb' products

These products are also far more expensive than similar things made from scratch. This way of eating does not require any special foods.

Plan your budget

Work out how much you want to spend on food each week and stick to it. Otherwise, you could be eating like a king at the start of the month and recycling teabags by the end of it.

Compare prices

Shop around. Find out whether your local greengrocer or market stall is better value than the supermarket. If you use a supermarket, buying their own brand products could save a significant amount over the heavily advertised big brands.

Chapter Four

Shop seasonally

In the middle of winter you'll pay more for summer produce flown in from a distant corner of the world. It's always cheaper to buy fruit and veg produced locally when it's in season.

Don't be seduced by special offers

Getting 20 p off, three for the price of two, or 15% extra is great if it's something you need. But don't fill the cupboards with stuff you don't need just because it's on special offer!

Cook in bulk

It can be expensive buying a different set of ingredients for every meal. It can also be expensive to use an oven for a small dish for one person, when it has room for ten, so it's a good idea to cook up a batch of food. Divided up into meal-sized portions, cooled and frozen, meals can be microwaved later as required. But make sure you reheat the food until it's hot all the way through.

Watch your waste

If you buy food that goes off quickly, plan your meals so it all gets eaten or frozen for future use.

Use 'sell-by dates'

Shops have to sell foods by their 'sell-by date'. If they have overstocked, there will usually be some items whose sell-by date has nearly expired and the item is being sold off cheap. Look out for these. Be aware that the sell-by or use-by dates are purely arbitrary and there is plenty of leeway for safety. I have often drunk cream more than a month after its use-by date has expired, and it has always been perfectly edible.

Fatty meat is cheaper

Most people today don't want fat meat – that's why it's not easy to find – but you do. This not wanting fatty meat can work to your advantage, because it is either cheaper so the shops can sell it more easily or, if you are cheeky enough and see a piece of nice fatty meat, you can usually get the price reduced. So ask for a particular piece of meat – but ask also for the price to be reduced because of the fat on it. It's amazing how often this will work. The only thing you have to watch is that the shop assistant doesn't cut the fat off, thinking that you won't want it!

Offal – liver, kidney, heart, tripe, et cetera – has fallen out of fashion. This is a shame as it is these parts that are the most nutritious. But, for us, this is a godsend, for offal is remarkably cheap. You can get enough ox liver to feed a family of four for under a pound, for example (2005 prices).

Sources of foods

Fruit and veg

This is a *low*-carb way of eating, not *no*-carb. But there is no health benefit from eating more than two or three portions of fruit and veg each day – that's a total, by the way, not that much of each. As vegetables are much more nutritious than fruits, I recommend two portions of vegetables and one of fruit. Fresh fruits and veges are best but they could be frozen, tinned or dried. I don't recommend fruit juice as this is usually highly processed and one glass, which will contain the juice and sugars of several fruits, is too much..

To get the most out of vegetables, they must be properly cooked to break down the cell walls and enable the body to absorb the nutrients inside, but be aware that much of the vitamin content ends up in the cooking water. Cook them in as little water as possible and use the water in soups or gravy. You can also season it and use it as a drink. If you have the freezer space, try buying frozen vegetables. These are economical because you can take just what you need out of the freezer and then there isn't any waste.

Carrots and onions are among the cheapest vegetables around when bought loose although baby carrots can be expensive. Add them to soups or casseroles as they add colour and flavour as well as nutrients.

Frozen peas are inexpensive and easy. All you need is a pan of water to cook these from frozen in a few minutes. Adding a few spoonfuls to a meal is an easy way to boost your vegetable quota.

Proteins

Eggs are undoubtedly the best source not only of protein but most other nutrients as well, and they are not expensive. Three large eggs, scrambled in butter, make a very filling meal for very little money, and you can cut the cost even further if you scramble them in lard. You could also make them into an omelette with leftover vegetables, or chop up hard-boiled egg to add to salads.

Canned meat and fish are also good and relatively inexpensive. All are good sources of protein. But beware: mackerel, tuna and sardines are good sources of omega-3 fatty acids if they are fresh, but the omega-3s are practically non-existent in some tinned fish: tuna is particularly fatless. Beware also of added sugar in canned meats.

Fresh meat and fish are better and should be cheaper. Cuts such as brisket are very cheap because they tend to be either fatty (which we want) or tough. But cooking them in a slow cooker or crockpot makes them marvellously tender and succulent. Put it on in the morning before you go to work and in the afternoon when you get home, yummy! Fresh fish is also better than canned, but it degrades quickly and really must be eaten on the day of purchase.

Chicken and bacon from supermarkets are a waste of money. They are both 'pumped' with water and a concoction of gunge. A 2003 news report (*Daily Mail* 21 May) found that as much as 45% of the weight of supermarket chicken wasn't chicken! Bacon isn't much better. If you want bacon, it is better to cure your own, but you do need fridge space to do it. You will find instructions in the Recipes section. Alternatively, farmers' markets can usually be relied upon for dry-cured bacon.

Dairy products. Milk is a good drink at any time of day, but it is expensive for what it has in it. It seems a waste to buy what is really mostly water. The most nutritious part of the milk is its cream. So why not just buy cream? This is a better and a cheaper option for drinks of tea, coffee or cocoa. Cheese is a better supplier of the other nutrients.

Offal. Liver, kidney, heart, faggots, liver sausage, and so on, are rich in nutrients and, as few people today eat them, fantastic value for money. Liver is the best multi-vitamin/mineral source I know.

Fats

The cheapest fat is lard, which is clarified pork fat. This is only about one sixth the price of butter, but contains the highest amounts of the anti-cancer vitamin D after cod liver oil. Beef dripping is also inexpensive. It too contains an anti-cancer agent – conjugated linoleic acid (CLA). Both of these can be used for the frying you will do a lot of. If you have friends who can't kick the low-fat habit, ask for the dripping that they would otherwise throw away from a roast goose or duck. These fats are really nice, but expensive if bought from a supermarket.

General tips

Sugar and artificial sweeteners

There are going to be occasions when you do need to sweeten something, even when you have lost your sweet tooth. I believe in using real foods as much as possible. For all its faults sugar is still a relatively natural product. Don't get obsessive about the sugar. It might not be good for you, but it is still better for you than the artificial alternatives. One of my clients told me that she had discovered the oddest thing about sugar: she didn't crave sweet things after she ate a small amount of it – but she did when she ate artificial sweeteners.

There may be a good reason for this. It's a bit like waving a cigarette in front of somebody who is trying to give up smoking. If you eat sugar you satisfy the craving, but by using an artificial sweetener, you are giving your body the taste and reminding it of what it's missing, without satisfying the craving.

I have never stopped eating 'sweets'. And, although fruit is not healthy in large quantities (as Chapter 13 shows, '5 portions of fruit and vegetables a day' as the establishment tells us in UK, is too much), I see no need to give it up altogether unless you are diabetic.

The sweetness of most fruit is generally a mild sweetness which does not lead to addiction. I would also use sugar rather than artificial sweeteners to sweeten other foods – rhubarb, for example, or sweet desserts – but I wouldn't use much. The secret is to get your liking or 'need' for sweet things down to where this sort of sweetness feels right.

Another thought: even if you crave sweeter things than this now, I guarantee that you can always cut the sugar in any 'normal' recipe by half and not notice the difference. The problem is that you can't do this with bought food, which is loaded with sugar to keep you addicted, so that you will continue to buy it.

So I would use sugar where necessary and cut the amount as low as possible. Apart from other health concerns, all the artificial sweeteners have a more intense sweetness that perpetuates the taste for oversweet things.

When buying prepared, packaged foods, beware of foods that boast 'no-added sugar', or 'sucrose-free'. Read the label carefully. Many foods, particularly jams and fruit drinks, are sweetened with concentrated grape or apple juice, or high-fructose syrups, which yield the same carb and calorie count as sugar, and have the same deleterious effects on your body.

However, there is one aspect of sugar that must be taken into account: sugar is addictive. Although other starchy foods may have a greater immediate effect on blood sugar levels than sugar, you are not likely to yearn after, say, a parsnip. But sugar, and foods that contain it in large quantity including sweet fruits, are craved. To ensure that you become addicted and your craving is maintained, food manufacturers now put sugar in just about everything that comes in a packet, tin or bottle. Just look at the labels even on tinned meat, for example, and try to find one that does not contain sugar.

A large part of learning to eat for health and weight loss is concerned with beating the sugar habit. When you can walk past the sweets at a checkout without the desire to buy some, you will be cured. It may take time, but it is well worth it.

Don't disguise the fat with carbs

Experiments show that our bodies are very sensitive to fat in the sense that, as soon as they have had enough, they switch off the appetite for it. Try to eat more fat and you will feel sick. And when the appetite for fat is switched off, it switches off the appetite for other things as well. In this way, eating fat controls the total amount of food eaten and, thus, it limits total calories eaten. On a high-fat diet, you cannot eat so much that you put weight on.

However, there is a proviso. If you disguise the fat with a sweetener or other concentrated carb, this dulls your body's ability to recognise the fat. In this way, a sweetened, fatty food can be eaten to excess and you may gain weight.

Boring meals?

I have heard 'experts' say that eating this way is boring. It's nonsense spoken by people who have never tried it. Don't worry about the food appearing boring in the early days; this is more perception than reality. Think of what you eat now. Most people generally tend to eat the same foods day in and day out – cereal for breakfast, sandwiches for lunch, and a few variations on dinner in the evening. When you switch to this plan, if you think it is boring and has less variety than your old way of eating, think about what you actually ate before and you will probably find that the old way of eating was not so varied after all.

Fatty foods are always more succulent than low-fat foods, and you can also jazz up your food with different spices, herbs, cream sauces, and so on. Select different vegetables and try cutting them in different ways; cook them in different ways with fats and cheese and cream. Look for different cuts of meats, fatty ones are best, and try to vary the ones you are buying. And don't forget about offal: not only does it really make a very nice change, it is far more nutritious and, thus, better value, than plain muscle meat.

Cravings

I said earlier in this book that nothing is forbidden. I meant it. If you crave a food, have it. If you don't, you will continue to want it until that wanting becomes an obsession, a fixation that takes over your mind. So, if you really need to eat chocolate, for example, have some – but have only a small piece, not the whole bar. Nine times out of ten this will take the edge off your craving. Problem solved?

If not, try another approach: increase the thing you crave. For example, I had a woman client who craved bread. So I told her to eat only bread for two or three days – nothing else. It didn't take that long. By the end of the first day, she was so stuffed with bread she couldn't continue eating it any more. She now no longer wants bread.

It works with children too. When Diane's mother changed her chubby daughter's diet to low-carb some years ago, Diane kept on nagging for sweets. So I suggested to her mother that she let her daughter have as many sweets as she wanted – but that was all. While she had sweets she couldn't have any other food. Diane thought this was great. She stuffed herself with sweets for two whole days. On the third day, she asked her mother for a banana. It was refused. The bargain was she could only have sweets or real food, not both. On the fourth day Diane was pleading for food and was prepared never even to look at another sweet. She is now a lovely slim girl, the envy of her girl friends and much sought by the boys.

But it might not be easy at first

Be aware that sugar is addictive and other sweeteners prolong the addiction. As with any other addiction, you may suffer withdrawal symptoms. Here is an example of what may happen. Terry wrote to me:

> 'Just like to say thanks for the info about Splenda, what an eye opener. I have to say that having been on low carbs for about 10 months, my last link to the old ways was to allow myself artificial sweeteners in my decaf coffee, chewing gum, and on raspberries and blackberries, all of which I consume daily. After your comments re getting rid for good of the desire for sweetness, I decided to bite the bullet and quit completely about 3 weeks ago. Well blow me, it was like going cold turkey, I have never taken drugs or smoked, but it is how I imagine it must feel. I became irritable and angry and had physical reactions ranging from headaches and neck/shoulder tension to palpitations and dizziness, and of course a strong desire for anything sweet. I persevered and am now sweetener free. The desire for sweetness has gone and I feel great.'

Don't eat your entire carb allowance at one meal

A question I am often asked is similar to this one which Polly asked me: 'Does it matter if I don't have many carbs during the day and eat most of them in the evening? I find that's when I want them, and I eat a big portion of veg and maybe some fruit for dessert. At breakfast or lunch I'm happy to just have meat, eggs etc.'

The answer is that it really depends on how much you are thinking of eating. Your body doesn't have the ability to look at the carbs and average them out over the day. It looks at the instantaneous level, and then produces the insulin needed to process it. Any excess will be stored as fat. It is this fat storing hormone that does all the damage. If you have a moderate level of carbs, three times a day, it is much better than a high level once a day, even if the total carbs in the one high-carb meal is less than the total eaten at three meals. That minimises the insulin spikes and you avoid storing glucose as fat.

How to get enough fibre

Jo told me: 'I find I just cannot get enough fibre in my diet. I am permanently constipated. This never used to be the case, only happened in the last year or so. I thought it would improve after my operation, but I'm still struggling! Should I eat more wholemeal bread?'

Most people have been led to believe that only cereals such as wheat contain fibre. But fibre is found in all plant foods. If the muscles in your gut have not had to work because you have been stuffing large amounts of waste through, it can take a while for those muscles to start working again. But if you do feel the need to increase your fibre intake, eat more raw leafy veges rather than bran. That is much healthier. Increasing your water intake will also help.

Being one with the crowd in the office

You are sitting at your desk at the office and one of your colleagues comes in laden down with left over food from a lunchtime meeting he has just been to. There are sandwiches, biscuits, savoury pastries and cakes! Everyone is gathering round his table helping themselves and someone from the office next door has come in with a huge piece of cheesecake to share around. The problem is: How do you not accept what people are offering round without feeling like a total outcast? And even though no one may be pushing you to have anything how do you stop feeling left out?

If no one is pushing, there shouldn't be a problem. You can join in with a cup of tea, and not eat. Probably, no one will notice. If the temptation is difficult to overcome, just think of the food as 'leftovers' and maybe they will not be so tempting.

The psychology of being not one of 'the crowd' is quite another thing. We humans are not comfortable with being different. But, if you think about it, the greatest humans were those who didn't mind being different.

However, if you do feel uncomfortable in these situations, pick out just one scrumptious thing, something you feel is truly worth it, and eat a very small amount. Savour it thoroughly, then put it behind you (not literally) and get on with your normal diet.

Chapter Four

Have you checked your thyroid?

Thyroid hormones control a wide spectrum of metabolic functions. If your thyroid isn't working properly, this can make weight loss more difficult, raise cholesterol levels, raise blood pressure; indeed there are a whole host of adverse effects. So check it. For this a doctor is not necessarily the best option in the first place. This is because a doctor will take a blood test, normally for TSH (thyroid stimulating hormone) only, and if this is within a 'normal' range, you are okay; except you might not be.

The 'normal' range was determined many years ago by checking the thyroid hormone levels of people who visited their doctors with an illness. So, it is reasonable to assume that these were not healthy people. Thus, the question is: Is the 'normal' range also a normal range for healthy people? There is much controversy over this.

The easiest and quickest way to determine if your thyroid is behaving itself is to check your temperature. This should be 37°C or 98.6°F. If it is one degree Celsius or two degrees Fahrenheit below these figures, then your thyroid is definitely not working properly.

Two things that have a harmful effect on the thyroid are foods that contain soya and water and medications containing fluoride. See Chapter 3 for more detail.

Miscellaneous tips

Don't buy foods you shouldn't eat

To help you to stay with this way of eating, it is a good idea not to have any illicit foods in the house to tempt you. You cannot have biscuits with your mid-morning cup of tea if there are none in the biscuit barrel.

However, that doesn't mean you can't have chocolate as a treat. If you are going to treat yourself to a bar of chocolate at the weekend, don't buy it on the previous Monday – you are bound to be tempted to eat it sooner than you planned.

Shopping

When you shop, make a list and stick to it. If you are held up at the supermarket checkout, next to the sweets, don't be tempted. You will be less tempted if you aren't hungry, so have a good breakfast before shopping.

When eating

Be aware of the signals your body gives you. If you carry on a conversation over a meal you may not notice when your appetite is satisfied and it's time to stop. Then you may eat too much. You should stop when satisfied, not stuffed. And if there is some left at this stage, leave it. You can perhaps save it to have later, or freeze it for another day. But whatever you do, don't use your body as a dustbin.

Don't drink 'food'

There is one other signal that your body will give you that you should respond to in the correct way: when you feel thirsty your body is telling you it needs water – *not food*. When you are thirsty, drink water or a beverage that contains no calories. Having a sweetened drink, fruit juice or alcohol is one of the best ways to put weight on – without apparently eating anything! Try to wean yourself off sweetened drinks, even the low-cal ones. Eating excessively sweet things is one habit you are better off without. You should reckon on drinking around six to eight 8-ounce glasses of water a day, more if it is hot and you sweat, or if you get thirsty. The water in coffee, tea and other drinks counts towards this.

If you like sweetened tea or coffee there are two ways to kick the habit: the first is to cut down over a period of time until you can drink it unsweetened; the second is to go cold turkey.

Don't weigh yourself every day

Resist the temptation to weigh yourself daily. Your weight will fluctuate from day to day (and throughout the day), and for women, throughout the month. Weighing yourself once a week is quite sufficient. When you weigh yourself, do it on the same day, at the same time, and in the same clothes (or, preferably, no clothes) each time.

Have 'fast foods' in reserve

Don't be caught short on quick snacks when you have to go out in a hurry. Make sure you have some hard-boiled eggs made in advance for emergencies. Date them with a felt-tip pen – that will also tell you that they are cooked ones. They will keep for a week in the fridge.

Cheeses are also quick and easy. With a huge variety, cheese is an absolute must-have in my household.

For diabetics

Don't buy diabetic foods. They have no advantages; and in most cases they aren't suitable for diabetics. The following list is adapted from the British Diabetic Association's discussion paper on the role of 'diabetic' foods[1]:

- Most diabetic foods provide slightly, but not substantially, less energy than comparable non-diabetic products.
- In percentage terms, the greatest difference between diabetic and non-diabetic foods remains that of carbohydrate content, particularly carbohydrate other than fructose or sorbitol. On a per portion basis (for instance, per teaspoon of jam) the difference is relatively small and likely to be of minimal practical significance.
- Diabetic foods cost between 1.5 and 4 times as much as their non-diabetic equivalents.
- The promotion and widespread availability of diabetic foods tend to delude patients into believing that these products are advantageous, or even necessary. Their existence also undermines current dietary teaching by implying that people with diabetes cannot eat normal foods.
- Diabetic foods offer no significant physiological or psychological benefits to diabetic patients and can even be counterproductive to good diabetic control. There is no longer a need for special diabetic foods in the modern dietary management of diabetes.

How to survive Christmas

My wife and I usually have goose at Christmas. It is a fatty meat and we get lots of goose fat to use for cooking. We have the goose with the usual trimmings but with limited root vegetables and a stuffing made without flour (see Recipes section). We don't have mince pies, but we do have Christmas pudding with cream and/or brandy butter.

In the evening we usually don't have very much; we have Christmas cake (see Recipes section), with cream as it isn't iced.

Because of the tradition of the occasion, we also have dark chocolates and nuts during the day.

If we have guests, we do very little different because it's easy to end up with lots left over and only us to eat it. The lack of mince pies isn't a problem as most people are full by that stage anyway. There will be plenty of green vegetables: Brussels sprouts, et cetera, but only one carrot, one parsnip and a couple of roast potatoes per person. Surprisingly, we always have some left over as some people have one but not the other.

If people drop in later, they have usually eaten and don't want much: a light salad, fruit and cream, and Christmas cake in the afternoon is plenty. We don't bother with crisps but there are usually nuts available.

Don't forget that food made with fat not only tastes good, it's much more filling and satisfying.

Other party tips

- When going to a party with friends, try to make sure you are the designated driver. This gives you the perfect excuse not to have lots of alcohol.
- Unless you know that low-carb foods will be available, have something to eat before you go.
- Where possible stock up on the chicken legs and cold meat, and give the potato salad a miss.
- If there are only carb-rich foods, pick an especially nice one and enjoy it – but make it last.
- If there is no way to avoid eating carb-rich foods without hurting your hostess's feelings, then eat them. Any weight you put on will soon be gone when you are back to eating properly.

Reference

1. Thomas BJ. British Diabetic Association's discussion paper on the role of 'diabetic' foods. Nutrition Subcommittee of the British Diabetic Association's Professional Advisory Committee. *Diabet Med* 1992; 3: 300–306.

Chapter Five

The ideal diet for diabetics

A very high-fat, low-carbohydrate diet has been shown to have astounding effects in helping type 2 diabetics lose weight and improve their blood lipid profiles.

Dr James Hays

I have included this chapter about diabetes as many people who are overweight or obese are diabetic or go on to develop diabetes.

You may not be able to tell that you have the condition as there are no symptoms for raised blood glucose levels, which is what determines whether you are diabetic or not. The condition is not normally picked up until you visit your doctor with one of the complications. As these can be serious it is better to try and avoid the condition. The way of eating recommended in this book will help to prevent diabetes developing as well as being a successful treatment for the condition.

In the 1990s I wrote a nutritional column for an international archery magazine. The first article I wrote was about the benefits to archers of eating a proper cooked breakfast. I sent it to the editor and he called me the next day to say he couldn't publish it as it flew in the face of 'healthy' advice. While we discussed the problem, I learned that he was a type-2 diabetic. In that case, I suggested, he should try it himself. That was on Saturday.

Early the following Monday morning the editor called me. He couldn't contain his delight. He had started on Sunday and after just one day his blood glucose levels were normal – for the first time in years. This is a story I often see, because diabetes must be the easiest disease to cure in the shortest time.

Diagnosis and cure

The diagnosis of diabetes is based solely on a number – the level of fasting blood glucose. Above 7.0 mmol/L (126 mg/dL) you are diabetic, below it you are normal. So, get your glucose level down and, essentially, your diabetes is cured. As glucose is raised almost entirely by dietary carbs, a switch to a low-carb, high-fat diet, as recommended in this book, is an instant cure for type-2 diabetes and also greatly helps with type-1. However, as type-1 is more difficult to treat without one-to-one consultation and guidance, this book will concentrate on type-2.

Types of diabetes

People with diabetes fall into two broad groups:

- In type-1 diabetes, the pancreas doesn't produce enough insulin.
- In type-2 diabetes, the pancreas does produce insulin but that insulin is ineffective or the amount of insulin produced is insufficient to deal with chronic high levels of blood glucose as the result of a carbohydrate-based diet.

Type-1 diabetes

Type-1 is generally believed to be an inherited form of the disease as it is more likely to occur in people who have close relatives with diabetes. However, this is unlikely; as this disease is wholly restricted to peoples of Western industrialised civilisation, it cannot have a genetic origin, although family dietary traits and lifestyle can play a major part in its appearance within families.

Maternal diet

If a pregnant woman eats too much carbohydrate, this will raise her insulin levels. It is not thought that insulin itself crosses the placenta from mother to unborn child. However, insulin produces antibodies that do.[1] Once in the fetus these increase glycogen and fat deposits resulting in an abnormally large baby. It may also predispose that baby to type-1 diabetes.

Infant diet

Human patients with type-1 diabetes show an unusually high frequency of sensitivity to gluten, a protein found in wheat. Wheat gluten, the most potent diabetes-inducing protein source, is closely linked with the autoimmune attack in the pancreas and is strongly associated with pancreatic islet inflammation and damage.[2] It is no real surprise, therefore, that early weaning to a diet which contains a gluten-containing cereal such as wheat, as well as barley, rye or oats is likely to increase the risk of type-1 diabetes.[3]

Type-2 diabetes

People who are overweight often go on to develop type-2 diabetes. For this reason, the accepted wisdom is that diabetes is caused by obesity. It isn't. Both obesity and diabetes are caused by the same thing: a low-fat, high-carb, 'healthy' diet. The only reason that diabetes appears to follow obesity is that obesity is more easily detected.

This type of diabetes is much more common: 90% or more of diabetics have type-2. In the same way that type-1 diabetes is not found in the wild animal kingdom or in primitive man eating a traditional diet, neither is type-2.

Symptoms of type-2 diabetes include:

- High blood glucose level (*hyperglycaemia*)
- Glucose in urine (*glycosuria*)
- Frequent thirst
- Increased urination
- Fatigue, drowsiness
- Blurred vision
- Infections that will not heal quickly
- Sometimes nausea and vomiting
- Women may also complain of urinary tract infections or vaginal itching.

You will not usually be aware of the first two, but your doctor should pick them up during a routine medical test. If you have any of the other symptoms, and particularly if you are overweight, then you should suspect and be tested for diabetes. Diabetes is usually first diagnosed when complications occur, but it is much better to find out before this to avoid the complications.

If you are diagnosed as diabetic, you should take it seriously, but don't think it's all doom and gloom. The good news is that there's plenty of evidence that with a low-carb, high-fat diet, you will have no symptoms and can live a normal life without ever having to resort to drugs.

Carbs raise glucose

All carbs are digested very quickly – within a few minutes. This means that within a very short time after a carb-rich meal, the level of glucose in your bloodstream will rise rapidly. This is shown graphically in Figure 1. This graph is the result of a test with either 100 g of glucose or 40 g of fat.[4] As you can see, the carbs increased blood glucose dramatically whereas the fats had practically no effect at all.

Carbs also raise insulin

Let us not forget that diabetes is a chronic disorder of carbohydrate metabolism. It is only carbs that raise blood glucose levels and blood insulin levels. This has been

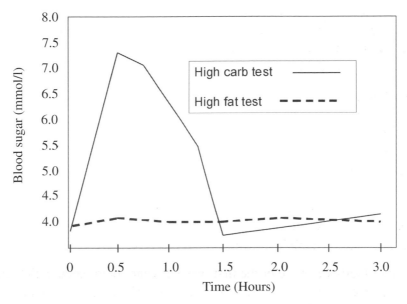

Figure 1   Blood glucose after 100 g of glucose or 40 g of fat

known since 1935.[5] High blood glucose levels are dangerous and, as levels of glucose rise rapidly in the bloodstream, your pancreas produces a large amount of insulin to take the excess glucose out. This can be seen clearly in Figure 2, a graph from the same test as that in Figure 1.

Not surprisingly, a 'healthy' carbohydrate-based diet, whether or not it is low-GI gives by far the worst control of blood glucose and insulin levels. You will note that insulin levels after a carb-rich meal don't return to normal for some four hours. Note again that fats have little or no effect on blood insulin levels.

Protein reduces glucose – but increases insulin

Over the years, there has been considerable uncertainty about the effects of protein intake on blood glucose levels. Recently a well-conducted study of people with type-2 diabetes showed clearly that protein improves overall glucose control.[6] In this study, protein intake was doubled while carbs were reduced proportionally. It produced impressive results by reducing twenty-four hour blood

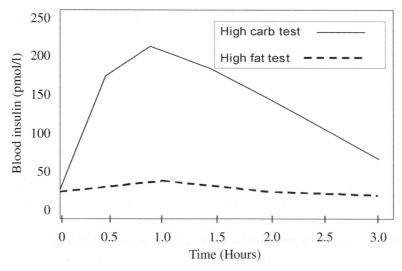

Figure 2   Blood insulin levels after high-carb and high-fat meals

glucose by a massive forty percent. There were also significant decreases in glycosylated haemoglobin and triglycerides after just five weeks. This was all to the good. However, the addition of 50 grams of beef had one drawback: it caused a prompt three-fold rise in blood insulin levels. Insulin was still at a maximum after two-and-a-half hours, and it did not return to a fasting value until more than six hours after the meal.

Fat gives the best control

Diabetics are generally told that eating fat increases glucose and insulin levels. Like most dietary advice today it is quite wrong as the graphs above demonstrate.

A healthy insulin level is one below 40 pmol/L. Figure 2 shows that is precisely the effect of a low-carb, high-fat diet. The one thing that studies in this area have consistently shown clearly is that eating fat gives by far the best control over blood glucose and insulin levels. I cannot stress this point strongly enough.

Lower GI diesn't mean lower blood glucose

Diabetics are told to eat high-fibre foods such as wholemeal bread as, having a 'lower glycaemic index', they don't raise insulin levels so quickly. But, like so many other recommendations, it doesn't work very well in practice.[7] Wholemeal flour is only marginally better than white flour: the GI of white bread is 71 and wholemeal bread's GI is 69, an insignificant difference. The real answer is to cut out bread altogether.

The same is true of other bran-rich foods. For example, a recent study compared blood glucose responses to either cornflakes or a bran cereal, both of which contained 50 g of carbohydrate.[8] As the fibre-rich bran cereal had a glycaemic index less than half of the cornflakes' GI, you might expect the bran to have to have been beneficial. But you would be wrong: there was no significant difference between the two. What actually happened was that although the cornflakes raised glucose more, 20 minutes after the meal the bran had raised insulin levels almost twice as much as the cornflakes. This removed glucose from the blood more quickly. Thus the lower GI of bran was not because it had a lower effect on raising glucose, but because it caused an earlier and bigger release of insulin. So, if you are insulin deficient, high-fibre foods such as bran might not be such a good idea.

Fruit is worse

Lastly, just like everyone else, diabetics are also told to eat '5 portions of fruit and vegetables a day', but fruit contains the fruit sugar, fructose.

The belief is that glucose raises levels of insulin quickly, but as fructose doesn't require insulin, it is healthier. However, it isn't that simple. A major part of the dietary advice to diabetics is aimed at reducing the risk of heart attacks which, we are told, is increased by cholesterol, particularly low-density lipoproteins (LDL; the 'bad' cholesterol). In this respect fructose does not seem to be a good choice because according to established evidence:

- 'Fructose glycosylates haemoglobin seven times faster than glucose.'[9] 'Glycosylates' means that it coats with sugar, rather like icing a cake. A significant protein in the blood that is glycosylated in this way is haemoglobin, the protein in red blood cells that carries oxygen around the body. When haemoglobin is glycosylated, this stops it from performing its function properly. Glycosylation also makes the blood 'sticky' which makes it more likely to clot, to stick to the artery walls and to block the small capillaries in the eyes, kidneys, brain and lower legs so that blood does not reach these parts. This is the cause of the damage to eyes, kidneys, and so on, that is so prevalent in diabetics.
- This tendency to glycosylation is also important because glycosylation of proteins such as low-density lipoprotein (LDL) and high-density lipoprotein (HDL) particles increases the growth rate of atheroma, that's the 'furring up' of the arteries generally believed to cause heart disease.[10]
- Fructose also appears to increase total cholesterol primarily by raising LDL.[11] Increasing dietary fructose from 3% to 20% of calories and reducing starch *increased* blood cholesterol by 9% and LDL by 11%. Researchers say 'There is now reason to believe that dietary fructose will increase the risk of atherosclerosis.'[11]

For these reasons, one of the first things that should go, if you are diabetic, is fruit. This makes a nonsense of the Glycaemic Index, unless it is used by someone who knows and understands its limitations.

Let's get some sanity back into diabetes treatment

Diabetes treatments are all aimed at getting glucose out of the bloodstream. Conventional diabetes advice is that patients should eat high-carb meals. Diabetes UK's website (http://www.diabetes.org.uk/About_us/Our_Views/Position_statements/Diabetic_foods/) says under the heading 'Healthy eating':

> 'Like the rest of the population, . . . They [diabetics] are encouraged to eat plenty of fruit and vegetables, and meals based on starchy carbohydrate foods such as bread, chapatti, rice, pasta and yams'.

These high-carb meals raise glucose in the blood to dangerous levels. To lower it, they are then given a variety of drugs that:

- Reduce glucose uptake from the gut after a high-carb meal
- Force muscle cells that don't want more glucose to take it
- Make body fat cells take in more fat so that weight is put on
- Force the pancreas to produce ever more insulin
- Make the pancreas release more insulin to remove the excess glucose.

Doesn't it make more sense not to get too much glucose into the bloodstream in the first place? Well, that means reducing your carb intake. It's that simple.

In 1999, Dr James Hays, an endocrinologist and director of the Limestone Medical Center in Wilmington, DE, proved this approach when he presented the results of three studies of men and women with type-2 diabetes involving such a diet at the annual meeting of the Endocrine Society.[12] His study reported that 'a very high-fat, low-carbohydrate diet has been shown to have astounding effects in helping type-2 diabetics lose weight and improve their blood lipid profiles'.

Patients were able to eat all the meat and cheese they wanted, but as for carbohydrates, they were restricted to eating unprocessed foods, mainly fresh fruit and vegetables. Whereas in a normal diet 60% of calories would come from carbohydrates and 30% from fat, patients in this diet were encouraged to get 50% of their caloric intake from fat, and just 20% from carbohydrates.

A whopping 90% of the fat content in their diets was saturated fat, compared with just 10% that was mono-unsaturated fat. Over the course of one year, the subjects achieved:

- A mean decline in total cholesterol of between 231 and 190 mg/dL.
- LDL (the 'bad' cholesterol) fell from 133 to 105 mg/dL.
- HDL (the 'good' cholesterol) increased from 44 to 47 mg/dL.

- Triglycerides declined from 229 to 182 mg/dL.
- HbA1c, which at the start of the study averaged 3.34% above normal, declined to just 0.96% above normal
- Average weight loss was in the order of 40 lbs (18.2 kg).

By the end of the one-year study 90% of the patients had achieved ADA (American Diabetes Association) targets for HbA1c, HDL, LDL and triglycerides.

As for the response from cardiologists who see a high-fat diet as anathema to what they have been instructing their patients for years now, Dr Hays said he has three cardiology patients who are now on the diet.

Sanity for type-1 diabetes

The medical profession generally regards type-1 diabetes as incurable. It is managed conventionally with a low-fat, carbohydrate-based diet. As the carbohydrates in such a diet inevitably put large amounts of glucose in the bloodstream, daily insulin injections have to be administered to bring these high levels of glucose in the blood down to normal. This means walking a tightrope for life, as exactly the right amount of insulin must be given or it will either reduce glucose levels too much or not enough.

However, the human body rarely produces no insulin at all. At diagnosis of type-1 diabetes, some 5 to 15% of pancreatic beta cells are usually still producing insulin. If these are relieved of the burden of continually having to reduce excessive levels of blood glucose, they will usually produce sufficient insulin for the variety of other metabolic processes that need it, and supplementation with injected insulin is not needed.

A study reported in 2005, also provided evidence that the pancreas continues to make insulin-producing beta cells even after many years with type-1 diabetes. Dr Peter C. Butler from the University of California in Los Angeles told the audience at the American Diabetes Association Scientific Sessions, 'The implication is that type-1 diabetes could, theoretically, be cured if we could stop the new insulin-secreting cells being destroyed.'[13]

Until now, the only hope of reversing the disease seemed to be replacement of beta cells by transplantation. Butler's team showed that, among individuals who'd had type-1 diabetes for decades – in some cases up to 60 years – the majority still had detectable insulin-producing beta cells in their pancreas.

This amount may be sufficient for type-1 diabetics to live a normal life without having to inject insulin, says Polish doctor Jan Kwaśniewski, who has successfully treated type-1 diabetics for over 30 years merely by reducing their carbohydrate intake to 'an amount dictated by the insulin-producing capacity of the sufferer'.[14] This amount, he says, typically equates to 1.5 grams of carbohydrate per kilogram body weight for a growing child and between 40 and 50 grams for an adult per day. With this regime, the main energy source is dietary animal fat. On such a diet, his type-1 diabetic patients no longer needed to use insulin.

I, too, find that merely reducing carbohydrate intake, particularly from fruit and cereals, may be all that is required to reduce the symptoms of type-1 diabetes from a serious health hazard to a mere annoyance. Even if it is still necessary to inject insulin, the amount needed can be reduced substantially.

Sanity for type-2 diabetes

There is a wealth of evidence that type-2 diabetes is easily treated without the need for any drugs at all. It is also very easily prevented. In a nutshell, you should drastically reduce your carb consumption – particularly from grains, sugar and fruit and replace the energy lost with fat. This will lower your carbohydrate load and slow your blood glucose rise. Problem solved – or at least made substantially better.

As such a diet is also the best to reduce excessive weight and obesity, it kills both birds with the one stone.

Beware of hypos

If you are a type-1 diabetic injecting insulin, or a type-2 taking a drug that increases your pancreas's insulin production, then you *must* reduce the dose as you reduce your carb intake to compensate for the lower levels of glucose in your blood to avoid a hypo. The way to do this is to lower carbs and drug in small amounts over a few weeks. Remember, if you make only small changes, you can make only small mistakes.

References

1. Menon RK, Cohen RM, Sperling MA, et al. Transplacental passage of insulin in pregnant women with insulin dependent diabetes mellitus: its role in fetal macrosomia. *N Eng J Med* 1990; 323: 309–315.

2. MacFarlane AJ, Burghardt KM, Kelly J, et al. A type 1 diabetes-related protein from wheat (*Triticum aestivum*): cDNA clone of a wheat storage globulin, Glb1, linked to islet damage. *J Biol Chem* 2003; 278: 54–63.

3. Ziegler A-G, Schmid S, Huber D, et al. Early infant feeding and risk of developing type 1 diabetes-associated autoantibodies. *JAMA* 2003; 290: 1721–1728.

4. Robertson MD, Henderson RA, Vist GE, Rumsey RDE. Extended effects of evening meal carbohydrate-to-fat ratio on fasting and postprandial substrate metabolism. *Am J Clin Nutr* 2002; 75: 505–510.

5. Given HDC. *A New Angle on Health*. John Bale, Sons and Danielsson, London, 1935.

6. Gannon MC, Nuttall FQ, Saeed A, et al. An increase in dietary protein improves the blood glucose response in persons with type 2 diabetes. *Am J Clin Nutr* 2003; 78: 734–741.

7. Jenkins DJ, Kendall CW, Augustin LS, et al. Effect of wheat bran on glycemic control and risk factors for cardiovascular disease in type 2 diabetes. *Diabetes Care* 2002; 25: 1522–1528.

8. Schenk S, Davidson CJ, Zderic TW, et al. Different glycemic indexes of breakfast cereals are not due to glucose entry into blood but to glucose removal by tissue. *Am J Clin Nutr* 2003; 78: 742–748.

9. Bunn HF, Higgins PJ. Reaction of monosaccharides with proteins: possible evolutionary significance. *Science* 1981; 213: 222–229.

10. Bierman EL. George Lyman Duff Memorial Lecture. Atherogenesis in diabetes. *Arterioscler Thromb* 1992; 12: 647–656.

11. Swanson JE, Laine DC, Thomas W, Bantle JP. Metabolic effects of dietary fructose in healthy subjects. *Am J Clin Nutr* 1992; 55: 851–856.

12. Hays J. *Diabetics Improve Health with Very High-Fat, Low-Carb Diet*. ENDO 99: Annual meeting of The Endocrine Society, San Diego, 15 June 1999.

13. Butler PC. *Beta-Cells Regenerate Even in Type 1 Diabetes*. ADA 57th Scientific Sessions, June 2005.

14. Kwaśniewski. J, Chyliński M. *Homo Optimus*. Wydawnictwo WGP, Warsaw, 2000; 163–166.

Chapter Six

Prevention is better

Long-term planning is not about making long-term decisions. It is about understanding the future consequences of today's decisions.

Gary Ryan Blair

Most diet and health books are usually concerned with helping those who have succumbed to diseases after the event, to undo the damage caused by previous faulty dietary practice. However, it must be self-evident that it is far better not to court ill-health in the first place. This relies on correct nutrition from the start; that is from a child's conception, for our nutritional status at our beginning has a profound effect on our health throughout life.[1] During the time the unborn child is forming, it requires an adequate supply of the right nutrients. If these are not supplied in the right quantity and at the right time, a damaged baby is the inevitable result.

Today, most of us in the West have access to, and can afford, almost any food we choose, yet most of us seem to choose a diet composed of highly refined and concentrated starches and sugars. For our offspring, such dietary practice may spell disaster.

In her book, *Let's Have Healthy Children*,[2] the world-renowned nutritionist, Adele Davies, tells how, when pregnant and nursing mothers ate a proper diet, not only did they have more normal pregnancies and easier labours, their babies were born with no congenital abnormalities. Davies also found that children of well-nourished mothers, who were themselves well-nourished, suffered no colic, were more intelligent, more attentive, and less prone to hyperactivity, allergies, colds and other ailments. On the other hand, expectant mothers who were malnourished to the point where they had small babies could expect their offspring to be more trouble to them and to have considerable difficulties in childhood and later life.

Birth-weight depends on what and how much the expectant mother eats

A study of diet towards the end of the first three months of pregnancy and subsequent birth-weights found that mothers of premature or low birth-weight babies ate significantly fewer essential nutrients than mothers of larger babies. The missing or deficient nutrients associated with premature births were salt, magnesium, phosphorus and iron; those associated with low birth-weight were thiamine (vitamin B1), salt, iron and magnesium, niacin and riboflavin (vitamin B2). These are all abundant in meat and other high-protein foods of animal origin. It is not surprising, therefore, that the worst cases were always found in children born to mothers who were either eating vegetarian diets or on slimming diets while they were pregnant.[3]

There is also a growing body of research that demonstrates that high levels of insulin in an overweight mother's bloodstream have a fattening effect in her unborn baby.[4] This is thought to be caused by leakage of insulin antibodies across the placenta. However, the real cause is the high levels of insulin in the mother, which is ultimately the result of a high-carb diet.

This book does not pretend to be the definitive book on paediatric diet and nutrition, but if its principles are followed from before conception, many of the trials and tribulations of infancy and of health in later life, as well as obesity, can be avoided.

Diet for pregnancy

Prepare in advance for children. A healthy child is dependent in the first place on being the product of a healthy egg and a healthy sperm.

Difficulty in conceiving is often the result of poor nutrition. Overweight women and those on low-calorie diets will find that the diet recommended here will frequently solve their problem.[5,6] Note also that it is equally important that the father has good nutritional status prior to conception.

Once pregnancy has been determined, the expectant mother will be subjected to all sorts of strong pressures: the forces of commercial interests; of folklore; and, on occasion, nutritional ignorance within the medical profession. These can have a seriously detrimental effect on her health and that of her child.

Before conception

Pregnancy, and a proper diet for it, should always be planned. You may not realise that you are pregnant until after you have missed a period. By that time, your fetus could have been developing for four to eight weeks. It is during these weeks that all your baby's internal organs, limbs and face begin to develop. Damage at this sensitive time through unsuitable diet, smoking or drugs contributes to many malformations such as cleft palate, malformed limbs, and defects to eyes, hearing, heart or brain.

Obesity makes delivery more difficult for the mother and increases the risks for her baby. Babies born to obese women are twice as likely to need intensive care. But, as rapid weight loss dieting is very harmful during pregnancy, excess weight should be lost before conception. What you eat immediately before and during pregnancy will also affect the amount of fat your baby will carry through life.

During pregnancy

During pregnancy you really are eating for two. A poor diet during pregnancy is a major cause of low birth-weight babies, who have a much increased risk of perinatal death, of other health problems throughout life and a reduced life-expectancy overall.

The ideal diet during pregnancy is the one advocated here: one that has a high nutrient density with foods such as meat, fish, milk, and dairy products, and fresh vegetables and a little fruit. Professor David Barker and colleagues at the Medical Research Council, University of Southampton, found that 'Mothers who had high carbohydrate intakes in early pregnancy had babies with lower placental and birth weights. Low maternal intakes of dairy and meat protein in late pregnancy were also associated with lower placental and birth weights' which 'could have long-term consequences for the offspring's risk of cardiovascular disease'.[7] Professor Barker's group has provided overwhelming evidence that malnutrition at a very early age in Britain in the last century resulted in earlier and more severe adult chronic disease. Dietary carbohydrates raise insulin levels.

The mother's size during pregnancy doesn't seem to matter; what matters is what a mother has eaten during pregnancy.

During pregnancy there is an inevitable weight gain. This should be about ½–1 kg (1–2 lb) in the first ten weeks, 3–5 kg (6–10 lb) by week 20 with about ½ kg (1 lb) a week after that to the end of pregnancy; a total weight gain of about 13 kg (28 lb) over the nine months.

If weight gain is substantially greater or less than this you should try to determine why. Excessive weight gain is usually caused by excessive intake of 'convenience food'.

The milky way

The Jesuits say that if they have a child for his first seven years, they have him for life. Similarly the way children are fed during these first formative years determines their eating patterns throughout life. Dietary habits learned during childhood are usually retained throughout life. Set them early, as trying to change them later is not easy.

The way to good nutrition for your infant should not be difficult. There is one product that alone will provide your baby with all the nutrients she requires for at least the first six months or more of her life. That product, consisting of all the proteins, fats, carbohydrates, vitamins, minerals and trace elements your growing infant needs, formulated in exactly the right proportions, available when required at exactly the right temperature and germ free, is mother's milk. Not only is it the right food for growth, it will protect your baby from allergies, gastric and bowel disturbances, and many other diseases.

Given free access to the breast, your baby will not overeat, taking only as much as she needs. One bonus for you as a nursing mother is that you will be less stressed by a colicky child. Both you and your baby are emotionally bonded and gain pleasure from the experience, and unlike most things today, this amazing product is free.

Breast-feeding for your baby's health

Breast-feeding has been shown to have profound and long-lasting benefits to health throughout life.

- Breast-feeding provides best protection against diseases and allergies such as acute or prolonged diarrhoea, respiratory tract infections, otitis media, urinary tract infection and neonatal septicaemia.[8]
- Babies who had been exclusively breast-fed for at least the first four months of life had only half the amount of wheezing of those who were wholly bottle-fed. Children who had been partly breast and partly bottle-fed were little better than those wholly bottle-fed.
- Blood pressure was also significantly higher in children who had been bottle-fed.
- Breast milk growth factor reduces skin problems in children.[9]
- Breast-feeding reduces leukaemia risk. The effect was strongest in those children who were breast-fed for more than six months.[10]
- Breast-feeding improves heart health. Professor Alan Lucas and colleagues at the Medical Research Council's Childhood Nutrition Centre in London found that adolescents who had been breast-fed in infancy had healthier cholesterol levels than those who were given formula milk.[11]
- Breast-feeding gives babies an average three-point advantage in IQ over bottle-fed babies.[12] All studies but one in the analysis were based on breast-fed and not just breast-milk-fed children.
- Breast-feeding fights the fat. The risk of obesity is reduced by more than 40% in children breast-fed exclusively for at least six months; bottle-fed children are nearly twice as likely to be obese when compared with breast-fed children.[13]

These positive and striking factors were observed in children during breast-feeding. If breast-feeding were carried out for longer, protection was improved.

Breast-feeding helps mother too

Breast-feeding makes motherhood much less of a traumatic experience as the breast-fed baby will suffer fewer illnesses, will smile more at one end and be less messy at the other.

Another bonus, in terms of weight, is that you will regain your figure more easily and quickly.

Many women are dismayed that they have large hips and thighs, but there is a very sound reason for this fat. Nature put it there for energy storage for lactation and to safeguard the food supply of offspring.

An infant consumes large amounts of energy in the first six or nine months of life, so nature guarantees this supply of energy in women's hips and thighs and has locked it up during the non-lactating phase. However, you can lose it by breast-feeding. Dr Carol Janney and colleagues at the University of Michigan found that women who breast-fed their babies exclusively for at least six months regained their original weight much more easily and quickly than those who bottle-fed or only partly breast-fed their babies.[14] There is no doubt that a mother's best 'hip and thigh diet' is the one she feeds to her baby.

Breast-feed immediately

Success with breast-feeding depends on how soon and how much a baby sucks. The breast produces milk only on demand: if your baby doesn't suck, you won't produce any milk.

Your baby should be put to your breast immediately after birth. Under one hour old, a baby is responsive and alert, and will suck easily. When a baby is born, her blood-sugar level is usually low. In nature, the first food a baby gets from the breast is colostrum. It may look a thin watery fluid, but it has a high protein content. This amazing food, for which there is no substitute, is the start that all babies should have.

Bottle-feeding is inferior to breast-feeding both in the quality of the milk and for the mother–baby bonding process. Cow's milk is not suitable for a baby human. It is designed for a calf that must double its weight in a few days. Formula milks are nearer to human milk, but looking round the pharmacy at baby milk formulas I note that, without exception, they are now all made with polyunsaturated vegetable oils. These are not healthy.

Disincentives to breast-feeding

Today, society conspires against breast-feeding. It is still the practice in some maternity hospitals for the newborn baby to be given a glucose drink to raise her blood-sugar level. This not only taxes her immature pancreas unnecessarily; it makes her less likely to suck as vigorously to start the milk flow. More than this, it is the start of the road to obesity, for the child will more rapidly develop a taste for sweet things.

Beware also that baby-food manufacturers seem to have arrangements whereby they are told of all new babies. If you get a deluge of promotional literature from them, bear in mind the monetary interest of those who sent it to you. I would advise you to throw it away.

If you use a dummy, do not dip it in a sweetened liquid first. Never feed a sweetened liquid in a bottle. Both these practices lead to a liking for sweet things and, thus, to obesity in later life. Preferences for sweet things can cause lack of appetite, and poor weight gain and growth, and diarrhoea and behavioural disorders, most noticeably irritability and aggressiveness.

Weaning

The point of weaning is to make the transition from milk to ordinary family food. It is at this phase in a child's life that the most care must be taken, for the foods that a child is introduced to at this stage will govern its choices of foods throughout its life.

Appetite is a conditioned attitude to foodstuffs. An infant brought up on a diet of ants' eggs and worms, knowing no other, will be quite happy to eat them – although he might get some strange looks from his school pals if he takes these for his midday lunch. Similarly, if a child is taught to like sweet things, that is what he will prefer. Once the appetite is programmed in infancy it's very difficult to change later.

Weaning should not be started before four months for the reasons stated earlier. Indeed there are advantages in not starting to feed solids until six months as avoiding them until this age dramatically reduces allergies,[15] but it should be started by six months. Breast-feeding may still continue simultaneously for two years or more.

It is important that you don't sweeten anything. Don't worry if these foods do not taste sweet enough to you, your baby doesn't know the difference. If she does not become used to sweetened foods, she will not develop a taste for them.

Don't wean to carbs

Traditionally, the first weaning food given is a milled cereal but there is no nutritional reason for this. When a baby is born, she has a store of iron that will last for several months but it will gradually be depleted. It is safer, therefore, to begin weaning with a little egg yolk. It is advisable to avoid the egg white at this stage, in case of possible allergy problems.

Other than that, the best foods are liquidised meat, eggs and fish, vegetables and a little fruit should be introduced as they provide not only a variety of tastes but also a full range of vitamins and minerals. Dairy products are a common cause of allergies at this age. It is better, therefore, to delay their use and use sparingly at first. By all means add cereal products, but be careful not to overdo these and steer clear of any that have added bran. And I repeat: do not sweeten anything.

A study published in 1990 showed that babies who were prematurely weaned to a high-carbohydrate diet were more likely to develop high blood cholesterol levels, but if babies were weaned to a high-fat diet, it normalised blood cholesterol. Getting back to obesity, breast-fed infants are always slimmer than formula-fed infants at one year.[16] Not surprisingly, perhaps, study found that 95% of obese people had not been breast-fed.

Lastly, dietary fat and cholesterol are needed to insulate nerve cells and prevent short circuits between nerves and subsequent brain damage. There is concern that infant formula milks do not provide the necessary long-chain fatty acids necessary for proper brain development. For proper growth and brain development children under the age of two need fat and cholesterol every day – even if they are chubby. Never forget that Nature has designed breast milk to be the perfect food for babies – and 50% of the energy in breast milk is in the form of fat. It is also very high in cholesterol.

Proteins

A baby's body – muscles, skin, internal organs, hair, nails, brain and bones – is made largely of proteins. Only when complete proteins of excellent quality are given every day, can every cell function properly and grow normally. It is vitally important, therefore, that a baby's stomach is not filled with foods such as breakfast cereals, fizzy drinks, potato chips, and so on. A child's stomach just hasn't got room for all that junk and real food as well.

You can tell easily whether a baby has enough of the right proteins. Strong, well-formed muscles hold the body erect automatically. If muscles have had insufficient protein they lose their elasticity and posture is poor. A mother who has to tell her child: 'Stand up straight', is actually admitting her own failure to provide the proper nourishment.

But not to worry. If you do find this happening, it is surprising how quickly faulty posture can be improved with a diet containing adequate protein.

Commercial baby foods

It is important that babies are introduced to high quality foods from the start. Jars of commercial baby food are best avoided for a number of reasons:

- Using commercial foods usually means that the child's first solids are very different from the foods you will want her to eat a few months later.
- These foods also contain large quantities of sugary or starchy fillers. Even those with 'no added sugar' usually contain fruit syrups, other sugars and starch thickeners to make them appear more like solid food. These not only predispose to obesity but also damage teeth.
- There is no requirement that baby foods which contain meat have either their meat content, the species from which it comes or which parts of the animal is used stated on the jar. Only 5% of one 'Turkey Dinner' tested was actually meat.
- Baby foods are highly processed and, as a consequence, nutrients may be destroyed. To make up this shortfall, manufacturers add vitamins. There is considerable evidence that taking vitamin supplements in this way is not a good idea.
- Baby foods also tend to be stored for a considerable time before being eaten. Lacking freshness and nutritional quality, they are the infant equivalent of junk food.

It is almost inevitable, I suppose, that you will want to use commercial baby foods for convenience from time to time. In which case, scrutinise the labels and reject any that contain ingredients that are not 'food' in the accepted sense, or that you wouldn't want to eat yourself.

Making baby foods

Making foods yourself for weaning is not difficult. A whole month's supply can easily be made in one go, puréed, divided up into ice-cube trays and frozen in the freezer or refrigerator's ice box to be thawed out as required.

All food should be nutritious. A child has a lot of growing to do and only a small stomach. She must have the building blocks for bone, teeth, muscle and brain in the form of protein, fats, vitamins and minerals. She also will use an inordinate amount of energy. The most concentrated energy source is the fat. Don't cut it off; your child needs it.

Drinks

When your child is thirsty, it means that her body is becoming dehydrated and requires water. Avoid fizzy drinks. The 'pop' rot can start early and quite subtly. Many baby drinks too are little better than sugared water; a single beaker of blackcurrant drink can contain 6–9 spoons of sugar! Also avoid low-calorie diet drinks. The best drink of all is water. Tap water is preferable to bottled water; the bottled water industry is not as well regulated and, for safety reasons, bottled water is not recommended by the medical profession for infants.[8] If you live in an area where the tap water is fluoridated, however, you should not give it to your child. Although fluoride is prescribed to combat dental decay, it is a powerful enzyme disruptor which has many serious, long-term, adverse effects and should be avoided at all costs.[19]

Teething

At the age of about six months your baby will be grasping things and taking them to her mouth to suck. Later she will begin teething. At this time it is usual to give baby something to chew on.

The old-fashioned bone teething ring is probably the best for her. Your baby can also chew on celery sticks or slices of carrot, swede or any other hard vegetable. These should be cut into chunks large enough to prevent their being inadvertently swallowed. Rusks are bad news; even the low-sugar rusks tend to contain a considerable amount of sugar. The first effect is that newly emerging teeth are bathed in the food of teeth-rotting bacteria and, secondly, your baby will develop a taste for sweet things.

As the weaning period ends, milky and puréed foods will be replaced by more solid foods and your infant will eat more like you do. Baby-food manufacturers make a wide range of foods for this period as well as the weaning period. But beware; carbohydrates – cereals and sugars – are cheap. For this reason, pre-cooked jars of food are liberally laced with them.

If you can keep your child away from sugar and sugary sweets before she goes to school, it is likely that she will not develop the taste for them at all. With this upbringing and experience, it is equally unlikely that she will ever become overweight. She will also be much less likely to catch the infections that plague most children.

Growing up

Childhood is a critical stage in any person's development. The way that children relate to their peer group is very important to them. Most important, particularly among girls and young women, is the way in which they perceive their own bodies.

Children generally follow the examples set by their parents. If a mother is preoccupied with dieting, she will set an example that can profoundly affect the whole of her child's life. The pre-school years are the most effective period in which to establish healthy eating patterns. Habits formed at this time are likely to persist. It is important, therefore, to instil the right attitudes at this time.

The parent who stays at home, bringing up the children, can teach them food preparation techniques and shopping. This is not just educational, but can be great fun for both parent and child. On the other hand when parents let their children fend for themselves or delegate their responsibilities to another, they must give clear guidance on diet and what is acceptable for their children to eat. It is essential to take and keep control of the situation, not just to let it go.

Don't force feed

Children should be allowed to be aware of and follow the dictates of their bodies' natural signals. That way, not only will they enjoy eating, they will learn to control food rather than have food control them. If they leave food, do not make so much next time, so don't force food on your child. There is no need to worry about an apparent lack of appetite unless they are not growing as they should, both physically and mentally. When they are hungry, they will eat. And if you are anxious about your infant's weight, don't give in by letting her eat junk-food. One parent told me that her first child was so skinny she was off the bottom of the weight charts. 'To my shame,' she said, 'I used to give her two of those horribly sugary baby yoghurts at a meal. No wonder she then didn't want to eat anything else.'

Don't use food as a reward

Do not reward good behaviour with food, particularly sweets. This encourages bad eating habits. It is much better to use praise. Similarly, do not use food as a comforter. It also sends the wrong message to praise a child for 'eating it all up'.

After all, she is only satisfying her hunger – a perfectly natural event. The danger here is that, if occasionally she is not so hungry and the praise stops, she will feel she has to eat more than she wants to earn the praise. This leads to overeating.

The early school years

Once your child starts school you lose control for a large part of the day. Other children will have sweets; she will be influenced by advertisements on television, the sweet counters at supermarket checkouts. It is at this time that your earlier efforts will pay off.

A friend of mine brought up three daughters. She stayed at home with them in their pre-school years. They had no sugar in their diets at all. The girls' grandmother was appalled. I remember she told us that her daughter-in-law 'even makes custard without sugar'. The girls didn't mind for they knew nothing else. When they started school, and came into contact with other children eating sweets, they knew that their mother did not want them to eat sweets and being well-brought up little girls they observed their mother's wishes.

Friends and relatives were discouraged from giving them sweets. However, if someone did give them sweets as a present, they were allowed to have a small piece. The rest was saved for another day, when again they had just a small piece. If it would not keep, it was quietly disposed of.

Before your child starts nursery school, if she is to eat there, look at the menu. Let the organiser know that you do not want your child to eat sweets, sugar or soft drinks. The National Children's Bureau recommends that nurseries should not disrupt a child's established eating patterns, so you should have no difficulty. If you wish to supply your own foods, the nursery should accommodate you.

Birthdays at school

Birthdays are special for children. At home you can control what food is served (see below). In the playschool environment, however, where there may be a birthday several times a week, there is little you can do other than suggest that only fruit is served: satsumas, apples, pineapple cubes, pink melon, strawberries, raspberries, peaches can be served on their own or with cream. Both at home and at nursery school, why not have a pretend cake? This can be built around a tin or a box and have candles to blow out. It doesn't have to be edible. Although I think it is better if children are not introduced to sweet cakes, if a pretend cake will not do, make a real but lower-carb cake by cutting the recipe's sugar by half and using a nut flour instead of wheat flour.

When leaving your child in the care of a childminder, make sure they understand what you want or do not want your child to eat. Better still, provide the food yourself.

Other tips

- **Beware of additives** that can cause a variety of adverse reactions. And avoid also foods with 'added vitamins'. This is a sign that the food is highly processed and nutritionally inadequate.
- **Shopping.** Supermarkets know that children watch television and are influenced by what they see and hear. They know that children have a big influence on what their parents buy – the way children force parents to buy unsuitable food. They even have a name for it – 'pester power'. This is why sweets are put at the checkouts, so when shopping do not let your child choose. Most children will choose the one advertised on TV – designed to appeal to them, but the most advertised foods are usually the worst. Not only are they invariably laced heavily with sugar, they are invariably more expensive (all that advertising has to be paid for).
- **Do not forget that the responsibility for choosing food is a serious matter** and that responsibility is yours. It should not be delegated to an impressionable child.

Here are some tips for shopping:

- **Make out a shopping list** and, when you shop, stick to it. Not only is it quicker, it's usually cheaper too. It also has the added advantage that if your child asks for something that you don't want her to have, you can say quite truthfully 'It's not on the list'.
- **Have a good meal** before you go shopping. You and your child are more likely to be tempted if you are hungry.
- **Use the information** that manufacturers have to put on their products. If the label on a food your child fancies contains just a list of chemicals, educate your child. Say: 'Ugh, look! There aren't any real strawberries in that, it's just red

colouring'. Make her aware that manufacturers make the packet pretty in the hope that you won't look too closely at the label. Taking this approach is both a good way to avoid buying products you do not want your child to eat, and a good consumer education for her future.

- **Don't 'diet'.** If you are dieting, don't let your child know. It teaches her to be faddy.

- **Suitable snacks.** Include pieces of cheese, natural, whole-milk yogurt (not fruit yogurt), raw vegetables or fruit. The best drink is water. Full-cream milk is also acceptable, but bear in mind that milk is more than a drink, it is a food.

- **Gifts.** Ask friends and relatives not to give sweets as gifts, and the same goes for you! If sweets are given, restrict them to, say, two only and then only once a week. And have them only after a meal, when they will do the least damage. If sweets accumulate, get rid of them quietly. No child needs to know about sweets before she starts playschool. Let your friends and relatives know that you prefer presents such as crayons, felt-tipped pens, books, sketch pads, bat and ball, knitting pins and wool, computer games – educational, of course. These will give more pleasure for longer, and they are not fattening!

- **Family meals.** Make sure that the family always sits down to meals together, particularly at breakfast time. If the child always has a good breakfast, she will be less likely to err later to boost flagging blood-sugar levels.

- **Cooking and helping.** Teach your child to cook – these days she won't learn it at school, and children love it. But best of all, it could stop your child living out of packets, tins and TV dinners in the future.

It's never too late

If your child is already eating sugar and sweets, slowly begin to reduce the amounts so that it is not noticeable. With sugar, you will find that you can cut amounts in some recipes by half without a noticeable difference to the taste. If you need to change eating patterns, try not to make it seem a punishment. One client's 11-month-old daughter, Lily, took to her healthier lifestyle very quickly. With some trepidation, her parents threw out all her 'high-carb rubbish' and changed her to a good, meat-based, eating regime. Lily loved the change; she quickly sampled and liked sausages and black pudding, and she loves to lick the butter off her toast. Her father told me 'then the bread goes on the floor!'

Parties

- **Make party foods mainly savoury.** You may be surprised to learn that many children actually prefer these.
- **Make open sandwiches.** These have two advantages: they are easier and quicker to make, and they use only half as much bread. After buttering the bread, top with any soft cheese, tinned fish, peanut butter, mashed egg, salad vegetables, or a combination of these. Make faces on some with tomato strips, red and green peppers, pieces of carrot or celery, with cress for hair and sultanas for eyes.
- **To save mess, make sandwiches bite-sized.** Cut out rounds of bread with a pastry cutter or build upon slices of cucumber or carrot. These are difficult to butter, but soft cream cheese will stick. Top them with sliced ham, tuna, salmon, mackerel, tomato or grated carrot.
- **Make cheesy dips with pieces of raw vegetables.** Fill unsightly gaps on plates with cherry tomatoes, satsuma or Mandarin orange segments, *et cetera.*
- **Build sweet courses around fresh fruit,** or fruit canned in natural juice (not in syrup and not sweetened). Sweeten puddings with fruit. There are some ideas in the Recipes section.

Of course if your child goes to another child's party, you lose control to some extent, but if you have followed the guidelines so far, it might not matter.

Ciaran was brought up from birth on a no-sugar way of eating. He did eat fruit, but nothing had sugar or other sweeteners added. He wasn't given sweets. Ciaran went to his first party when he was one year old. While he was there, he was given a Cadbury's Button. Ciaran put it in his mouth – and promptly spat it out again. It was so sweet it tasted horrible to him. This story illustrates how effective teaching from birth can be. I have little doubt that Ciaran will grow into a healthy and slim adult, as he is unlikely to be seduced by the disgustingly sweet foods that abound in the junk food market.

Conclusion

You will devote a great deal of time, money and effort into bringing up your children. Don't let it go to waste.

Health patterns for life are set in early childhood. Not only childhood diseases such as rickets and colds, but the likelihood of heart disease and cancers in adulthood are also determined at this time as, of course, is obesity. Feed and teach your child good nutritional practices in the first months and years and you lay the foundation for a long, healthy (and slim) life.

References

1. a. Barker DJP, et al. Weight in infancy and death from ischaemic heart disease. *Lancet* 1989; ii: 579.

   b. Barker DJP. The intrauterine origins of cardiovascular and obstructive lung disease in adult life. *J R Coll Phys* 1991; 25(2): 129.

   c. Barker DJP, Godfrey KM, Osmond C, Bull A. The relation of fetal length, ponderal index and head circumference to blood pressure and the risk of hypertension in later life. *Paed Perinat Epidem* 1992; 6: 35.

2. Davies A. *Let's Have Healthy Children.* Unwin Paperbacks, London, 1981.

3. Doyle W, Crawford MA, Wynn AHA. Maternal nutrient intake and birthweight. *J Hum Nutr Dietet* 1989; 2: 415.

4. Menon RK, et al. Transplacental passage of insulin in pregnant women with insulin dependent diabetes mellitus: its role in fetal macrosomia. *N Eng J Med* 1990; 323: 309–315.

5. Barton M, Weisner BP. The role of special diets in the treatment of female infecunditis. *BMJ* 1948; 2: 847–851.

6. Smith CA. The effect of wartime starvation upon pregnancy and its produce. *Am J Obstet Gynecol* 1947; 53: 599–608.

7. Godfrey K, Robinson S, Barker DJP, Osmond C, Cox V. Maternal nutrition in early and late pregnancy in relation to placental and fetal growth. *BMJ* 1996; 312: 410–414.

8. Hanson LA. Breast-feeding provides passive and likely long-lasting active immunity. *Ann Allergy Asthma Immunol* 1998; 81: 523–33; quiz 533–534, 537.

9. Kalliomaki M, Ouwehand A, Arvilommi HK, et al. Transforming growth factor-beta in breast milk: a potential regulator of atopic disease at an early age. *J Allergy Clin Immunol* 1999; 104: 1251–1257.

10. Shu XO, Linet MS, Steinbuch M, et al. Breast-feeding and risk of childhood acute leukemia. *J Natl Cancer Inst* 1999; 91: 1765–1772.

11. Singhal A, Cole TJ, Fewtrell M, Lucas A. Breastmilk feeding and lipoprotein profile in adolescents born preterm: follow-up of a prospective randomised study. *Lancet* 2004; 363: 1571–1578.

12. Uauy R, Peirano P. Breast is best: human milk is the optimal food for brain development. *Am J Clin Nutr* 1999; 70: 433–434.

13. Arenz S, Ruckerl R, Koletzko B, von Kries R. Breast-feeding and childhood obesity – a systematic review. *Int J Obes Relat Metab Disord* 2004; 28:1247–1256.

14. Janney C, Zhang D, Sowers M. Lactation and weight retention. *Am J Clin Nutr* 1997; 66: 1116–1124.

15. Fomon S. *Infant Nutrition*, 2nd edn. WB Saunders, Philadelphia, 1974, p. 455.

16. Dewey KG, et al. Breast-fed infants are leaner than formula-fed infants at 1 y of age: The DARLING Study. *Am J Clin Nutr* 1993; 57: 140–145.

17. Makrides M, Neumann M, Simmer K, Pater J, Gibson R. Are long-chain polyunsaturated fatty acids essential nutrients in infancy? *Lancet* 1995; 345: 1463–1468.

18. Richards J, Stokely D, Hipgrave P. Quality of drinking water. *BMJ* 1992; 304: 571.

19. Groves BA. *Fluoride: Drinking Ourselves to Death?* Newleaf, Dublin, 2001.

Chapter Seven

Dealing with doctors

They say 'You really need a high level of proof to change the recommendations,' which is ironic because they never had a high level of proof to set them.

Dr Walter Willett

Over the past few years all sorts of concerns have been raised about what are perceived as 'unhealthy' diets – the ones that don't conform to the tenets of 'healthy eating'. So let me put your mind at rest. In this chapter are answers to typical concerns that have been raised by doctors, nutritionists and sceptics of low-carbohydrate diets recently, to show how we are misinformed and misled. These concerns are explained more fully in Part Two of this book.

This book allows all foods – including carbs, fruits and vegetables – and, while carbs are restricted somewhat, there is no restriction on the total amount of food you can eat. That should be enough to stop anyone objecting to it. However, not only the public but nutritionists and doctors, too, have been so brainwashed over the past couple of decades that no doubt someone will.

The hardest ones to convince are the 'experts'. You will not be surprised to learn, therefore, that I am often asked how to deal with doctors. It really can get annoying after a while, can't it? So if you have the same problem, you may find it comforting to know that you're not alone. You might also like some ammunition with which to retaliate. Here it is:

Q: *Won't eating more fat raise my cholesterol and triglycerides and increase my risk of heart disease?*

A: *No, quite the opposite.* The whole vexed question of fatty diets, cholesterol and heart disease is a biggie. As this is the whole basis for cutting fats down in the first place, this book has a full chapter devoted to it (see Chapter 12).

Q: *Will eating more protein increase my risk of heart disease?*

A: *No, quite the reverse!* I should make clear that the way of eating recommended in this book is not high-protein, merely moderate or adequate protein. Having said that, however, researchers at the Harvard School of Public Health answered this question when they studied 80,082 women aged between 34 and 59 without any previous indication of heart disease.[1] When all other risk factors for heart disease were controlled for, and irrespective of whether the women were on high- or low-fat diets, the results showed that both animal and vegetable proteins contributed to a *lower* risk of heart disease. The researchers concluded:

> 'Our data do not support the hypothesis that a high protein intake increases the risk of ischemic heart disease. In contrast, our findings suggest that replacing carbohydrates with protein may be associated with a lower risk of ischemic heart disease'.

Q: *Will everyone's blood fats respond the same way to reducing carbohydrates and increasing protein and fat?*

A: *Why not?* Although we do have slightly different reactions to different foodstuffs because of our different evolutionary backgrounds in different parts of the world, we are all one species and all designed to eat essentially the same foods. All the trials of low-carb diets, for over a century, have found dramatic benefits wherever, and on whom, they have been conducted. But if you are concerned about this, have a blood test before you begin this way of eating and another three or four months into it to reassure yourself.

Q: *Will eating more protein and less carbohydrate damage my kidneys?*

A: *No.* The claim that protein intake leads to kidney disease is another popular myth that is not supported by the facts and there is not one study in which kidney damage has been demonstrated – not one. Although protein restricted diets may be helpful for men who already have kidney disease, eating meat does not cause kidney problems.[2] With women the situation is different: it doesn't seem to matter whether women have kidney disease or not, protein neither causes nor worsens the condition. Furthermore, the fat-soluble vitamins and saturated fatty acids found in animal foods are necessary for properly functioning kidneys.[3] In an Israeli study, the kidney function of a group of healthy individuals consuming an *ad libitum* high-protein diet was compared to a group of healthy vegetarians eating a low-protein diet. At the end of the study, the authors concluded that protein did not affect kidney function in normal kidneys, and it did not influence the deterioration of kidney function with age.[4] They say 'These results suggest that, in contrast with the important therapeutic effect of low-protein intake on the progressive deterioration of kidney function in diseased kidneys, such a diet does not significantly affect kidney function with "normal aging" in healthy subjects.'

On the other hand, sugar *has* been implicated in kidney disease,[5] so the answer is to give up simple sugars – table sugar, honey and fruits.[6]

If you're unsure whether your kidneys are healthy, consult your doctor before changing your diet.

There is one other point. This is not a high-protein diet. So this question is not really relevant.

Q: *Can a reduced-carbohydrate/higher-protein plan lead to osteoporosis?*

A: *No, a low-carb diet reduces the risk of osteoporosis.* In certain sections of the nutritional world, there seems to be a belief that if we eat animal protein this will cause our bones to lose calcium. This question is of particular interest in the light of Palaeolithic diet research for two related reasons. The first is because estimates of the levels of animal protein in the hominid diet during at least the last 1.7 million years of human evolution (from the time of *Homo erectus*) are much higher than is considered 'healthy' in some sectors of the nutritional research community today. The second is because the fossil evidence shows that Palaeolithic humans had a higher bone mass that would have been more robust and fracture-resistant than modern Western human's bones.

When studies were done with people eating meat together with its fat, no calcium loss was detected, even over a long period of time.[7] Other studies confirmed that meat eating does not adversely affect calcium balance[8] and that protein actually promotes stronger bones.[9]

For example, researchers at Tufts University in Boston studied the bone density of elderly men and women who were taking calcium and vitamin D and found that bone density improved most in the participants who ate the most protein, including animal proteins.[10] The lead researcher, Dr Bess Dawson-Hughes, said: 'Excess protein intake should be bad for bone, but the results of the study suggest that concerns about protein intake are probably unfounded.' She admitted that the study and other published research 'go a long way toward refuting' concerns that animal protein is bad for bones.

A year later researchers at the Bone Metabolism Unit, Creighton University School of Medicine, Omaha, looked again at this question and concluded that 'the results of the present study in postmenopausal elderly women suggest that a higher protein intake as a percentage of energy is associated with higher BMD [bone mass density] in the presence of an adequate calcium intake. . . Our results suggest that in the elderly, who are at the highest risk of osteoporosis, a higher protein intake is important for the maintenance of good bone health.'[11]

Other evidence shows that men and women who ate the most animal protein had better bone mass compared to those who avoided it.[12] The evidence also showed that vegan diets containing no foods from animal sources placed women at a greater risk for osteoporosis.[13] My wife, Monica, is the only woman I know to have lived with this way of eating as long as I have. Just before her 67th birthday Monica had a bone scan as part of a clinical study. The results showed that her bones are as good as someone less than half her age.

Protein powders

The studies that purported to show that calcium loss from bone was greater in people who ate lots of protein were not conducted with real, whole foods but with isolated amino acids and fractionated protein powders. The reason why the amino acids and fat-free protein powders caused calcium loss while the fat meat diet did not, is because protein, calcium and other minerals require the presence of other nutrients such as the fat-soluble vitamins A and D before they can be used by the body. When protein is consumed without these other nutrients, it upsets the normal biochemistry of the body and mineral loss may be the result.[14] True vitamin A and full-complex vitamin D are only found in animal fats. Furthermore, saturated fats that are present with meat are essential for proper calcium deposition in the bones.[15]

What the protein-causes-osteoporosis hypothesis really teaches us is avoid special 'low-carb' foods such as whey powder, soya protein isolates, high-protein smoothies and protein bars – and to eat meat in its natural state – with its fat.

Q: *Does the plan in this book contain all the nutrients I need to protect my bones?*

A: *Yes.* This eating plan is high in protein and in calcium- and magnesium-rich foods like cheese, fish, green leafy vegetables and nuts.

There is just one caveat: vitamin D is needed to metabolise calcium and there is very little vitamin D in any foodstuffs. Our bodies make it from the action of sunlight on the skin. It is also made in other animals the same way. Vitamin D is a fat-soluble vitamin. It is found in the fat of animals that have been allowed to graze in sunshine, but you won't find any in plant foods. This is why the best foods are animal fats and full-fat dairy products – as long as animals that supply these have been kept outside. These days, that is not guaranteed, so it is also a good idea to get out in the sun often so that your body can make vitamin D naturally.

Q: *I have heard that you can eat more meat on a reduced-carbohydrate plan. I am concerned about eating more meat because I've also heard that there is a link between meat and cancer. Is this true?*

A: *No.* The evidence suggesting that meat-eaters have more cancer came largely from just one study that looked at vegetarian Seventh Day Adventists.[16] They did have less cancer than the average American population. But a similar study among meat-eating Mormons found that, in them, cancer was even lower than that of Seventh Day Adventists.[17] It seems that stress plays a large part in cancer and many other conditions. What the various studies show is people who belong to supportive groups, such as tightly knit religious groups, have a lower incidence of these diseases regardless of what they eat. Traditional Inuit and Maasai, eating nothing but meat, have no cancer at all. This is probably because cancer is a response to a high-carb diet.

Q: *But doesn't the latest research prove that a high animal fat diet increases the risk of breast cancer?*

A: *No, it doesn't.* If eating animal fat increased the risk of breast cancer, one would expect that populations that eat more animal fat would have more breast cancer. Yet they don't. Populations from the Maasai in the tropics to the Inuit in the Arctic, who eat diets where eighty percent of the calorie intake is in the form of animal fats, don't get breast cancer or any other form of cancer.

The evidence shows that the fats which increase cancer risk are the 'healthy' polyunsaturated vegetable margarines and cooking oils (see Chapter 13).

Q: *Does restricting carbohydrates reduce energy and cause fatigue?*

A: *Quite the reverse.* Fatigue and energy loss are usually signs of low blood sugar (hypoglycaemia). The correct low-carb approach will keep your blood sugar levels stable. Carbs are usually thought of as 'energy foods', and it is true that carbs do provide energy. But they don't provide the best energy. Fats do that. And fat is what you should eat to replace the energy lost from carbs.

The people who experience fatigue at the beginning are those on other plans which cut carbs too low to start with – levels as low as 20 grams are common. This is why I recommend 60 grams (the equivalent of five slices of bread in a day). At this level these symptoms are avoided. That means cutting down on carbs – but not cutting them down too much.

Q: *Does restricting carbohydrates cause headaches?*

A: *Not if you don't cut down too much.* It was thought that the brain used only glucose as an energy source. But recent research from Japan has demonstrated that it can also use fats just as well.[21] All the reports of headaches are associated with diets which cut down drastically on carbs at the start. The transition from one kind of fuel to another can cause problems if that change it too drastic. This is another reason not to cut carbs below 60 grams to begin with.

Q: *Is my breath going to smell funny on this diet?*

A: *No.* The 'badger's breath' associated with one popular low-carbohydrate diet is not a problem on this plan because the carbs are not as restricted. This book advocates a *lower*-carb approach by avoiding concentrated carbohydrates such as sugars and cereals. It is only very severe carb restriction that triggers the extreme 'ketosis' which causes smelly breath.

Q: *But doesn't any low-carb diet cause ketosis?*

A: *Yes and no.* 'Ketones' are a class of compounds that are quite normal products of fat metabolism. With this and other low-carb, high-fat plans, ketones are used in the body to provide a source of energy for the cells that would otherwise use glucose. However, raising levels of ketones in excess of what is needed is not a good idea.

When glucose appears in the urine of a diabetic, it is their body's way of getting rid of excess glucose – which is why giving diabetics even more carbs is such a ridiculous protocol. Raising ketones in body tissues to such high levels that they have to be disposed of by excretion in urine, as is advocated on one popular low-carb plan, is exactly the same; the body is getting rid of something it has too much of. In a similar way to feeding diabetics more carbs when they are already getting rid of excess glucose, feeding fats to people whose bodies are already rejecting ketones, is equally stupid in my opinion.

There is also an economic side to this. Ketones are made from foods that you buy. You have paid for these – and the foods they came with are relatively expensive. Why flush them down the toilet?

So while a ketogenic diet is healthy, I do not believe overt ketosis is desirable, and I have not found it necessary, to go to such extremes. The 60 grams of carbohydrate a day that are included in this plan are more than enough to avoid this.

NOTE: A condition called *ketoacidosis* may occur in diabetics. This should not be confused with ketosis, which is quite different.

Q: *Should I expect to be constipated?*

A: *No.* The liberal use of green, leafy vegetables, both cooked and as salads, will ensure that you are not constipated. Drinking at least 2 litres (3½ pints) of water will also help to avoid the condition.

Q: *My friend had to have a gallstone operation and was told to go on a low-fat diet. I have also been told that eating lots of fat causes gallstones. Will I develop gallstones eating this way?*

A: *Quite the reverse – a fatty diet actually prevents gallstones.* Elaine was told by her doctor that her gallstones were caused by following a low-fat diet. John was told that his gallstones were caused by eating a high-fat diet. Isn't it infuriating when doctors give out such contradictory advice? So let me put the record straight.

Fair, fat and forty. That is the general perception of someone with gallstones. For this reason, gallstones, often found in fat people, are usually attributed to a diet high in fats. In fact this is the opposite of the truth: gallstones are caused by eating too little fat rather than too much.

Before dietary fat can be digested, it has to be emulsified, using bile. The liver makes bile continuously and stores it in the gallbladder until needed. So gallstones can be formed when the gallbladder is not emptied regularly – because you aren't eating fat.

Low-fat slimming diets are probably the major cause. All such diets restrict fats. In people who eat a low-fat diet, bile is stored for long periods in the gallbladder – and it stagnates. In time – and it can be really quite a short time – a 'sludge' begins to form. This then coagulates to form small stones, called 'gravel' which then become bigger. The speed with which this happens was dramatically demonstrated in a trial at several American university hospitals.[22] None of the subjects had any sign of gallbladder disease at the start of the study. However, after only eight weeks of low-fat, weight-reduction dieting, more than a quarter had developed gallstones. Where they were fed intravenously, half developed gallbladder sludge after 3 weeks, and *all* had developed sludge by six weeks. Nearly half of those who developed sludge also developed gallstones. This is an alarming finding as gallstones are not only painful, the operation to remove them is potentially life-threatening. The more one uses low-fat diets, the greater is the risk.

The pain that someone with gallstones gets is when these are passed with the bile in response to a fatty meal and get stuck in the bile duct.

So, it is a low-fat diet which causes the gallstones, but it is eating a high-fat diet that makes them apparent. If you eat a low-fat diet and never eat fat again, then you probably won't get the pain, even though the stones are there.

If someone suffers from gallstones, a low-fat diet 'prevents' the symptoms, so doctors often suggest such a diet, but it makes the *cause* of the symptoms (gallstones) worse. Doctors are often loath to operate to remove the stones, so just preventing you knowing about them seems to them to be a good compromise – despite the fact that you will then be miserable and hungry as a result!

Q: *But how can a diet that cuts out a whole food group be a balanced diet?*

A: *There is no concept so dear to a nutritionist's heart as that of a balanced diet.* Those who complain that this way of eating is not a balanced diet, or that it cuts out a whole food group, simply don't understand what a balanced diet is. You will realise just how necessary a 'balanced' diet is when you consider that in many parts of the world large groups of hunters live quite healthily on nothing but a small part of one group: fat meat. There is an enormous body of evidence from all over the world that people can and do remain entirely fit and healthy on diets that are restricted to meat alone. Obviously, the 'balanced' diet so beloved of dieticians is not so important after all.

The truth is that a balanced diet is any diet that supplies all the nutrients the body requires, in the correct proportions. A diet of fresh meat alone, if fat is included, can do just that. And offal helps too: liver, for example, contains four times as much vitamin C as either apples or pears, and kidney is nearly as good. This plan, however, goes much further in that carbohydrate intake is not cut out, merely reduced. It is, in all respects, a balanced diet.

Q: *But eating a lot of fat makes me queasy*

A: *Some people say that they find a high-fat diet nauseating.* They associate the word 'fat' with blubber or greasy food. It is noticeable, however, that they usually have no difficulty eating fat if that fat is called 'butter' or 'cream'. And the person who cannot stand 'greasy food' usually has no problem eating chocolate.

Strangely, although people have been professing to want leaner meat since the end of food rationing in 1954, the actual consumption of fat in Britain has been rising steadily throughout this century. The problem with this, as far as health is concerned, is that the increase has not been of healthy animal fats but of unhealthy hydrogenated vegetable oils.

If you really cannot stand the sight of visible fat on a succulent piece of meat, you can avoid offending your palate by choosing foods that are high in invisible fats, or the acceptable fats that you eat now. After a while you will find that you will come to relish the crackling on pork, the skin on chicken or the fat on a piece of roast beef and you will be back to the ideal way of eating. At this stage fat will only make you feel nauseous if you try to eat more of it than your body wants. And that is what we want it to do: it's your body's signal that it has had enough. Listen to your body, stop eating when it tells you, and fat will not be a problem – either in your food or on your body.

You may even find that your diet is 'healthier' in the conventional sense. One client told me that before she started to eat this way she didn't like vegetables. She did eat them but only because she was told that '5 portions' of vegetables were 'healthy', not because she liked them. Now that she can fry vegetables or put olive oil or butter on them, she enjoys vegetables so much that she is actually eating more than she did before. 'It's opened up a whole new world to me,' she said.

Q: *But doesn't this way of eating cost more?*

A: *It can actually work out cheaper!* Carbohydrate foods such as potato crisps or bread and jam tend to be more readily available for snacks than meat and cheese. This can be a problem when you are eating what you are used to, and when well-meaning friends press such food on you. Sweet and starchy foods are also cheaper to buy as far as bulk is concerned. But you have to eat a lot more of these to supply the nutrients your body needs.

Eating this way can actually cost less. For example, at the time of writing, three peppers – one red, one yellow and one green, which is how supermarkets seem to sell them – cost the same as six extra-large eggs or six duck eggs. The better value in the eggs is demonstrated below:

	Peppers	Eggs
Energy	150 cal	480 cal
Protein	5.7 g	43.2 g
Carb	35.4	3.2 g
Fat	0.0 g	28.8 g
Calcium	61.5 mg	170.4 mg

In other words, in energy terms and the length of time you can keep going until you start to get hungry, you would need to spend over three times as much on peppers as you would on eggs. In addition to the nutrients listed, the eggs will also provide all the other nutrients your body needs.

There is another aspect: do you spend good money on slimming clubs and magazines? You would be better advised to spend that money on good wholesome food. It need not cost more than the membership fees. By eating properly, you will not get hungry and are much less likely to snack on sweets – which will again reduce your costs.

Q: *But can I be sure it's safe? There are no long-term clinical trials of your diet.*

A: There are no clinical trials of parachutes preventing the death of a person falling from an aeroplane, but surely it is obvious that parachutes prevent deaths due to hitting the ground at high speed. Do we really need a clinical trial to prove it?

Observations over the past couple of centuries have shown that where humans live with a natural diet such as recommended here, they get none of the 'diseases of civilisation' we do. Do we really need more evidence? Would a dietary trial, artificially conducted in a clinical environment with artificial foods be as relevant as looking at real people in a natural environment?

Incidentally, the nutritionists who complain that there are no long-term trials of low-carb diets have it completely wrong. It is their low-fat, 'healthy' diet that has no long-term evidence of either safety or effectiveness. Judging by the dramatic rises in a range of diseases since its inception, there never will be!

Q: *But could your diet lead to other diseases?*

A: *There is no evidence of it.* In fact, the opposite is true. The low-carb, high fat way of eating recommended here significantly reduces the risk of a wide range of modern, chronic degenerative diseases. These are listed at Appendix A.

Conclusion

Over the past century or so, many studies have looked at possible adverse effects from eating a low-carb, high-fat diet. Not one has ever demonstrated that it is anything but beneficial.

References

1. Hu FB, Stampfer MJ, Manson JE, et al. Dietary protein and risk of ischemic heart disease in women. *Am J Clin Nutr* 1999; 70: 221–227.
2. Dwyer JT, Madans JH, Turnbull B, et al. Diet, indicators of kidney disease, and late mortality among older persons in the NHANES I Epidemiologic Follow-up Study. *Am J Pub Health* 1994; 84: 1299–1303.
3. Enig M. Saturated fats and the kidneys. *Wise Traditions* 2000; 1:3:49. Posted at http://www.westonaprice.org.
4. Blum M, Averbuch M, Wolman Y, Aviram A. Protein intake and kidney function in humans: its effect on 'normal aging'. *Arch Intern Med* 1989; 149: 211–212.
5. Yudkin J, Kang S, Bruckdorfer K. Effects of High Dietary Sugar. *BMJ* 1980; 281: 1396.
6. Blacklock NJ. Sucrose and idiopathic renal stone. *Nutr Health* 1987; 5: 9–17.
7. Spencer H, Kramer L. Factors contributing to osteoporosis. *J Nutr* 1986; 116: 316–319; Further studies of the effect of a high protein diet as meat on calcium metabolism. *Am J Clin Nutr* 1983; 37:6: 924–949.
8. a. Hunt J, et al. High- versus low-meat diets: Effects on zinc absorption, iron status, and calcium, copper, iron, magnesium, manganese, nitrogen, phosphorus, and zinc balance in postmenopausal women. *Am J Clin Nutr* 1995, 62:621–632;
   b. Spencer H, Kramer L, Osis D. Do protein and phosphorus cause calcium loss? *J Nutr* 1988; 118: 657–660.
9. Cooper C, et al. Dietary protein and bone mass in women. *Calcif Tiss Int* 1996; 58: 320–325.
10. Dawson-Hughes B, Harris SS. Calcium intake influences the association of protein intake with rates of bone loss in elderly men and women. *Am J Clin Nutr* 2002; 75: 773–779.
11. Rapuri PB, Gallagher JC, Haynatzka V. Protein intake: effects on bone mineral density and the rate of bone loss in elderly women. *Am J Clin Nutr* 2003; 77: 1517–1525.
12. a. Munger RG, et al. Prospective study of dietary protein intake and risk of hip fracture in postmenopausal women. *Am J Clin Nutr* 1999; 69: 147–152;
    b. Hannan MT, et al. Effect of dietary protein on bone loss in elderly men and women: The Framingham Osteoporosis Study. *J Bone Min Res* 2000; 15: 2504–2512.
13. a. Chiu JF, Lan SJ, Yang CY, et al. Long-term vegetarian diet and bone mineral density in postmenopausal Taiwanese women. *Calcif Tissue Int* 1997; 60: 245–249;
    b. Lau EM, Kwok T, Woo J, et al. Bone mineral density in Chinese elderly female vegetarians, vegans, lacto-vegetarians and omnivores. *Eur J Clin Nutr* 1998; 52: 60–64.
14. Fallon S, Enig M. Dem bones – do high protein diets cause osteoporosis? *Wise Traditions* 2000; 1: 4: 38–41. Also posted at http://www.westonaprice.org
15. a. Watkins BA, et al. Importance of vitamin E in bone formation and in chondrocyte function. *American Oil Chemists Society Proceedings* 1996, at Purdue University;

b. Food lipids and bone health. In: McDonald and Min, eds. *Food Lipids and Health.* Marcel Dekker, NY, 1996.

16. Phillips RL. Role of lifestyle and dietary habits among Seventh-Day Adventists. *Cancer Res* 1975; 35: 3513.

17. Lyon JL, Klauber MR, Gardner JW, Smart CR. Cancer incidence in Mormons and non-Mormons in Utah, 1966–70. *N Engl J Med* 1976; 294: 129–133.

18. Cho E, Donna Spiegelman, Hunter DJ, et al. Premenopausal fat intake and risk of breast cancer. *J Natl Cancer Inst* 2003; 95: 1079–1085.

19. Holmes MD, Colditz GA, Hunter DJ, et al. Meat, fish and egg intake and risk of breast cancer. *Int J Cancer* 2003; 104: 221–227.

20. Bingham SA, Luben R, Welch A, et al. Are imprecise methods obscuring a relation between fat and breast cancer? *Lancet* 2003; 362: 212–214.

21. Takenaka T, Hiruma H, Hori H, et al. Fatty acids as an energy source for the operation of axoplasmic transport. *Brain Res* 2003; 972: 38–43.

22. Liddle RA, Goldstein RB, Saxton J. Gallstone formation during weight-reduction dieting. *Arch Intern Med* 1989; 149: 1750–1753.

Part Two

The evidence

Chapter Eight

Mr Banting's diet revolution

If we do not learn from the past, we remain in the infancy of knowledge.
Cicero

Introduction

Whether you want to lose weight or not and whether you have any interest in diets or not, you will almost certainly have heard of 'the Atkins diet'. However, unless you are extremely old or live in Scandinavia, you may not have heard of the Banting diet.

There seems to be a general belief that the rash of low-carbohydrate, high-fat diets are 'new' or 'revolutionary' in some way. Popular diet books certainly give that impression, but nothing could be further from the truth. I started eating a low-carbohydrate diet in 1962 when a doctor advised me that this was the best way to lose weight. You may also think that these 'new' low-carbohydrate regimes were pioneered by far-seeing and learned medical men. Again, this is incorrect. The truth is that we would probably never have heard of diets where people could lose weight eating that most calorific of foods, fat, if it had not been for a 19th century English carpenter by the name of William Banting and one of the most famous books on obesity ever written.

It was Banting's work that inspired me to write this book. It is also the basis of all the other low-carb plans around today.

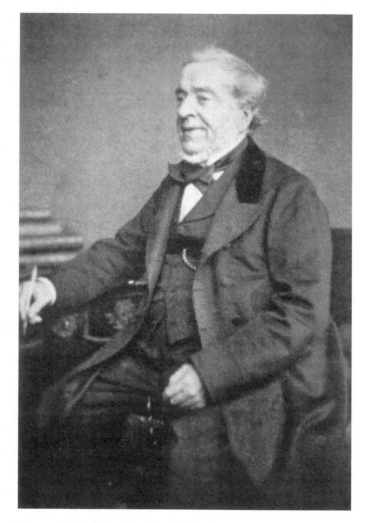

Figure 3   William Banting 1796–1878

William Banting was well-regarded in 19th century society; he was an undertaker to the rich and famous. If he had remained only that, his name would probably be remembered today merely as the Duke of Wellington's coffin maker, if indeed it were remembered at all.

None of Banting's family on either parent's side had any tendency to become overweight. Nevertheless it was a condition he dreaded. When he was in his thirties, he started to become overweight and he consulted an eminent surgeon, a kind personal friend, who recommended 'increased bodily exertion before any ordinary daily labours began'. Banting had a heavy boat and lived near the river so he took up rowing the boat for two hours a day. All this did for him, however, was to give him a prodigious appetite. He put on weight and was told to stop.

Another physician advised him that he could remedy his obesity by 'moderate and light food' but didn't tell him what was intended by this. Banting says he brought his system 'into a low, impoverished state without reducing his weight, which caused many obnoxious boils to appear and two rather formidable carbuncles for which he was ably operated upon but also fed into increased obesity'.

Banting went into hospital 20 times in as many years for weight reduction. He tried swimming, walking, riding and taking the sea air. He drank 'gallons of physic and liquor potassae', took the spa waters at Leamington, Cheltenham and Harrogate, and tried low-calorie, starvation diets; he took Turkish baths at a rate of up to three a week for a year but lost only 6 lb in all that time, and had less and less energy.

He was assured by one physician ('one of the ablest physicians in the land') that putting weight on was perfectly natural; that he, himself, had put on a pound for every year of manhood and he was not surprised by Banting's condition – he just advised 'more exercise, vapour baths and shampooing and medicine'.

Banting tried every form of slimming treatment the medical profession could devise but it was all in vain. Eventually, discouraged and disillusioned – and still very fat – he gave up.

By 1862, at the age of 66, William Banting weighed 202 lb (14 st 6 lb) and he was 5 ft 5 in tall. He says that, although he was of no great weight or size, still I 'could not stoop to tie my shoes, so to speak, nor to attend to the little offices humanity requires without considerable pain and difficulty which only the corpulent can understand. I have been compelled to go downstairs slowly backward to save the jar of increased weight on the knee and ankle joints and have been obliged to puff and blow over every slight exertion, particularly that of going upstairs.' He also had an 'umbilical rupture', and other bodily ailments. If this were not bad enough he found that his eyesight was failing and he was becoming increasingly deaf.

Because of this last problem, he consulted a hearing specialist who made light of his case, sponged his ears out and blistered the outer ear without the slightest benefit and without enquiring into his other ailments. Banting was not satisfied; he left in a worse plight than when he went to the specialist.

Eventually, in August of 1862 Banting consulted a noted Fellow of the Royal College of Surgeons, an ear, nose and throat specialist, Dr William Harvey. It was an historic meeting.

Dr Harvey had recently returned from a symposium in Paris where he had heard Dr Claude Bernard, a renowned physiologist, talk of a new theory about the part the liver played in the disease of diabetes. Bernard believed that the liver, as well as secreting bile, also secreted a sugar-like substance that it made from elements of the blood passing through it. This started Harvey's thinking about the roles of the various food elements in diabetes and he began a major course of research into the whole question of the way in which fats, sugars and starches affected the body.

When Dr Harvey met Banting, he was interested as much by Banting's obesity as his deafness, for he recognised that the one was the cause of the other, so Harvey put Banting on a diet.

Banting's diet to that date had followed this pattern:

- **Breakfast:** bread and milk for breakfast, or a pint of tea with plenty of milk and sugar, and buttered toast (this was before the invention of breakfast cereals, but it is actually very similar to the modern cereal breakfast).
- **Dinner:** meat, beer, bread and pastry for dinner.
- **Tea:** a meal similar to breakfast.
- **Supper:** generally a fruit tart or bread and milk.

Banting says he had little comfort and far less sound sleep. Harvey's advice to him was to give up bread, butter, milk, sugar, beer and potatoes. These, he told Banting, contained starch and 'saccharine matter' (sugar) tending to create fat and were to be avoided altogether.

When told what he could not eat, Banting's immediate thought was that he had very little left to live on. Harvey soon showed him that really there was ample and Banting was only too happy to give the plan a fair trial. Within a very few days, he says, he derived immense benefit from it, the plan leading to an excellent night's rest with six to eight hours' sleep per night.

For each meal, Harvey allowed Banting:

- up to six ounces of bacon, beef, mutton, venison, kidneys, fish or any form of poultry or game;

- the 'fruit of any pudding' – he was denied the pastry;
- any vegetable except potato;
- and at dinner, two or three glasses of good claret, sherry or Madeira.

Banting could drink tea without milk or sugar. Champagne, port and beer were forbidden and he could eat only one ounce of toast. There was no restriction on the total amounts of food Banting could eat.

On this diet Banting lost nearly 1 lb per week from August 1862 to August 1863. In his own words he said: 'I can confidently state that quantity of diet may safely be left to the natural appetite; and that it is quality only which is essential to abate and cure corpulence.' He went on: 'These important desiderata have been attained by the most easy and comfortable means . . . by a system of diet, that formerly I should have thought dangerously generous.'

After 38 weeks, Banting felt better than he had for the last 20 years. By the end of one year, not only had his hearing been restored, he had much more vitality, had lost 46 lb (21 kg) in weight and 12¼ inches (310 mm) off his waist. He was also able to come downstairs forward naturally with perfect ease, go upstairs and take exercise freely without the slightest inconvenience, could perform every necessary office for himself, the umbilical rupture was greatly ameliorated and gave him no anxiety, his sight was restored, his other bodily ailments had 'passed into the matter of history'.

Banting was delighted. He would have gone through hell to achieve all this but it had not been necessary. Indeed the diet allowed so much food, and it was so easy to maintain, that Banting said of it: 'I can conscientiously assert I never lived so well as under the new plan of dietary, which I should have formerly thought a dangerous, extravagant trespass upon health.'

He says that this present dietary table is far superior to what he was eating before – 'more luxurious and liberal, independent of its blessed effect, but when it is proved to be more healthful, the comparisons are simply ridiculous.' 'I am very much better both bodily and mentally and pleased to believe that I hold the reins of health and comfort in my own hands.' 'It is simply miraculous and I am thankful to Almighty Providence for directing me through an extraordinary chance to the care of a man who worked such a change in so short a time.'

It is obvious from these comments that Banting didn't need the strength of willpower that today's dieter needs; that he found his weight loss diet very easy to maintain.

He wished that the medical profession would acquaint themselves with the cure for obesity so that so many men would not descend into early graves, as he believed many did, from apoplexy, and would not endure on Earth so much bodily and mental infirmity.

Banting was so pleased with his progress that on top of Harvey's fees, he gave the doctor £50 to be distributed amongst Harvey's favourite hospitals, although despite this, he still felt deeply obligated in a way that he could never hope to repay.

Fortunately for us today, Banting was quite a remarkable man. It is for this reason alone that we can know today what this miraculous diet was. In May 1863, after just 38 weeks on the diet, Banting published and gave away 1000 copies of his now famous *Letter on Corpulence* at his own expense. Banting charged nothing for the first two editions of his book as he didn't want to be accused of doing it merely for profit. The second edition numbered 1500; he gave this away although each copy cost him 6 d (old pence). Copies of the third edition, still in 1863, were sold at one shilling each.

When Banting's booklet, in which he described the diet and its amazing results, was published, it was so contrary to the established doctrine that it set up a howl of protest among members of the medical profession. The 'Banting Diet' became the centre of a bitter controversy and Banting's papers and book were ridiculed and distorted. No one could deny that the diet worked, but as a layman had published it, and medical men were anxious that their position in society should not be undermined, they felt bound to attack it. Banting's paper was criticised solely on the grounds that it was 'unscientific'.

Dr Harvey had a problem too. He had an effective treatment for obesity but not a convincing theory to explain it. As he was a medical man, and so easier for the other members of his profession to attack, he came in for a great deal of ridicule until, in the end, his practice began to suffer.

However, the public was impressed. Many desperate, overweight people tried the diet and found that it worked. Like it or not, the medical profession could not ignore it. Its obvious success meant that the Banting Diet had to be explained somehow.

To the rescue came a Dr Felix Niemeyer from Stuttgart. He managed to make the new diet acceptable with a total shift in its philosophy. At that time, the theory was that carbohydrates and fat burned together in the lungs to produce heat. The two were called 'respiratory foods'. After examining Banting's paper, Niemeyer came up with an answer to the doctors' problem: All doctors knew that protein was not fattening, only the respiratory foods – fats and carbohydrates. He, therefore, interpreted 'meat' to mean only lean meat with the fat trimmed off and this subtle change solved the problem. The Banting Diet became a high protein diet with both carbohydrate and fat restricted. This altered diet became enshrined in history and still forms the basis of some slimming diets today.

Banting's descriptions of the diet are quite clear, however. Other than a prohibition against butter and pork, nowhere is there any instruction to remove the fat from meat and there is no restriction on the way food was cooked or on the total quantity of food which may be taken. Only carbohydrate – sugars and starches – were restricted. The reason that butter and pork were denied him was that it was thought at the time that they, too, contained starch.

Banting, who lived in physical comfort and remained at a normal weight until his death at the age of 81, always maintained that Dr Niemeyer's altered diet was far inferior to the one that had so changed his life.

The Banting diet is confirmed

Banting's *Letter on Corpulence* travelled widely. In the 1890s, an American doctor, Helen Densmore, modelled diets on Banting.[1] She tells how she and her patients lost an average 10–15 lb (4.5–6.8 kg) in the first month on the diet and then 6–8 lb (2.7–3.6 kg) in subsequent months 'by a diet from which bread, cereals and starchy food were excluded'. Her advice to would-be dieters was: 'One pound of beef or mutton or fish per day with a moderate amount of the non-starchy vegetables given above [tomatoes, lettuce, string beans, spinach and such] will be found ample for any obese person of sedentary habits'.

Dr Densmore was scathing of those others of her profession who derided Banting's diet. She says of them: 'Those very specialists who are at this time prospering greatly by the reduction of obesity and who are indebted to Mr Banting for all their prosperity are loud, nevertheless, in their condemnation of the Banting method'.

In 1898 a German doctor, N. Zuntz, reported a case of a man who gained weight on a high-carbohydrate diet and lost weight on a high-fat diet, both of which had similar calorific values. Two American doctors clinically confirmed Zuntz's observation in 1907 with a subject who did uniform amounts of work each day on a bicycle ergometer.[2]

Real-life tests

In 1906, Dr Vilhjalmur Stefansson, a young Harvard anthropology teacher who later became a world-famous explorer and anthropologist, revolutionised polar exploration by crossing the Arctic alone and living off the land with the Eskimos. It was not quite what had been planned. Stefansson had gone on ahead of the Leffingwell-Mikkelson Expedition and had missed a planned rendezvous at Herschel Island. He was left to spend an Arctic winter with the Eskimos eating a diet composed only of meat and fish. Unlike the diet he had been brought up on, it contained no plant material whatsoever.[3]

It was a golden opportunity for the young scientist to conduct an experiment into the effects of an Eskimo diet on a European unaccustomed to it. The usual Eskimo meal consisted of briefly stewed fish washed down with water. It was so different from what he was used to that at first Stefansson was repelled by it. To try to make the fish more palatable, he tried broiling it. This resulted in his becoming weak and dizzy, with other symptoms of malnutrition. Stefansson reasoned that with such a restricted diet the body had to have not just the fish but the other nutrients that had been leached out into the water, and so he tried harder. Eventually he became so accustomed to the primitive diet that, by the time he left the Eskimos, Stefansson managed as well as them. On this regime, Stefansson remained in perfect health and did not get fat.

The experience had a profound effect on Stefansson. Like Banting before him, he became interested in the possibilities of diets high in proteins and fats, and low in carbohydrates. It seemed to him that a balanced diet in which there was relatively little meat, 'balanced' by larger amounts of potatoes, bread, rice and other starchy foods followed by sweet desserts and sugared coffee might be balanced in the wrong direction, and so like Banting, Stefansson questioned the established ideas on diet. Unfortunately, he had no more success than Banting. Although he became famous and his position as an anthropologist was unassailable, still no one took any notice of his ideas on nutrition.

Some years after his first experience with the Eskimos, Dr Stefansson returned to the Arctic with a colleague, Dr Karsten Andersen, to carry out research for the American Museum of Natural History. They were supplied with every necessity including a year's supply of 'civilised' food. They didn't take it, deciding instead to live off the land. In the end, the one-year project stretched to four years, during which time the two men ate only the meat they could kill and the fish they could catch in the Canadian Arctic. Neither of the two men suffered any adverse after-effects from their four-year experiment.

It was evident to Stefansson, as it had been to Banting, that the body could function perfectly well, remain healthy, vigorous and slender if it used a diet in which as much food was eaten as the body required, only carbohydrate was restricted, and the total number of calories was ignored.

The first clinical trial

In 1928, Stefansson and Andersen entered Bellevue Hospital, New York, for a controlled experiment into the effects of an all-meat diet on the body. The committee which was assembled to supervise the experiment was one of the best qualified in medical history, consisting as it did of the leaders of all the branches of science related to the subject. The experiment was directed by Dr Eugene F. DuBois, Medical Director of the Russell Sage Foundation (subsequently chief physician at the New York Hospital, and Professor of Physiology at Cornell University Medical College). The study was designed to find the answers to five questions about which there was some debate:

1. Does the withholding of vegetable foods cause scurvy?
2. Will an all-meat diet cause other deficiency diseases?
3. Will it cause mineral deficiencies, of calcium in particular?
4. Will it have a harmful effect on the heart, blood vessels or kidneys?
5. Will it promote the growth of harmful bacteria in the gut?

The results of the year-long trial were published in 1930 in the *Journal of Biological Chemistry* and showed that the answer to all of the questions was No! There were no deficiency problems; the two men remained perfectly healthy; their bowels remained normal, except that their stools were smaller and did not smell. The absence of starchy and sugary carbohydrates from their diet appeared to have only good effects.

Once again, Stefansson discovered that he felt better and was healthier on a diet that restricted carbohydrates. Only when fats were restricted did he suffer any problems. During this experiment Stefansson averaged about 2650 calories a day, 2100 calories coming from fat and 550 from protein. Andersen averaged about 2620 calories a day, 2110 from fat and 510 from protein.

One interesting finding from a heart disease perspective was that Stefansson's blood cholesterol level fell by 1.3 mmol/L while on the all-meat diet, rising again at the end of the study when he resumed a 'normal' diet.

However, the published results had little effect on the people trying to lose weight in 1930. A diet that allowed as much meat as one could eat and also allowed a large proportion of fat must contain lots of calories. To the average dieter, lots of calories meant putting on weight.

The evidence mounts

Drs D.M. Lyon and D.M. Dunlop of the Royal Infirmary, Edinburgh, noticed that healthy adults maintained an almost constant body weight over long periods in spite of considerable variations of physical activity and of food intake. They further noticed that those who regularly overate did not necessarily become overweight; neither did those who had a poor appetite necessarily become thin. During 1931 they conducted a controlled dietary trial using a wide variety of low- and high-calorie diets, ranging from 800 to 2700 calories.[4] So that comparisons would be more meaningful, all the patients were put initially on 1000-calorie slimming diets. On the low-calorie diets, average weight losses were found to depend not so much on the calorie content of the diets but on the carbohydrate content. The average daily losses on the 1000-calorie diets were:

- High-carbohydrate/low-fat diet: 49 g (like the modern slimming diet).
- High-carbohydrate/low-protein: 122 g.
- Low-carbohydrate/high-protein: 183 g.
- Low-carbohydrate/high-fat: 205 g (like *Natural Health and Weight Loss*).

It was expected that patients would not lose weight on the 1700 to 2700-calorie diets. In fact all but three did.

At the end of the trial, the average weight loss for those on the low-calorie diets was 145 grams per day but those on the high-calorie diets lost more at 157 grams per day. Lyon and Dunlop, in their conclusions say:

> 'The most striking feature . . . is that the losses appear to be inversely proportionate to the carbohydrate content of the food. Where the carbohydrate intake is low the rate of loss in weight is greater and conversely'.

In other words, the more carbohydrate there was, the less weight was lost.

In 1944, Dr Blake F. Donaldson carried out another famous experiment at the New York Hospital when very overweight patients were reduced on high-fat, low-carbohydrate diets.[5] Patients were encouraged to eat as much as they wanted and some of the sceptical ones certainly did – and they lost weight. High-fat, high-protein, low-carbohydrate diets were back. Dr Donaldson tells of this milestone in the history of slimming diets in his book, *Strong Medicine*. In Britain, deeply involved in a war and with food rationed, however, the experiment went largely unnoticed. Even in the USA, the average dieter went on counting the calories in her low-calorie salad oblivious of the harm that she was doing to her health.

After World War II, the E.I. du Pont de Nemours chemical company of America undertook a slimming programme with some of its overweight executives who'd had no success with the more usual low-calorie diets. Dr Albert W. Pennington and the director of Du Pont's medical division, Dr George H. Gehrmann, ran the programme. Pennington had sifted through all the available evidence and decided to try Banting's recommendations. Therefore, the subjects were allowed all the untrimmed meat they wanted, with only carbohydrates withheld, and the results were spectacular. Dieters each lost an average 10 kg (22 lb) in three months while their energy intakes averaged 3000 calories per day.

This time the public was interested and *Holiday* magazine published a series about the project. For a while, the 'Holiday Diet' became a household phrase in the USA. But the regimen offered so many calories, and the general public had been so brainwashed for so long, that most found it impossible to believe that such a diet could work.

In 1956 Professor Alan Kekwick and Dr Gaston Pawan conducted a clinical test of Banting's diet at the Middlesex Hospital in London.[6] (It was this study that Dr Robert Atkins says started his interest in low-carb diets for his patients.) They opined that if weight loss in overweight persons were merely a case of reducing dietary calorie intake to below the amount the body needed, then the lower the intake of calories, the greater should be the weight loss. To demonstrate this they used diets of 500, 1000, 1500 and 2000 calories made up of constant proportions of carbohydrates (47%), proteins (20%) and fat (33%). This first series of tests, not surprisingly, did find a definite relation between the deficiency of calories and the amount of weight lost – the less the patients ate the more weight they lost.

It is at this point that dieticians today seem to stop. Kekwick and Pawan were more intelligent.

They went on to reason that if a deficiency in calorie intake alone were responsible for weight loss, then diets of equal energy value, no matter what they were composed of, should produce equal loss of weight. To test this they set up a second series of tests, where all the diets were 1000 calories, but made up of different constituents. Four 1000-calorie diets were formulated. These were 90% carbohydrate, or 90% protein or 90% fat respectively, plus a fourth which was a normal mixed diet. So different were the rates of weight loss in this series of tests that it was obvious that what the diet contained was far more important than simply how many calories it had. Subjects on the high-fat diet lost much more weight than those on the others – while some on the 1000-calorie high-carbohydrate diet actually put weight on.

As it was the composition of the diet that had the most profound effect on weight loss when the diets were restricted to *below* what the body needed, a third series of tests was performed with diets that were less restricted. Patients were put first on 2000-calorie diets with a normal composition of protein, fat and carbohydrate. During this test, the patients either stayed at the same weight or gained slightly. Calorie intakes were then *increased* to 2600 by increasing the amounts of fat and protein, while at the same time the amount of carbohydrate was reduced. This time patients lost weight. There was only one possible explanation: carbohydrates put weight on while fats took weight off.

These findings were no surprise as far as dietary protein was concerned. That protein had a role in weight loss had been known for many years. It was a surprise, however, that fat also worked in this way, particularly as the slimming action of dietary fat appeared to be greater than that of protein.

In 1959, Dr John Yudkin, Professor of Nutrition and Dietetics, Queen Elizabeth Hospital, University of London, confirmed Kekwick and Pawan's findings when he showed that a diet with unlimited protein and fat, but with little or no carbohydrate was far more effective in causing weight loss than a calorie-controlled, low-fat diet.

During the 1950s, another British physician, Dr Richard Mackarness, found that the low-carb, high-fat diet was so successful with his overweight patients that he wrote a book that was in print for nearly 20 years – a feat almost unheard of in the slimming book industry. It was Dr Mackarness who introduced this concept to me in 1962 and so dramatically changed the lives of my family and me. In more than 40 years since, none of my family has been overweight, although we were before that date.

In 1972, Dr Robert Atkins published *Dr Atkins' Diet Revolution.*

'Healthy eating' is fattening

As time passed and praising the value of fat became politically incorrect, it became more difficult to get such trials published. Nevertheless, it did happen occasionally.

Published in the year 2000, a prospective study was conducted to evaluate the effect of a low carbohydrate, high-protein/fat diet in achieving short-term weight loss.[7] Researchers at the Center for Health Services Research in Primary Care, Durham, North Carolina, reported data from a six-month study that included 51 individuals who were overweight, but otherwise healthy. The subjects received nutritional supplements and attended bi-weekly group meetings, where they received dietary counselling on consuming a low-carbohydrate, high-protein/fat diet. After six months, they had lost, on average, more than 10% of their weight and (remember this for later) their total cholesterol dropped by an average 10.5 mg/dL (0.27 mmol/L).

Twenty patients chose to continue the diet after the first six months, and after 12 months, their mean weight loss was 10.9% and their total cholesterol had decreased by 14.1 mg/dL (0.37 mmol/L).

Dr William S. Yancy, M.D. admitted that:

> 'This study of overweight individuals showed that a low carbohydrate, high-protein/fat diet can lead to significant weight loss at one year of treatment.'

All these recommendations and evidence could have saved a great deal of grief, trauma and ill-health if two other doctors had been listened to in 1994. Writing in the *British Medical Journal*, Professor Susan Wooley and Dr David Garner highlighted the role of the professional in people's increasing weight.[8]

They recognised that for fat people weight loss was the one thing they wanted 'above all else'. They pointed out that blaming the overweight for their problem and telling them they were eating too much and must cut down, was simply not good enough. The profession must recognise, they said, that an overweight person's failure to lose weight was not their fault, but a failure 'of the methods of treatment that are used'. In other words, it was the dieticians' advice and treatment offered that were wrong. Wooley and Garner went on to say that health professionals should admit that their treatments are 'ineffective' as that would be the only way to begin 'to undo a century of recruiting fat people for failure'. They concluded: 'Researchers who think they have invented a better mousetrap should test it in controlled research before setting out their bait for the entire population.'

But of course there is a 'better mousetrap'. William Banting wrote of it nearly a century and a half ago. Now we need to know how and why it works.

References

1.   Densmore H. *How to Reduce Fat.* H Densmore, Los Angeles, 1895.
2.   Benedict FG, Milner. *US Dept Agr Office Exp Sta Bull* 1907; 175: 225.
3.   Stefansson V. *The Fat of The Land.* Macmillan, New York, 1956; and Change your diet: eat like an Eskimo. *Daily Mail* 8 June 1999; 42.
4.   Lyon DM, Dunlop DM. The treatment of obesity: a comparison of the effects of diet and of thyroid extract. *Quart J Med* 1932; 1: 331.
5.   Donaldson BF. *Strong Medicine.* Cassell, London, 1962.
6.   Kekwick A, Pawan GLS. Caloric intake in relation to body-weight changes in the obese. *Lancet* 1956; ii: 155.
7.   Yancy WS. New research examines effectiveness and weight loss maintenance of the low carbohydrate diet. *NAASO 2000 – Annual Scientific Meeting*, Long Beach, California, 30 October 2000.
8.   Wooley SC, Garner DM. Dietary treatments for obesity are ineffective. *BMJ* 1994; 309: 655.

Chapter Nine

It's in our genes

The mountain sheep are sweeter,
But the valley sheep are fatter;
We therefore deemed it meeter
To carry off the latter.

Thomas Love Peacock

Introduction

'I hear', said one diner to his companion, 'that "you are what you eat".' 'In that case' replied his friend, 'we'd better order something rich'.

'You are what you eat.' Dr Magnus Pike coined the expression in his book, *Food for all the Family*, in 1980. We now hear the expression frequently. It may, or may not, be true of what we eat today but it is certainly true that we are what our ancestors ate. It is that which explains why Banting's diet works. But why? The answer lies in the way Nature has designed us. To be healthy, we need to eat a diet that is natural to us as a species. What we need to determine, therefore, is what that diet is.

Consider this: how many wild animals, in their natural environment require instruction or frequent bulletins from a Department of Health to guide them in their choice of food? The answer, of course, is none. The grazing animals seek and eat plant food; the carnivorous animals hunt and devour the plant eaters. Nature is as simple as that. Wild animals are perfect examples of optimum nutrition resulting from their respective correctly balanced diets. That applies equally to humans. Have you ever heard of a primitive tribesman consulting a calorie chart before deciding what and how much he should eat? They, too, eat what comes naturally to them, in the quantities they want and at the times they want.

We 'civilised' people forget that we, too, were also in this situation for millions of years before we began to acquire the 'assets' of civilization. It is certain that Nature gave us a similar innate wisdom to choose foods best suited for us. So long as they remained nutritionally ignorant and uninformed our ancestors did a pretty creditable job of selecting their diet. If they hadn't, we wouldn't be here today.

Many claims are set forth stating what the 'natural' diet of humans is or should be. They vary widely from carnivore to vegetarian, fruitarian, even breatharian. (Breatharians believe it is possible to live without eating anything at all – yes, honestly, they really do exist.) To decide which is correct we must look at human diets from the earliest times to the present day, and at cross-cultural dietary comparisons of primitive and modern societies. It is also useful to consider the diets of mankind's nearest relatives, the primates.

Primates

Apart from humans, there are 192 other species of primate.[1] Many believe that we are the only one that is carnivorous; that all of them except us are herbivorous. Some with this belief suggest that we too are really a vegetarian species, but several studies have revealed that all the other primates also eat small animals.[2]

The National Zoo in Washington attempted to breed the Amazon Golden Marmoset monkey in captivity, but failed until animal protein was added to its diet.[3] It had been assumed – wrongly – that marmosets were completely herbivorous, but we now know that they must have some animal protein in order to be fertile. With the addition of animal protein, they reproduce rapidly in captivity.

Until Jane Goodall published her research in the 1960s,[4] it was assumed that chimpanzees ate only plant foods, but Goodall discovered that they kill and eat monkeys, baby baboons, and other small animals. Dian Fossey and Richard Perry also showed that gibbons, orang-utans, and baboons kill and eat small animals regularly.[5] And the most primitive primate of all, the tree shrew, is entirely carnivorous. Studies such as these have led to the reclassification of primates from herbivore to omnivore.

Homo carnivorous

So, if every other primate eats meat, why not us? There is no reason at all. Indeed the evidence is overwhelming that we took meat eating to the extreme, by eating little or nothing else for most of our existence, and we know that many human cultures still do today.

The archaeological and climate records tell us clearly what prehistoric Man ate. It was a diet largely of meat and fat, supplemented at certain times of the year with berries and leaves. It could not have been otherwise for, over at least the last two and a half million years, our ancestors lived, evolved and adapted during a series of Ice Ages. The last Ice Age began to end a mere 9000 years ago, but it didn't end everywhere at the same time. As the Earth warmed up, the ice cleared from the equatorial regions towards the poles over a period of five or six thousand years. It was only after this that agriculture even started to be practised.

The further our ancestors lived from the equator, the later came the domestication of grains. Modern man consumes just eight major cereal grains: wheat, rye, barley, oats, maize (corn), rice, sorghum, and millet.[6]

All of these grains were derived from wild grasses whose original ranges were quite localised. Wheat and barley began to be cultivated only about 9,000 years ago in the Fertile Crescent of northeast Africa and the Near East; rice and maize were domesticated approximately 7,000 years ago in southeast Asia and Central and South America respectively; millet and sorghum were first cultivated in Africa some 5,000–6,000 years ago; rye was domesticated around 5,000 years ago in southwest Asia; and oats were domesticated only about 3,000 years ago in Europe. Today, the major grain in Britain is wheat. But, although wheat was probably the first edible grass seed to be cultivated, it simply would not have been available in Britain until several thousand years later. We must also remember that the seeds of the wild grasses were much smaller than the domesticated versions of today. This would have made them extremely difficult to harvest. These seeds would also have required substantial amounts of energy to gather and process. All these constraints suggest that cereals would only have been eaten under conditions of prolonged dietary shortages. It is extremely likely, therefore, that our ancestors would never have consumed grass seeds when and where large mammals abounded.

The significance of this is that, if you are like me – a blond-haired, blue-eyed individual – whose long-term ancestry is in northern Europe, your genes, which are essentially the same as those of your early ancestors and control every function of your body, were developed during a long period of weather patterns that are not unlike those of present day Greenland. Even if your ancestry is in southern Europe, your genes will be very much the same.

Therein lies the problem, for your genes are concerned only with the foods that they have been programmed over millions of years to recognise as 'food'. They care nothing for what we place in our mouths today; they simply won't recognise many of them as 'food'.

If they are fed properly these genes will do their job of keeping us healthy, but give these genes nutrients that are unfamiliar or in the wrong ratios, and they malfunction.

According to Dr S. Boyd Eaton, one of the foremost authorities on Palaeolithic (prehistoric) diets, late 20th/early 21st century diets are quite unlike anything our genetic makeup has prepared us for. Eaton makes the point that 99% of our genetic heritage dates from before our biological ancestors evolved into modern *Homo sapiens* about 40,000 years ago, and that 99.99% of our genes were formed before the development of agriculture. The less we eat like our ancestors, the more susceptible we will be to coronary heart disease, cancer, diabetes, and many other 'diseases of civilisation'.[7]

As we have seen, studies show that eating an unrestricted diet, composed mainly of proteins and fats, helps in the battle of the bulge; that cutting calories, and, particularly, cutting fats, does not. But fats contain the most energy, so how can this be so? The answer lies in the way our bodies have evolved to deal with the different foods.

Our natural diet

Books written by nutritionists and dieticians today tend to be contradictory, often reflecting current fads. As they cannot all be right, how are we to determine what is our natural diet?

The answer lies in our past, but not the immediate past; the way we live now is based on advanced agriculture and the domestication of plants and animals, recent innovations to which we cannot yet have become adapted. To determine what foods are likely to make up a natural diet for mankind as a species, we must look further back, at our evolutionary history. For the food we are genetically programmed to eat is determined by what has been coded in our genes over millions of years.

We can trace human evolution from remains and artefacts of early hominids found in Africa and other parts of the world dated as long as four million years ago; we have fossilised bone records of both our hominid ancestors and of animals; we have stone tools and implements that must have been used for killing and cutting flesh or for grinding plants; we even have hominid faeces. These findings have led to a great deal of speculation about our diet. Are we a carnivorous, omnivorous or a herbivorous species?

We call our ancestors and the various modem primitive tribes 'hunter-gatherers'. In the world today, some tribes live exclusively on meat and fish; others live on fruit, nuts and roots, although meat is also highly prized; still more live without eating anything derived from animal sources. It is obvious, therefore, that as a species we can survive on a wide variety of foods. Which, if any, is the diet that we have evolved to eat?

In our hunt for an answer, the first evidence to consider lies in the fossil sites of Africa, widely accepted as our birthplace. Here, where hominid remains are found, so also are animal bones – sometimes in their thousands.[7] If those hominids were not meat-eaters, why is that? Second, although many modern hunting tribes do eat plants, they have fire. There were very few plant foods with sufficient calorific value that our prehistoric ancestors could have digested without fire. There were fruits, of course, but there is not one prehistoric site in all Africa that indicates forests extensive enough to have supplied sufficient fruit to meet the needs of its inhabitants. Furthermore, there is agreement that our ancestors did not dwell in forests at all but on the savannah, where there were vast plains of grass. However, grass is of no value whatsoever to the human digestive system. Even to live off the fleshier leaves would require the much more highly specialised digestive systems found in some other primates.

The walls of all plant cells are made of cellulose, a form of dietary fibre which is indigestible. There is no enzyme in the human digestive system that will break it down, neither do we have the bacteria and nutrient-absorbing colons of other primates. With no means of breaking down the plant cell walls, the nutrients those cells contain cannot be digested. Passing unaffected straight through the gut, they would be ejected as waste.

Neither is it likely that the seeds of the savannah grasses could have supplied early humans with the energy they required. Seeds are naturally indigestible, designed to pass through an animal's body, to be defaecated and take root elsewhere. There are two means whereby seeds can be made digestible: cooking and grinding. Seeds could have been pounded to break down the plant cell walls, but no archaeologist has ever found a Stone Age tool suited to this task.

If seeds had been ground down by chewing, fossilised teeth would show a great deal more wear than they do; in addition, a very large proportion of the seeds would have escaped and, passing through the body undigested, ended up in the faeces. Fossilised hominid faeces, known as coprolites, have been studied in detail and almost none contain any plant material.

Homo erectus began to appreciate the value of fire around 350,000 years ago. If our ancestors had started cooking grains then, we could have evolved and adapted to them by now. But, to process grains and other seeds, you need either to crush them and make the flour into a paste, or a container of some sort to cook them in. The absence of suitable tools makes the former unlikely, and the latter can be discounted because the oldest known pot is just 6800 years old. In evolutionary terms, that was yesterday.

Cooking also requires a controlled fire. Although hearths have been discovered that are 100,000 years old, these are very rare. European Neanderthal coprolites dating from around 50,000 years ago, before fire was used, contain no plant material.[9] It was not until the Cro-Magnon colonisation of Europe, some 35,000 years ago, that hearths became universal. Even then the evidence suggests that they were not used for cooking plants but merely for warmth. At the time, Europe was in the grip of a succession of ice ages. For some 70,000 years there were long, cold winters and short, cool summers. Cro-Magnon man and his Eurasian ancestors cannot have been plant eaters then – for most of the year there weren't any plants! They ate meat or died, and they ate that meat raw.

It's difficult to do now, but if you get the opportunity to tour the sites of Palaeolithic caves in Spain and southern France, including those of Les Eyzies, Lascaux and Trois-Fréres, you will see depicted wild horses, bison, aurochs, shaggy ponies and deer, all magnificently and realistically portrayed. These cave paintings are thought to have been done in the Palaeolithic period between 30,000 and 13,000 years ago. This was the coldest part of the last great Ice Age. Surely these were all game animals? Our Cro-Magnon ancestors must have depended on animals like these for their food and, given the climatic conditions that prevailed in Europe at the time, their diet must have consisted almost entirely of meat and meat fat. The fact that these animals are depicted in hunting scenes proves that they were the main food of these ice-age nomads, and played a vital role in these people's lives. There are no pictures at all of any plants, vegetables, fruits or nuts.

The evidence that we could not be a vegetarian species was already overwhelming and in 1972 the publication of two independent investigations confirmed this.[10] They concerned fats.

About half our brain and nervous system is composed of complicated, long-chain, fatty acid molecules. These are also used in the walls of our blood vessels. Without them we cannot develop normally. These fatty acids do not occur in plants, although fatty acids in a simpler form do. This is where the plant-eating herbivores come in. Over the year, herbivores convert the simple fatty acids found in grasses and seeds into intermediate, more complicated forms. By eating the herbivores we can convert the herbivores' store of the less complex fatty acids into the ones we need.

Our brain is considerably larger than that of any ape. Looking back at the fossil records from early hominids to modern man, we see a remarkable increase in brain size. This expansion simply could not have happened without large quantities of the right kinds of fatty acids.[11] It would never have occurred if our ancestors had not eaten meat. Human breast milk contains the fatty acids needed for large brain development; cow's milk does not. It is no coincidence that, in relative terms, our brain is some 50 times the size of a cow's.

Carbs signal us to store fat

It is abundantly clear that early man hunted and ate meat primarily but, if meat were in short supply, he would eat almost anything – so long as it did not require cooking. This still precluded some of the roots and most of the seeds we eat today.

We also have a sense of taste for sweet things, a tendency we are unlikely to have developed if it served no function; thus it is possible that fruit formed part of our ancestors' diet. As fruit contains no essential nutrients that cannot be better obtained from meat sources, perhaps it had another function: a signal to store fat.

During winter, when food is scarce, many animals – bears, dormice and others – stock up with food, store it as fat in their bodies, and hibernate. Many other species don't hibernate, but given the seasonal unavailability of most food sources in the world, their bodies also need some ability to store energy for when food is scarce. These species are also programmed to store fat – and significantly these include us. We all have a mechanism that determines when to store fat and when to use that stored fat. By varying our body's overall metabolic rate, energy is conserved to store fat when the signal is given *regardless of calorie intake levels.*

The signal to store fat in Man and other carnivorous animals is the presence of the largely carbohydrate vegetable foods available in spring and summer. (Herbivores also store fat this way against winter when the carbohydrate levels in their food falls dramatically.) Plant foods are much easier to get. They wait to be picked and don't run away. It is likely, therefore, that in the short, cool summers, our ancestors would have stocked up on carb-rich foods before the relatively more difficult period of winter set in. The plant foods, stored as fat, would have given us a large energy store for such times.

Periods of food shortage and starvation – and low-calorie dieting falls into this category – heighten the signal to retain fat against further hard times to come while, at the same time, signalling the body's energy-using mechanisms to slow down the body's metabolism to save energy.

Before agriculture, Eurasian Man's access to vegetable foods was restricted for much of the year as the winter cold killed most vegetation. Even in more temperate zones the dry season had a similar effect. Before the advent of the grains, beans, potatoes, dairy products and refined sugars we eat today, all that was available for Man to eat in winter was the meat and fat of animals that had stored fat against the winter. Eating these signalled the body that it was time to raise its metabolic rate. This higher metabolic rate kept us warm and allowed us to move faster, thus making game easier to catch.

Those are the conditions in which our genetic make-up evolved, but the world we live in today is vastly different. We live now in a permanent supermarket summer and can eat as much as we want of what we want. It is unfortunate that we seem to want carbohydrates as they signal our bodies to store fat. It is no wonder civilised Man is so overweight by hunter-gatherer standards. Don't forget that this is our own history. We have inherited and still carry the same genes; and our bodies are adapted to the same diet our ancestors ate during that last Ice Age.

What we should be doing, then, is eating fewer carbohydrate-rich foods, convince our bodies that winter has arrived, and watch it do what it has evolved and is genetically programmed to do.

Agriculture and the first diet revolution

It was not until the last Ice Age came to an end about 9000 years ago and the ice receded, that there was sufficient surplus food for some to be stored, and some previously nomadic tribes were able to develop stable settlements. The cultivation of wild seeds began. From these are derived the cereals we know today, such as wheat, barley, maize, and rice. These had the advantage that they could be stored for long periods against winter famines. Cooking solved the problem of their indigestibility.

This development caused a dramatic change in Man's lifestyle. The capacity to store controlled quantities of higher-energy starches meant that population numbers could grow. As numbers grew, it became more difficult to maintain food supplies through hunting alone. Thus our ancestors' basic diet changed from a high protein/fat diet to one containing more starchy carbohydrates.

There is no evidence of nutritional diseases before the invention of agriculture, but post-agriculture there is. Cereals that became the modern staples, together with root crops which began to be cultivated, are all relatively deficient in protein, vitamins and several minerals, notably iron and calcium. Additionally, all cereals contain a substance called phytate that binds with some minerals and other nutrients and reduces the ability of the body to absorb them. As a consequence, the coming of agriculture gave rise to nutritional diseases such as rickets, pellagra, dental caries, beriberi, obesity, allergies and cancers: the so-called 'diseases of civilisation'.

Even after this dramatic change, the preference for meat, and fat meat in particular, continued. This is evidenced in written records over the last several thousand years. We'll start with the Bible. While I do not regard the Bible as a scientific work, it does tell us what the peoples of the Middle East believed and what they liked to eat.

The first indication that fat was prized in the Middle East comes in Genesis, with the story of Cain and Abel and the account of the first recorded offering to Jehovah.

> 'And Abel was a keeper of sheep, but Cain was a tiller of the ground.
> 'And in process of time it came to pass, that Cain brought of the fruit of the ground an offering unto the Lord.
> 'And Abel, he also brought of the firstlings of his flock and of the fat thereof. And the Lord had respect unto Abel and to his offering.
> 'But unto Cain and to his offering he had not respect.'

This story tells us two things: first, it represents the preferences of Jehovah and the preferences of the Hebrew people themselves when they were living in the region of Babylonia and Egypt 3000 or 4000 years ago – meat and fat was regarded as far superior to vegetables; second, the inclusion of the words 'and of the fat thereof' means that Abel didn't only bring fat meat but also fat separately as an added, superior, gift.

Further on in *Genesis* 45:17–18 we learn by inference that both Jews and Egyptians thought well of a high-fat diet: 'And Pharaoh said unto Joseph . . . "Take your father and your households, and come unto me; and I will give you the good of the land of Egypt, and ye shall eat the fat of the land".' And in *Isaiah* 25:6: 'And in this mountain shall the Lord of hosts make unto all people a feast of fat things . . . of fat things full of marrow.'

From other passages of the Old Testament we know that Jews were thinking of fat mutton, or of mutton fat, when they spoke of 'the fat of the land'. The Bible tells us that mutton fat was considered the most delicious portion of any meat, and the tail and adjacent part the most exquisite morsel in the whole body. Biblical sheep were the fat-tailed variety, still found in Syria and Palestine today.

The New Testament also has similar references, and we learn that beef fat was also held in high esteem: when the prodigal son returned home, his father didn't welcome him with an ordinary calf, he 'slew a fatted calf'.

Across the Mediterranean from the Holy lands, the Greeks also liked their meat fat and believed that their heroes preferred it so. You won't find a kind word about lean meat in the poems of Homer, but they are larded with praise of fat meats. Take the case of Agamemnon, who 'slew a fat bull of five years to most mighty Kronion' (*The Iliad*, Book II). And in Book IX, 'Patroklos . . . cast down a great fleshing block in the firelight, and laid thereon a sheep's back, and a fat goat's, and a great hog's chine rich with fat.'

The same is true of the religious and profane classics of northern European peoples, preserved in the Scandinavian Eddas and sagas. One Icelandic poem reads 'There (in paradise) the feast will be set with clear wine, fat and marrow'. That's bone marrow, by the way, not the vegetable kind.

The Norwegian explorer and scientist, Dr Carl Lumholtz (1851–1922), reported that the same was true in the southern hemisphere. When he was with the tropical forest-dwelling Aborigines of northern Australia, Lumholtz tells how they lived mainly on animal food, and never ate anything from a plant source if flesh foods were available. Lumholtz also noted that the Aborigines ate their meals in the same way that children will: they ate the best things first – that was always meat; and the fatter the meat the better.

Sir Hubert Wilkins (1888–1958), Australia's most famous explorer, conducted a two-year expedition for the British Museum in northern Australia.[12] Wilkins confirmed Lumholtz's findings, and added certain observations along the same line.

The Aborigines were cannibals, and the missionaries were having some difficulty breaking them of this habit. Wilkins noted that when a thin man died, all that was needed was a stern word from the missionaries, but when a fat man was buried, the missionaries had to stand watch over the grave. Even after some months the Aborigines would dig up fat corpses. They either liked their cadavers high, or did not mind them being that way if they were fat enough.

Of course, it is no secret that peoples further north, the Lapps and Saami of northern Scandinavia, the peoples of Siberia, the Inuit of Greenland and the Canadian north live entirely on animals and fish even today, as do many peoples in the tropics: the Maasai, Samburu, Watusi, Marsh Arabs, Berbers, and many others.

When Christianity spread northward, the Biblical phrase 'to live on the fat of the land' was readily understood across Europe. In English speech fat food was called 'rich' food. This was the highest praise.

The fattest meat was regarded as the best in most religions and in all countries. Indeed ancient peoples around the world seem to praise fat meat and sweet wine – and nothing else. And that continued right up to modern times. Medical missionary, G.W. Harley MD PhD, who founded the Ganta Mission in Liberia in the 1920s wrote[13]:

> 'Meat-hunger is striking and constant among the tribes I have contacted. While meat of any kind is in great demand, it is interesting to note that the following are the favorite cuts:'

Harley then cites a long list of animals in order of preference. They are from the fattest to the leanest. For example, he starts with:

1. Brisket of beef with the fat and cartilages.
2. The skin and subcutaneous fat of a wart hog. Pig skin is never saved for rawhide and leather. It is too valuable as food, and is eaten after singeing off the hair, and prolonged boiling. Plump cow skin is similarly eaten. A lean cow skin will be saved for rawhide and leather.

And so on. Later he states:

> 'We had fresh vegetables every day from our own garden, whatever the season; but it was for meat and butter that we often felt hungry.
>
> 'On returning to the United States, I arrived during a heatwave, and hungrily devoured fat pork and country sausages in Washington, D.C. Was disappointed when I could not get sausages with pancakes in Boston because it was "too hot for sausages."
>
> 'Men who work in hot places (stokers) do not avoid meat and fats, rather the opposite.'

In 19th century Britain, the most esteemed part of the diet was the fat. Describing good meat, Mrs Beeton says, 'Beef of the best quality is of a deep red colour; and when the animal has approached maturity, and has been well fed, the lean is intermixed with fat, giving it the mottled appearance which is so much esteemed'.[14] If meat didn't have much fat, that was a sign of poor quality.

The industrial revolution and the second diet revolution

About 200 years ago the industrial revolution heralded a second dietary revolution which had two powerful but opposite effects on our health. Industrialised countries like Britain with their increased wealth no longer had to rely on home-produced, seasonally dependent foods; they could import what they wanted. They could look forward to going through life without ever being hungry. However, there were adverse effects.

Many of the imported foods were unnatural to those eating them. New fruits tasted nice and, as a consequence, people changed from eating what they needed to eating what they liked. Unaided by previous experience, the human autonomic nervous system has never learned when to stop.

As time went by, science made possible the production of synthetic foods that had the appearance, texture and taste of the real thing, but with few of the proteins and vitamins. Sugar became easy and cheap to produce, leading to a 30-fold increase in its consumption. The industrial revolution, therefore, was something of a double-edged sword: on the one hand it gave people a wider range of food than had ever before been possible, on the other, diabetes, peptic ulcers, heart disease and a whole host of other medical conditions were added to the list of new diseases. In the late 20th century, the pace at which our diet became increasingly unnatural quickened – and so did the numbers of people getting fat or diabetic.

Unnatural processing

Many packaged foods today contain substances with such names as 'modified starch' or 'maltodextrin'. These, too, are highly concentrated carbohydrates, in this case cereal starch. These sugars and starches are added to make foods cheaper or more attractive, or to create larger profits for the manufacturers, but they have detrimental effects on large sections of the population. Our bodies' natural nutrient-requirement signal, the appetite, has not evolved to cope with such unnatural foods. It knows when to stop us eating meat, but not when to stop us eating chocolate bars and cakes. It is also much easier to eat modern white bread than the stodgy, pre-industrial revolution bread.

The concentration of carbohydrate allowed a dramatic and rapid increase in its consumption. Annual sugar consumption in Britain in the middle of the 18th century was less than 2 kg (4 lb) per person; today it is more than 60 kg (130 lb). The same is true of cereals.

Food and disease

A study by Drs W.S. McClellan and E.F. Du Bois found that the Eskimos in Baffin Island and Greenland, who lived on a diet composed almost entirely of meat and fish and ate no starchy or sugary foods, were almost completely free from all disease.[15] This was not the case with the Labrador Eskimos. They had been 'civilised' and lived on preserved foods, dried potatoes, flour, canned foods and cereals. Among them the diseases of 'civilisation' were rife.

A comparison between the Maasai tribes of East Africa, who live alongside the Kikuyu, shows a similar pattern.[16] The Maasai, when wholly carnivorous, eating only the meat, blood and milk of their cattle, were tall, healthy, long-lived and slim. The Kikuyu, when wholly vegetarian, were stunted, diseased, short-lived and pot-bellied. During the middle of the 20th century the Kikuyu started to eat meat – and their health improved. Since 1960 the Maasai diet has also changed, but in the opposite direction. They are now eating less blood and milk, replacing them with maize and beans. Their health has deteriorated.[17]

Many explorers noted that the people they called 'savages' had excellent teeth and that civilised men had terrible teeth. It seemed to Dr Weston A. Price, a dentist, that we had been extraordinarily stupid in concentrating on finding out why our teeth are so poor, without ever bothering to learn why 'savage' teeth were so good. He travelled the world in a ten-year fact-finding mission.[18] What he found was that every tribe that had had contact with Western civilisation not only had worse teeth than those that hadn't, they all had worse health overall. There were no exceptions. A 'civilised', carbohydrate-based diet is inherently unhealthy.

The bottom line

What we are advised to eat today is far removed from the diet which we are genetically programmed to eat. We are designed to eat a high-fat diet – but we are told to eat a low-fat diet; we are designed to eat a low-carb diet, yet are told to eat a high-carb diet. Dieticians also tell us to eat foods that are quite unnatural to us: bread, breakfast cereals and pasta. High in refined carbohydrates, these are the sources of the carbohydrates in our diets which cause us harm and make us fat. Things like sugar, sticky sweets, soft drinks, pasta, cakes and white bread are the main culprits and we are rightly told to avoid these. However, others that can be harmful in sufficient quantity include fresh fruits, dried fruits such as raisins, and the starchier cereal grains and root vegetables. Cooked, refined carbohydrate foods are worse than raw. Green vegetables, which are generally low in carbohydrates, cooked or uncooked, present few problems.

There is no evidence that any foods from animal sources are fattening or in any other way harmful, and that includes their fats. We may need some carbohydrate in our diet – the evidence for this is unconvincing – but even if we do, we certainly do not need it in large quantities, and not in the form in which most carbohydrate is ingested today.

The best place to get the carbohydrate part of your diet is the greengrocer's shop – not at the baker's or the grocer's – and certainly not at the confectioner's.

References

1. Morris D. *The Naked Ape*. McGraw Hill, New York, 1967, p.9.
2. a. Abrams HL Jr. The relevance of Paleolithic diet in determining contemporary nutritional needs. *J Applied Nutr* 1979; 31: 43–59;

b. Vegetarianism: an anthropological/nutritional evaluation. *J Appl Nutr* 1980; 32: 53–87;

c. Chapman CA, Chapman LJ. Dietary variability in primate populations. *Primates* 1990; 31: 121–128.

3. Campbell S. Noah's Ark in tomorrow's zoo: animals are a-comin', two-by-two. *Smithsonian* 1978; 8: 42–50.

4. a. Goodall J. *Miss Goodall and the Wild Chimpanzees.* A documentary film of Jane Goodall's studies of wild chimpanzees in their natural habitat in a rain forest in Tanzania, Africa, National Geographic, 1966;

b. Van Lawick-Goodall J. *In the Shadow of Man.* Houghton Mifflin, New York, 1971, p.297.

5. a. *Search For the Great Apes.* A documentary film on the ethological research on gorillas by Dian Fossey and the ethological research of orang-utans by Birute Galdikas-Brindamour, National Geographic, 1975;

b. Perry R. *Life in Forest and Jungle.*Taplinger Publishing, New York, 1976, pp.165–185.

6. Harlan JR. *Crops and man.* American Society of Agronomy Inc, Madison, Wisconsin USA, 1992.

7. Eaton SB, Eaton SB III, Konner MJ, et al. An evolutionary perspective enhances understanding of human nutritional requirements. *J Nutr* 1996; 126: 1732–1740.

8. Hawkes JG. The hunting hypothesis. In: Ardrey R, ed. *The Hunting Hypothesis.* Collins, London, 1976.

9. Bryant VM, Williams-Dean G. The coprolites of Man. *Sci Am* January 1975.

10. Crawford M, Crawford S. *The Food We Eat Today.* Spearman, London, 1972; Leopold AC, Ardrey R. Toxic substances in plants and food habits of early Man. *Science* 1972; 176(34): 512–524.

11. Crawford MA, Cunnane SC, Harbige LS. A new theory of evolution: quantum theory. In: Sinclair A, Gibson R, eds. *Essential Fatty Acids and Eicosanoids.* American Oil Chemists Society, Champlaign, Ill, 1992, pp.87–95.

12. Wilkins H. *Undiscovered Australia.* Putman, London, 1928.

13. Harley GW, quoted in Stefansson V. *The Fat of the Land.* Macmillan, New York, 1957, pp.130–132.

14. Beeton I. *Mrs Beeton's Book of Household Management.*Ward Lock, London. 1869.

15. McClellan WS, Du Bois EF. Prolonged meat diets with a study of kidney function and ketosis. *J Biol Chem* 1930; 87: 651.

16. Orr JB, Gilks JL. *Studies of Nutrition: The Physique and Health of Two African Tribes.* HMSO, London, 1931.

17. McCormick J, Elmore-Meegan M. Maasai diet. *Lancet* 1992; 340: 1042.

18. Price WA. *Nutrition and Physical Degeneration: A Comparison of Primitive and Modern Diets and Their Effects.* Paul B. Hoeber, New York, 1939.

Chapter Ten

The Metabolic Syndrome

There is increasing evidence to indicate that the type of diet recommended in the USDA's food pyramid is discordant with the type of diet humans evolved with over eons of evolutionary experience.

Professor Loren Cordain

The importance of blood sugar levels

We now know that the cause of obesity and many other illnesses in the West is too high an intake of sugar and other sweet or starchy foods. When the body's energy and blood sugar levels are low, it signals the need to eat via the feeling of hunger. Then, if we are sensible, we eat a meal composed of food items which are natural to us and which are digested and absorbed at different rates. This way energy is released continuously over the period to the next meal. When eaten, carbohydrates are digested and absorbed quickly, within minutes; proteins are digested more slowly and fats are digested last. If we eat the three in the correct proportions, there will be no problems. If the meal is too high in carbohydrates, however, blood sugar levels rise rapidly. This blood sugar is metered in the brain by the hypothalamus. When blood sugar levels get too high, the hypothalamus stimulates the pancreas to produce insulin. The insulin converts the excess glucose for storage and reduces the level in the blood, but there is a time lag. By the time the pancreas finds that the blood sugar level has dropped sufficiently, it has produced more than enough insulin to reduce those high blood sugar levels. Blood sugar is driven down to a low level, making us feel hungry again. The effect is known as 'reactive hypoglycaemia'. So we eat more – and tend to snack on sweets! It is a vicious circle. We feel hungry even though we eat more, and become run down and depressed. In the mean time the excesses have been converted to fat for storage and we have gained weight.

The answer is to eat less carbohydrate so that your blood sugar level does not fluctuate so violently, and eat *more* fat. Because it takes a long time to digest, fat not only prevents those violent fluctuations in blood sugar levels, it gives a feeling of satiety, which stops that feeling of hunger.

As you will have realised, it is not just people wanting to lose weight who should beware of overeating carbohydrates. Apart from making us overweight, a number of other disorders are caused or exacerbated by too high an intake of sugars and starches – environmental diseases from diabetes and coronary heart disease to decayed teeth and fatigue. It even makes us more susceptible to bacterial attack and viral diseases such as the common cold. These will be discussed later in this book.

The cholesterol theory has it that blocked arteries prevent oxygen from reaching the heart muscle, but the majority of people who die of coronary heart disease do *not have blocked coronary arteries*. The blocked artery hypothesis cannot account for this. The oxygen used in muscles to oxidise glucose is only half the equation. Low utilisation of glucose by the heart muscle may be due not to lack of oxygen but to low blood glucose levels, and low blood glucose levels are caused by a *high*-carbohydrate diet.

Triglycerides are neutral fats found at high levels in many heart disease cases. Eating too much fat is usually blamed, but blood triglyceride levels have been shown to be proportional not to fat intake but to carbohydrate intake. Platelets, the agents which make blood clot when we are cut, also tend to clump together on a diet high in sugars and refined starches. It has been shown that a diet that contains a large proportion of carbohydrate can cause blood clots and reduce the flow of blood to the extremities. If such a clot reaches the heart, it can cause a blockage in a coronary artery. The best way to reduce the risk of a blood clot and, thus, a heart attack is, again, to reduce your carbohydrate intake.

Don't forget that carbs are addictive. One reason is because, in raising blood glucose, they give you an energy lift. But they also increase a brain chemical called serotonin. Serotonin plays a crucial role in controlling states of consciousness and mood by promoting sleepiness and also relaxation.

What has confused researchers is that serotonin is a 'feel good' chemical. Obese, premenstrual and depressed people usually report a temporary improvement in mood and depression after a high-carb meal. Researchers are still not sure whether this is because serotonin levels do not increase under these conditions or if serotonin is released, but some factor in these three conditions causes the serotonin to be mood elevating. It is these mood-enhancing properties that make carbs addictive.

What is insulin resistance?

Insulin is a hormone made in the beta cells of the pancreas. It helps the body utilise glucose (blood sugar) by binding with receptors on cells like a key would fit into a lock. This stimulates glucose uptake from the blood into body tissues. Once the insulin key has unlocked the door, the glucose can pass from the blood into the cell. Inside the cell, glucose is either used for energy or stored for future use in the form of glycogen in liver or muscle cells, or as fat in the body's fat cells (*adipocytes*). Its ability to do this varies greatly among individuals.

Most industrialised countries have seen a dramatic increase in the numbers of cases of obesity over the last 20 years. In the United States for example, the increase in obesity has reached epidemic proportions, and a 33% increase in diagnosed diabetes was reported between 1990 and 1998. And it's going to get worse.[1]

The reason is that the type of diet we are told to eat, and which is enshrined in the sorts of processed foods on supermarket shelves, increases the levels of glucose in our blood. This is harmful: it clogs our arteries and causes all the complications associated with obesity. Our bodies recognise this. They tell the pancreas to increase its production of insulin, a hormone that takes glucose out of the blood and stores it in muscle and fat cells, and so we put weight on. When insulin is excessive, the cells start reducing the activity of body cells' receptors. The cells then refuse to take so much glucose – they resist the action of the insulin. This is insulin resistance. If diabetics eat even more carbohydrates, as they are told to do by their doctors, this makes the situation even worse.

There is also a second, consequent effect: our beta cells can only make and secrete so much insulin, and our body cells can only store so much excess energy. Eventually the beta cells reach the point where they throw in the towel, say, 'blow this, I've had enough' and they pack up. At this stage, the non-insulin dependent diabetic becomes insulin dependent.

Sequence of events

In lay terms what happens is this: it's really a balancing act with a carb-based diet that doesn't happen with a high-fat diet. You may be told that being overweight causes insulin resistance. But this really is a true 'chicken and egg' situation because increases in body weight and insulin resistance actually occur at the same time. In simple lay terms the sequence of events is this:

- You eat carbs and your body uses the resultant glucose up. No problem.
- Then you start to eat a little more – '5 portions of fruit', et cetera.
- Now you start to get higher levels of glucose for which the body has no immediate use and these trigger higher levels of insulin to reduce them.
- This starts the process of fat deposition and you start to put on weight.
- So you go on a low-fat, carb-based diet. This means eating more carbs which continue the cycle, increasing levels of glucose and insulin in the blood.
- Eventually, your body cells, both muscle cells and fat cells (adipocytes) get to the point where they really don't want to know. They lose some of their insulin receptors. At this stage you are insulin resistant.
- As the excess glucose now has nowhere to go, this leads to uncontrolled increases in blood glucose and the onset of type-2 diabetes. And, of course, all the conditions associated with diabetes.
- Then you are prescribed drugs to lower glucose levels and, at the same time, told to eat even more carbs.
- Your pancreas finally gives up and you have to take insulin.

There are two ways to avoid this cycle: either you exercise – and that means running a marathon three or four times a week – or you keep your carbohydrate intake to less than 100 g per day. This is either one big potato or 800 ml of the richest ice cream per day. It's your choice!

But back to our story:

In 1976 Drs Kahn and Flier described two syndromes of severe insulin resistance, and research at the time began to focus on the newly described insulin receptor as the cause of insulin resistance.[2] It looked useful, but further studies showed that the insulin receptor was usually *not* the cause of insulin resistance.[3]

Diseases of insulin resistance, particularly diabetes, occur with greater frequency in populations that have recently changed dietary habits from hunter-gatherer to

Western grain-based regimes, compared to those with long histories of such diets. This is why obesity and diabetes are so much more common among Americans of African and Asian origin than among those whose ancestry is European. It has been suggested that insulin resistance in hunter-gatherer populations may be an asset, as it may facilitate consumption of high-animal-based diets – and I am sure that's true. But the down side of this is that when high-carbohydrate, grain-based diets replace traditional hunter-gatherer diets, insulin resistance becomes a liability and promotes type-2 diabetes.[4]

Insulin resistance occurs when the normal amount of insulin secreted by the pancreas is not able to unlock the door to cells and tissues have a diminished ability to respond to the action of insulin. To compensate for this and maintain a normal level of blood glucose, the pancreas secretes more insulin. Insulin-resistant persons, therefore, also have high blood insulin levels (*hyperinsulinaemia*). Many people who are insulin resistant produce large enough quantities of insulin to maintain near normal blood glucose levels, but in some cases (about one-third of the people with insulin resistance), when the body cells resist or do not respond even to high levels of insulin, glucose builds up in the blood resulting in high blood glucose. This is the definition of type-2 diabetes.

Several recent epidemiological studies have measured insulin levels in populations.[5] These have found higher insulin levels in people with high blood pressure and other vascular disease. For this reason, insulin resistance is now also considered a risk factor for heart disease. These studies have added a great deal of confusion to the field because many individuals with insulin resistance do not have diabetes.

People who are insulin resistant typically have an imbalance in their blood fats (lipids); they have an increased level of *triglycerides* which may be associated with the risk of heart attacks; and lower levels of HDL (high density lipoproteins).

Syndrome X

The term 'Syndrome X' we hear about today, was coined by Dr Gerald Reaven, head of the Division of Endocrinology, Gerontology and Metabolism at Stanford University School of Medicine, to describe the collection of symptoms – *hypertriglyceridaemia* (high blood fats), low HDL-cholesterol, *hyperinsulinaemia* (high blood insulin), often *hyperglycaemia* (high blood glucose), and *hypertension* (high blood pressure), elevated uric acid, and small, dense LDL (low density lipoproteins) molecules – that collectively appear to be caused by disturbed insulin metabolism. These symptoms appear in turn to increase the risk of heart disease, type-2 diabetes and many other conditions. Syndrome X may be responsible for a large percentage of the heart and artery disease that occurs throughout the world today. The term Syndrome X is often an expression interchangeable with insulin resistance.

Almost all individuals with type-2 diabetes and many with high blood pressure, cardiovascular disease, and obesity are insulin resistant. These diseases and conditions are predominantly found in countries with an improved economic status such as Britain and the USA, where it is thought that as many as a quarter of the apparently healthy population may be insulin resistant.

When body tissues become resistant to insulin the pancreas is frequently able to maintain normal glucose tolerance by sustaining a relatively high level of insulin in the blood to compensate for the raised glucose levels. The onset of impaired glucose tolerance or type-2 diabetes marks a failure of the pancreas to maintain this state of compensatory high insulin level. This state underlies several of the most common and deadly chronic diseases in western, industrialised nations. Because insulin resistance is now such a common phenomenon, it has been suggested that the various facets of Syndrome X are involved to a substantial degree in the cause and clinical course of the major diseases of Western civilisation.[6]

What are the symptoms of insulin resistance?

There is only one outward physical sign of insulin resistance, namely, the type of obesity known as 'apple shape' obesity. That is excess fat around the waist and upper half of the body. Other than that, a glucose tolerance test during which insulin and blood glucose are measured can help determine if someone is insulin resistant.

Syndrome X or insulin resistance is characterised by:

1. Resistance to insulin-mediated glucose uptake.
2. Fat cells releasing a hormone *resistin* that causes insulin resistance.
3. Glucose intolerance.
4. High blood insulin levels.
5. Increased levels of low density lipoproteins (LDL).
6. Decreased high-density lipoprotein cholesterol (HDL).
7. High blood pressure.
8. Overweight and obesity, particularly around the waist and upper part of the body.

One point that must be made is that, despite what you are told, obesity is a *consequence* of Syndrome X and all its associated conditions; it is *not* a cause of them. This is demonstrated in studies of peoples with different ethnic origins and evolutionary food habits. For example, since the differences in insulin resistance between Pima Indians and Europeans in the USA remain even after matching for obesity, the increased insulin resistance could not be blamed on their obesity.[7]

The mechanism whereby high insulin levels cause weight gain is not entirely understood, but the most important aspect seems the fact that insulin promotes fat storage and causes carbohydrates to be used as energy in preference to fat if meals are mixed.[8] It has also been suggested that high insulin levels may cause obesity by preventing the breakdown of fats for energy,[9] reducing the body-heating effect,[10] and increasing appetite.[11] If you eat carbohydrate-rich meals one after another, therefore, this would promote continued fat accumulation rather than body fat usage, and weight gain would be the outcome.

The importance of insulin resistance is that it is accompanied by a progressive deterioration of the small blood vessels supplying blood to many tissues, including the skeletal muscles that provide most of the body's insulin mediated glucose disposal. These changes in the blood vessels and circulation may cause a decline in muscle blood flow and increase the severity of the metabolic disorder.[12]

Conclusion

Too much glucose and insulin in the bloodstream lies at the root of obesity and all the other diseases associated with the Metabolic Syndrome. Our bodies have a hormonal system designed to protect us from too much sugar in our bloodstream. Insulin does this by promoting the storage of glucose as glycogen or as fat, or by encouraging its use in cells that would not use glucose as their first choice. However, there is a limit to how much these cells can use the constant stream of glucose being forced into them and, in the end, they put up a fight against it. This is insulin resistance.

It is very important that we do not see insulin resistance as the problem *per se*. This approach has led conventional medicine to attempt to suppress the resistance with drugs, but this is a mistaken approach. Insulin resistance is a symptom of the problem, not its cause. The best answer – the healthiest answer – is to take away the need for the cells to put up resistance by giving insulin less of a job to do in the first place. As *all* dietary carbohydrate, whether it is bread, pasta, breakfast cereals, sugar or fruit, and whatever its Glycaemic Index (which we will discuss in the next chapter), initially reaches the blood as glucose, the best way to reduce the need for increased insulin is to reduce dietary carbohydrate.

It is essential that we never lose sight of this fact, for it is a fundamental fact upon which all else depends.

References

1. Mokdad AH, Serdula MK, Dietz WH, et al. The continuing epidemic of obesity in the United States. *JAMA* 2000; 184: 1650–1651.
2. Kahn CR, Flier JS, Bar RS, et al. The syndromes of insulin resistance and acanthosis nigricans: insulin receptor disorders in man. *N Engl J Med* 1976; 294: 739–745.
3. Krook A, O'Rahilly S. Mutant insulin receptors in syndromes of insulin resistance. *Bailliers Clin Endocrinol Metab* 1996; 10: 97–122.
4. Brand-Miller JC, Colagiuri S. The carnivore connection: dietary carbohydrate in the evolution of NIDDM. *Diabetologia* 1994; 37: 1280–1286.
5. Despres JP, Lamarche B, Mauriege P, et al. Hyperinsulinemia as an independent risk factor for ischemic heart disease. *N Engl J Med* 1996; 334: 952–957.
6. Cordain L. Syndrome X: Just the tip of the hyperinsulinemia iceberg. *Medikament* 2001; 6: 46–51.
7. Lillioja S, Degregorio M, Ferraro R, et al. Insulin resistance and insulin secretion in Pima Indians. *Prog Obes Res* 1990: 56; 339–364.
8. Flatt JP. Importance of nutrient balance in body weight regulation. *Diabetes Metab Rev* 1988; 4: 571–581.
9. Arner P. Control of lipolysis and its relevance to development of obesity in man. *Diabetes Metab Rev* 1988; 4: 507–515.
10. Felig P. Insulin is the mediator of feeding-related thermogenesis: insulin resistance and/or deficiency results in a thermic defect which contributes to the pathogenesis of obesity. *Clin Physiol* 1984; 4: 267–273.
11. Jeanerauld B. Neuroendocrine and metabolic basis of type II diabetes as studied in animal models. *Diabetes Metab Rev* 1988; 4: 603–614.
12. Ganrot PO. Insulin resistance syndrome: possible key role of blood flow in resting muscle. *Diabetologia* 1993; 36: 876–879.
13. Brand-Miller JC. Glycemic load and chronic disease. *Nutr Rev* 2003; 61: S49–55.
14. Ludwig DS, Maizoub JA, Al-Zahrani A, et al. High glycaemic index foods, overeating, and obesity. *Pediatrics* 1999; 103: E26–E32.

15. Parilo M, Coulston A, Hollenbyck C. Effect of a low fat diet on carbohydrate metabolism in patients with hypertension. *Hypertension* 1988; 22: 244–248.

16. Liu S, Willett WC, Stampfer MJ, et al. A prospective study of dietary glycemic load, carbohydrate intake, and risk of coronary heart disease in US women. *Am J Clin Nutr* 2000; 71: 1455–1461.

17. Salmeron J, Ascherio A, Rimm EB, et al. Dietary fibre, glycemic load, and risk of NIDDM in men. *Diabetes Care* 1997; 20: 545–550.

18. Elliott SS, Keim NL, Stern JS, et al. Fructose, weight gain, and the insulin resistance syndrome. *Am J Clin Nutr* 2002; 76: 911–922.

Chapter Eleven

Glycaemic truth

In summary, lowering the glycemic load and glycemic index of weight reduction diets does not provide any added benefit to energy restriction in promoting weight loss in obese subjects.

Raatz SK, Torkelson CJ, Redmon JB, et al.[14]

At this stage I want to explain what has become quite a phenomenon: The Glycaemic Index (GI). It needs explanation because, since I wrote *Eat Fat, Get Thin!*, which was one of the first diet books to discuss GI, in 1999, this potentially useful aid has been badly misrepresented and taken over by the discredited, low-fat, 'healthy eating' camp to promote their low-fat cause.

Although it is widely believed that people get overweight because they take in more energy than they use – eat more, exercise less – there is no consistent evidence that this is the cause of the current epidemic. In fact, dietary studies conducted in many developed countries suggest that the average calorie intake for adults, particularly in the form of fats, is now much lower than in previous decades.[1] The reason we are getting fatter is not because we eat too much, but because we eat too much of the wrong foods. These are certainly mostly those with a high-GI, but there is more to it than that.

Here is the truth about GI.

Sugar and starch

All dieters know that sugar, above all else, is fattening. Every diet yet devised counsels, quite rightly, against eating sugar. At the same time, many modern dieticians also tell dieters that they should eat more starchy foods: bread, pasta or potatoes and, of course, 'five portions of fruit and vegetables a day'. However, you need to know that it doesn't matter whether you eat sugar and jam or pasta, bread, breakfast cereals and fruit, your digestion makes no distinction between them. *All* the carbohydrates you eat are destined to be converted and enter your bloodstream as the blood sugar, glucose.

What we tend to eat more and more of today are 'convenience foods' such as prepacked sandwiches and meals and TV dinners, but the manufacturers of these have only one goal: to make a profit in a very competitive market. They can't afford to use expensive ingredients, so backed by 'healthy eating' recommendations to base meals on carbs, these 'foods' are bulked out with refined, concentrated sugars and starches. So that you don't realise just how much of these their product contain, the sugar and starch content is frequently obscured by the manufacturers – sugar contents being variously described as sucrose, fructose, glucose, maltose, dextrose, corn syrup, maltodextrin, modified starch, and so on. There's no shortage of words they can use to disguise the contents.

It is easy to understand this and avoid such products, but bread, pasta, rice, and other cereals are also all high in similar concentrated carbs. From both a slimming and a health point of view, these may actually be worse than sugar because, during digestion, many starchy foods, particularly from cereals, produce even higher levels of glucose in the blood than sugar does.

The amount that carbs raise glucose in the blood is measured by the Glycaemic Index (GI), and according to the GI, sugar is actually lower than bread. You can see, therefore, that avoiding the more harmful foods is not as easy as it first appears.

GI blues

In March 2005, I was reading the latest copy of a popular woman's magazine, as you do when bored on holiday. It had a whole ten pages about the GI diet – billed on the cover as 'the healthiest low-carb plan around'. And it got it completely wrong!

The author correctly stated that GI is a measure of how much carbs raise blood glucose levels. But then, in lists of high-GI, medium-GI and low-GI foods they listed fatty foods as high-GI, when all fats, which have a GI of zero, are the lowest GI foods of all. They also listed 'omega-3 eggs' as low-GI, and 'eggs' as medium-GI, when both types of egg also have a GI of nothing; and low-fat cottage cheese was listed as low-GI, light cream cheese as medium-GI and full-fat cheese as high-GI when, yet again, their GIs are all zero. In fact because fats, meat, fish, cheese and eggs don't raise blood glucose at all, they don't have a GI – or they have a GI of 0, depending how you look at it. Lastly, diet fizzy drinks were listed as both low-GI and high-GI depending on whether they contained caffeine – yet caffeine plays no part whatsoever in the GI tables. It looked to me like a classic case of ignorance trying to cash in on the latest fad.

The magazine article gave a recommended reading list of six recently-published GI diet books. If the article was based on information from these books, then those authors had got it hopelessly wrong as well.

So what is GI?

The Glycaemic Index (GI) was originally designed as an aid for diabetics. It is a measure of how much carbohydrates raise blood glucose and, thus, insulin levels.

To compile this index, scientists fed 50 grams of glucose to their test subjects and measured how much this raised their subjects' blood glucose. That became their reference point, and they labelled it 100. Then they tested their subjects with other foods and measured blood glucose response relative to the glucose meal. If, for example, a food raised their test subjects' blood glucose level to 50% of the reference, then it had a glycaemic index of 50; if it raised blood glucose by 70%, then its GI was 70, and so on. So far, so good.

However, glucose is a bit too sweet for many people. The testers didn't like to drink 50 grams of the stuff and so, later, white bread was substituted. White bread has a GI of about 70 compared with glucose. The people doing the eating preferred this, but unfortunately it generated another index in which bread was rated at 100.

There were now two GIs: one based on glucose = 100; the other based on white bread = 100. This started the confusion as both indexes came into general use – and many publications failed to say which one they were using. It is the glucose = 100 that is generally used today.

GI has provided new insights into the relationship between foods and chronic disease, but GI should not be taken in isolation. While observational studies suggest that diets with a high glycaemic *load* – that is a food's GI *as well as* its carbohydrate content – is an important consideration, GI and carb content are both independently associated with increased risk of type-2 diabetes and other degenerative diseases.[2]

The height to which glucose rises after meals plays a direct role in the process leading to these diseases. Thus, either high-GI food or large amounts of carbohydrates, and particularly a combination of the two, significantly increases the risk of obesity,[3] hypertension,[4] cardiovascular disease,[5] and type-2 diabetes,[6] and all their associated complications.

If glucose and insulin levels are not allowed to go high after meals, this markedly lowers the risk. There is also limited evidence that a low-GI diet may also protect against colon cancer and breast cancer.

The flaws with GI

Considering the large amount of work that has been done on GI in different countries, it's disappointing that GI is not as useful as it was hoped to be. It has serious flaws, some of which are explained below.

Foods are arbitrarily divided into three bands: a GI of 70 or more is classed as high-GI; 56–69 is medium-GI; and 55 and below is low-GI. But that doesn't tell us much because:

- One grain of sugar has a GI of 64 – and a pound of sugar is also 64. So how much sugar can you eat? There is no way of telling. But as a parsnip's GI is 97, you can obviously eat a lot more sugar than parsnip – or can you?
- In the example above I have quoted the GI of sugar as 64 because that is the usually accepted figure, but 64 is really only the average of several tests which have been wildly different, with the GI of sugar ranging between a low of 58,[7] and a high of 110.[8]
- We are told that white bread is high-GI and that wholemeal bread is medium-GI, but the difference between their GIs is very little: white bread is 71 (on average); wholemeal is 69. That difference is hardly significant, and the only whole-wheat bread made in the UK which is listed in the official International GI data has a GI of 74 – which is actually higher than white bread!
- Another problem is that the same food, made by the same manufacturer but in a different plant, can have widely differing GIs. Take Kellogg's All-Bran, for example. This has a GI of 30 in Australia, 38 in the USA and 51 in Canada. I have

no idea what the GI of Kellogg's All-Bran is here in Britain – and neither has anyone else – as it hasn't been tested. Bürgen® Mixed Grain bread made in Australia has a two-fold variation with GIs ranging from 34 to 69.

- You might think that Kellogg's Special K, a cereal which is promoted as being high in protein, would have a lower GI, but it may actually by worse, depending on where you live. According to the official GI lists published in 2002, the GI of Special K varies between 54 (low-GI) in Australia, 69 (medium-GI) in the USA and 84 (high-GI) in France. Again, we don't know what GI the UK's version of Special K has as this hasn't been tested either.

- Then there is wholemeal flour. The GI of this can be anything between 52 and 72 in Canada, as high as 78 in Australia and 87 in Kenya. Yet again, the flour in the UK hasn't been tested, so its GI is anyone's guess.

- There are some strange anomalies. For example, you might assume that foods containing sugar would have a higher GI than the same food made without sugar. But 'Banana cake, made with sugar' is 47, while 'Banana cake, made without sugar' is 55.

- Here is another strange one: 'Gluten-free white bread, unsliced (gluten-free wheat starch) (UK)' is 71, while exactly the same bread, sliced, is 80. And similarly, 'gluten-free fibre-enriched, unsliced bread (gluten-free wheat starch, soya bran) (UK)' is 69 while the same bread, sliced, is again higher, at 76. Why should slicing bread raise its GI? I don't know, but it seems it does.

- Then again the way a food is cooked or processed makes a difference to its final glycaemic index according to a trial conducted at Department of Dietetics, Queen Elizabeth Hospital in Hong Kong.[9]

- The GIs for the same foods can be markedly different depending on where foods are grown, how they are produced and how they are stored.

- There is yet another problem, particularly as far as diabetics are concerned. The GI of fructose, the sugar found in fruit, is 22, which is very much lower than sucrose (table sugar) at 64. For this reason, diabetics are recommended to use fructose as a sweetener in preference to sugar, yet fructose is far more damaging to health than sucrose (see below and Chapter 5).[10–12]

- GI only applies to carbs and foods that contain carbs. This means that foods containing only fats and protein, such as meat, fish, cheese, eggs, butter, olive oil, lard, and so on, which have a GI of 0 because they don't raise glucose at all, are excluded from the GI lists. This might not matter if this fact was explained, but generally it isn't. And that allows authors with restricted knowledge – or a hidden agenda – to misrepresent these foods, as in the examples from the magazine article quoted above. In fact, the best way to lower the GI of any carb-rich food is to add fat to it, whereas the impression often implied is that adding fat makes it worse.

- The effects of the glycaemic index and glycaemic load (see below) of foods seems to depend on how old and what sex those eating the various foods are. A Danish study published in 2005 found that while GI and GL were positively associated with body fatness among Danish boys aged 16 years, there was no similar association found among younger boys or among girls of any age.[13]

- Lastly, there is generally a subtle, but important, distinction between what readers of diet books are told GI measures and what it really does measure. You are usually told something like 'Foods that lead to a rapid rise in blood sugar levels are known as high glycaemic index foods. Foods that lead to a slower rise in blood sugar levels are said to have a low glycaemic index'. However, GI is *not* a measure of the *speed* of a glucose rise but the height of the rise. Thus books that suggest that glucose from low-GI foods enters the bloodstream more slowly than from high-GI are misinforming their readers.

Glycaemic Load

When the glycaemic index had been established, it was thought that would make selecting carb-containing foods easier. As you can see from the above, it didn't.

Even if the anomalies above didn't exist, there was still another problem because increase in blood glucose levels is not just dependent on GI, but also on the amount of the food you eat and what it is eaten with. Therefore, yet another scale was created which tried to take this into consideration. That scale is the Glycaemic Load, or GL.

In Glycaemic Load tables, foods are listed with their carb contents and with both their Glycaemic Index and Glycaemic Load values. Then, as this produces very large numbers, these are divided by 100, but we now have a situation where trying to work it all out can be horribly complicated. Although I have included GI and GL lists at the back of this book to give you the whole picture, I think it is probably much easier in the long run to forget about GI and GL, and just to take note of the carb content, keeping the total for the day around 60 g, spread equally among three meals (see Appendix E).

Testing the hypothesis

In one of the most recent studies of the Glycaemic Index, researchers from the University of Minnesota wondered whether lowering the GI of a diet which was already low in calories would have any further effect on weight loss.[14] To test the idea, they assigned obese patients to one of three diets – high GI, low GI or high fat – all with the same number of calories.

After 12 weeks, all three groups lost weight. Those on the low-GI diet lost an average of 21.8 lb (9.9 kg), while those on the high GI diet lost 20.5 lb (9.3 kg). This difference is very little. The authors of the study conclude:

> 'In summary, lowering the glycemic load and glycemic index of weight reduction diets does not provide any added benefit to energy restriction in promoting weight loss in obese subjects.'

That the GI and GL are of little use was confirmed in a 5-year test published in 2006 by scientists at the University of South Carolina, the National Institute of Diabetes, Digestive, and Kidney Diseases, Bethesda, Maryland, USA, and the German Institute of Human Nutrition, Potsdam-Rehbruecke, Germany.[15] Starting in 1994–96 and following 1255 adults for five years, the researchers evaluated the GI and GL of foods eaten in relation to blood glucose levels measured before meals and 2 hours afterwards. When the dietary information was analysed, researchers found no association between Glycaemic Index levels and blood sugar levels. They concluded that: 'present results call into question the utility of GI and GL to reflect glycaemic response to food adequately, when used in the context of usual diet.'

These studies tell us that eating a carbohydrate-rich diet based on either Glycaemic Load or Glycaemic Index only helps with weight loss because many carbohydrate foods with a low Glycaemic Index are also low in calories. For example, most vegetables and fruits are low-GI, but you would have to eat many more pounds of low-GI, low-carb cabbage than you would from eating high-GI bread to get the same amount of energy, so these diets which rely solely on low-GI foods work by starving you. They are low-calorie, low-fat, which is exactly the diets that most people got fat on in the first place.

Low-GI fruit may be worse

So far we have been talking about glucose in the bloodstream, but the type of sugar found in fruit is *fructose*. Because fructose enters the bloodstream and is transported to the liver as it is and does not stimulate insulin secretion from the pancreas, foods such as fruit that contain fructose produce smaller glucose and insulin surges than glucose-containing carbohydrates such as bread and pasta, and have a much lower GI than those foods. So, on the face of it, it looks as if fruit may be healthier, but again it's not so simple. In fact, although the GI of fruit is low, it may actually be worse than higher GI foods for three main reasons.

The first problem concerns the way it increases the risk of heart disease and other complications associated with diabetes which I mentioned in Chapter 5.

The second is that low-GI fruit also compromises our immune system. This is discussed more fully in Chapter 14.

The third is that our bodies produce a hormone called *leptin* which controls weight gain: the more leptin produced, the less weight is put on. But the production of leptin is regulated by insulin responses to meals. As fructose does not raise insulin, it reduces circulating leptin concentrations. Dr Sharon Elliot and colleagues at the Universities of California and Pennsylvania, say that the combined effects of lowered leptin and insulin in individuals who eat diets that are high in dietary fructose could therefore increase the likelihood of weight gain and its associated disorders.[16] In addition, they point out that fructose, compared with glucose, is preferentially metabolised to fat in the liver. Fructose consumption has been shown to induce insulin resistance, impaired glucose tolerance and high blood levels of insulin and triglycerides, as well as raising blood pressure in animal studies, although the figures are not so clear in humans. Nevertheless, there are human data that suggest that eating more fructose may be detrimental in terms of increased fat storage and body weight and the illnesses associated with the metabolic syndrome.

We mustn't forget insulin

By the time all these studies had been published it was obvious that both the Glycaemic Index and Glycaemic Load tables had severe limitations. And there was one more aspect to factor in: because insulin promotes the storage of excess blood glucose as body fat, a diet with a low glycaemic index or load should make weight loss faster and easier – in theory at least. Nutritionists believed that a greater glycaemic response meant a greater insulin response. However, while the glucose/insulin link holds true with *some* foods, it doesn't hold true for all of them. As we know, insulin levels rise when you eat a food high in protein – even though blood sugar levels don't. Protein-rich foods or the addition of protein to a carbohydrate-rich meal can also stimulate a modest rise in insulin secretion without increasing blood glucose, particularly in people with diabetes.

Two studies considered the effect of adding fats to carbs.[17,18] In both, the result was a significant flattening of the glucose curves after meals but insulin responses were not so affected. In one study insulin rose slightly and in the other it stayed about the same. This is an important finding because adding fat to any carb lowers the overall GI.

These findings change the picture radically. GI and GL are concerned only with measuring the amount of glucose which carbohydrate-containing foods put in bloodstream, but raised insulin levels are just as important as they contribute both weight gain and the inability to lose weight, as well as other serious conditions such as heart disease and cancer. So while blood glucose is important, it is only half the problem.

The other half is the amount that blood insulin is raised, and so the scientists at the University of Sydney who gave us the GI later developed an 'Insulin Score' based on 38 common foods.[19] For this, subjects were given meals which all contained the same amount of energy (240 kcal). You will note some very unexpected results in the Table below.

These figures are not to be confused with the Glycaemic Index. Dr Susanne Holt, the leading researcher says, 'In the insulin index study, we measured glycaemic scores and insulin scores for 1000 kJ portions of foods. They are not GI values. In a healthy person that has fasted for more than 10–12 hours overnight, cheese and steak can cause a small rise in blood glucose in the second hour of our two-hour test periods due to gluconeogenesis. Also the normal fluctuations in blood glucose around the fasting value that our experiments start from produce some area above the fasting blood glucose level, which is used to calculate both GI and glycemic score values.'

Table 11.1   Insulin and glucose scores of common foods

Food	Insulin score	Glucose score
Peanuts	12	20
Beef (very lean)	21	51
Fish	28	59
All-Bran*	32	40
Oranges	39	60
Porridge (oatmeal)*	40	60
Muesli*	40	60
Eggs (poached)	42	31
White pasta	46	40
Apples	50	59
Potato chips (McCain's prefried)	52	61
Cheese (mature cheddar)	55	45
Cake	56	82
Grain [rye] bread	60	56
Popcorn	62	54
Lentils	62	58
Yogurt, (strawberry fruit)	62	115
Doughnuts	63	74
Special K*	66	70
Honeysmacks*	67	60
Brown pasta	68	40
Ice cream	70	89
Sustain*	71	66
French fries	71	74
Croissants	74	79
Grapes	74	82
Cookies	74	92
Cornflakes*	75	76
Bananas	79	81
Mars bar	79	112
Whole-meal bread	97	96
White bread (Reference)	**100**	**100**
Brown rice	104	62
White rice	110	79
Baked beans	114	120
Crackers	118	87
Jellybeans	118	160
Potatoes	141	121

*All cereals were served with semi-skimmed milk

Based on data from Holt, Brand-Miller & Petocz (1997).[19]

Limitations

Unfortunately, while a great deal of work has been done on carbs, proteins and fats separately, and on carbs plus proteins, and carbs plus fats, no-one has yet studied the effects of fats plus proteins which form the bulk of our traditional diets and which is recommended here. As fats on their own do not have any appreciable effect on either blood glucose or insulin levels, and as protein has no effect on glucose and only a modest effect on insulin, I am confident that the protein-plus-fat combination we have evolved to eat will turn out to be entirely harmless.

Conclusion

To sum up, the Glycaemic Index is a very weak index which is not only misrepresented in popular diet books, but is over-simplified, over-hyped and over-sold. While it has a use in a clinical setting, it is really of very little practical use to the general public; and the Glycaemic Load figures are far too complicated, as is the addition of an insulin score. Even if these were more useful, they really have little practical value because what matters as far as your body is concerned is not the GI of a carbohydrate, but the total amount you eat and absorb: A hundred grams of carbohydrate is a hundred grams of carbohydrate whatever its GI is. The reason Banting's diet worked was because he cut out things like bread. He didn't bother with counting anything particularly.

It is certainly a good idea to avoid foods listed as high-GI, but you should also still be wary of low-GI foods which have a high carb content. It's not that there is anything wrong with following a diet that has a low GI; it's certainly much better than following a high-GI diet. Despite the popularity of low-GI diet books, if you eat *more* carbohydrate-rich foods with a low GI and *fewer* carbohydrate-rich foods with a high GI – without making any other change to your diet – the chances are you'll end up feeling hungry, and frustrated because you're not losing any weight.

References

1. Bouchard C. Obesity in adulthood: the importance of childhood and parental obesity. *New Engl J Med* 1997; 13: 926–927.
2. Brand-Miller JC. Glycemic load and chronic disease. *Nutr Rev* 2003; 61: S49–55.
3. Ludwig DS, Maizoub JA, Al-Zahrani A, et al. High glycaemic index foods, overeating, and obesity. *Pediatrics* 1999; 103: E26–E32.

4. Parilo M, Coulston A, Hollenbyck C. Effect of a low fat diet on carbohydrate metabolism in patients with hypertension. *Hypertension* 1988; 22: 244–248.

5. Liu S, Willett WC, Stampfer MJ, et al. A prospective study of dietary glycemic load, carbohydrate intake, and risk of coronary heart disease in US women. *Am J Clin Nutr* 2000; 71: 1455–1461.

6. Salmeron J, Ascherio A, Rimm EB, et al: Dietary fibre, glycemic load, and risk of NIDDM in men. *Diabetes Care* 1997; 20: 545–550.

7. Gannon MC, Nuttal FQ, Krezowski PA, et al. The serum insulin and plasma glucose response to milk and fruit products in type 2 (non-insulin-dependent) diabetic patients. *Diabetologia* 1986; 29: 784–791.

8. Pelletier X, Hanesse B, Bornet F, Debry G. Glycaemic and insulinaemic responses in healthy volunteers upon ingestion of maltitol and hydrogenated glucose syrups. *Diabetes Metab* 1994; 20:291–296.

9. Chan EM, Cheng WM, Tiu SC, Wong LL. Postprandial glucose response to Chinese foods in patients with type 2 diabetes. *J Am Diet Assoc* 2004; 104: 1854–1858.

10. Bunn HF, Higgins PJ. Reaction of monosaccharides with proteins: possible evolutionary significance. *Science* 1981; 213: 222–229.

11. Bierman EL. George Lyman Duff Memorial Lecture. Atherogenesis in diabetes. *Arterioscler Thromb* 1992; 12: 647–656.

12. Swanson JE, Laine DC, Thomas W, Bantle JP. Metabolic effects of dietary fructose in healthy subjects. *Am J Clin Nutr* 1992; 55: 851–856.

13. Nielsen BM, Bjørnsbo KS, Tetens I, et al. Dietary glycaemic index and glycaemic load in Danish children in relation to body fatness. *Br J Nutr* 2005; 94: 992–997.

14. Raatz SK, Torkelson CJ, Redmon JB, et al. Reduced glycemic index and glycemic load diets do not increase the effects of energy restriction on weight loss and insulin sensitivity in obese men and women. *J Nutr* 2005; 135: 2387–2391.

15. Mayer-Davis, EJ, Dhawan A, Liese AD, et al. Towards understanding of glycaemic index and glycaemic load in habitual diet: associations with measures of glycaemia in the Insulin Resistance Atherosclerosis Study. *Br J Nutr* 2006; 95: 397–405.

16. Elliott SS, Keim NL, Stern JS, et al. Fructose, weight gain, and the insulin resistance syndrome. *Am J Clin Nutr* 2002; 76: 911–922.

17. Collier G, McLean A, O'Dea K. Effect of co-ingestion of fat on the metabolic responses to slowly and rapidly absorbed carbohydrates. *Diabetologia* 1984; 26: 50–54.

18. Gannon MC, Nuttall FQ, Westphal SA, Seaquist ER. The effect of fat and carbohydrate on plasma glucose, insulin, C-peptide, and triglycerides in normal male subjects. *J Am Coll Nutr* 1993; 12: 36–41.

19. Holt SHA, Brand-Miller JC, Petocz P. An insulin index of foods: The insulin demand generated by 1000-kJ portions of common foods. *Am J Clin Nutr* 1997; 66:1264–1276.

Chapter Twelve

Eat less, weigh more?

Nature has taken good care that theory should have little effect on practice.

Samuel Johnson

Introduction

The hormones that control our bodies' responses to internal and external events were conditioned by our environment over the past couple of million years. These set in motion different combinations of hormonal responses. We have several hormones that raise levels of glucose in our bloodstream: adrenaline (epinephrine), glucagon, cortisol, and growth hormone. All of these raise glucose levels in times of crisis as part of the 'fight-or-flight' reflex which prepares the body to confront danger or run away from it. If something is important, it makes sense to have more than one if possible, but we have only one hormone – insulin – to bring blood glucose levels down. This suggests that high-glucose levels were not a problem in earlier times, and that reinforces the theory that we must have eaten a low-carb diet in pre-historical times.

Insulin, the fattening hormone

Carbs are the only foods that increase body weight. I know this is heresy to the 'healthy eating' dictocrats, but it is demonstrably true. This is how it works:

All carbs are digested quickly. This means that within about half an hour after a carb-rich 'healthy' meal the level of glucose in your bloodstream will rise rapidly. High blood glucose levels are dangerous and, as levels of glucose rise rapidly in the bloodstream, your pancreas produces a large amount of insulin to take that glucose out. It does this by converting it and storing it first as glycogen and then as body fat.

This is the process of putting on weight. Not surprisingly, a high insulin response to glucose has been shown to be a risk factor for long-term weight gain, and this effect is particularly so in people who are insulin-resistant.[1] As we saw in the graph in Chapter 5, dietary fats do not raise insulin levels. They are not stored as body fat.

However, there is a further problem. There is an inevitable time delay between cause and effect. When your blood glucose level is back down to normal, your pancreas is still making insulin. As a result, the levels of glucose in your blood fall below normal, and you feel hungrier quicker. So you have a snack, usually of more carbohydrates – bread, sandwiches, biscuits or sweets – and start the whole process over again. Obesity is almost inevitable.[2]

There is yet a third problem. The action of insulin may account for the apparent contradiction between the paradoxical dietary effects of fat and carbohydrate on human weight, because insulin is a storage hormone – its job is to get energy out of the bloodstream, not to let more in. So the production of insulin inhibits hormone sensitive *lipase*, a fat-burning enzyme, thereby preventing your body's fat cells releasing their fat.[3] This effectively stops your body from burning your stored fat and makes it well nigh impossible for you to lose the weight you have put on. This is another reason why weight loss is more difficult on a carbohydrate-rich diet.

Lastly, insulin resistance in the brain may impair insulin's ability to satisfy a satiety centre which again could contribute to overeating, obesity, and diabetes.[4]

This is the first crucial problem with the 'healthy eating' dogma. Eating the 'healthy' way, you can eat far more calories than your body needs as energy for the day, yet still feel hungry – and eat more. You enter a vicious cycle of continuous weight gain combined with hunger. Under such circumstances it is almost impossible not to overeat.

So, if you are overweight, is it your fault – or theirs?

Conventional nutritionists will invariably tell you, if you are overweight, it's your own fault: you are eating too much or not exercising enough – usually both. But are they right? In my experience, nobody wants to be overweight. You get ridiculed, stared at, are embarrassed to be seen in a bathing costume on the beach. In other words, you live a generally less happy life.

It may not be your fault at all if you are doing what you are told. That's because the 'healthy' recommendation that a low-fat diet is the best way to lose weight bears no resemblance to what our evolutionary history and more recent evidence says we should be eating to lose weight. It must surely play a part as evidence from epidemiological studies and clinical, controlled hospital-based trials have consistently shown for the last 140 years that the best diet for weight loss, or not to get overweight in the first place, is one that is very high in fats and with not a lot of carbohydrate – the exact opposite of what you are told.

This has not gone unnoticed. According to a report published in 1997 by Drs Heini and Weinsier:

> 'Reduced fat and calorie intake and frequent use of low-calorie food products have been associated with a paradoxical increase in the prevalence of obesity.'[5]

You won't be surprised to hear that this study was not reported in the press!

So what went wrong?

With all the evidence that it is carbs that are the cause of obesity, why is it that those in nutritional authority can't see it? The answer seems to lie in their implicit belief in the First Law of Thermodynamics which states that energy cannot be created or destroyed, merely changed.[6]

Around the end of the 19th century, doctors devised a simple concept, based on the laws of thermodynamics. They likened the body to a tank, into one end of which energy is poured in the form of food. This, they said, is then either used up or stored. If you use up more than you pour in, you get thinner and if you pour in more than you use, you get fatter. The theory was easy to understand, made sense, obeyed the laws of physics, and for a while it seemed satisfactory. Dieticians could now say, apparently with scientific backing, that fat people must either be eating too much or working too little. By the start of the 1914–18 war, however, doubts were creeping in. For instance, diabetes is a defect of carbohydrate metabolism and the treatment for diabetics at that time involved completely depriving them of carbohydrate. In this case, scientists found that the energy input/energy output sums simply did not add up.

By the early 1920s, interest in the theory was renewed. It was found to be impossible to measure the total amount of water in a person at any one time. Therefore, water retention or loss was said to account for any discrepancy in the balance between energy input/output and excess weight. It was decades before this convenient theory was disproved.

In the 1950s, isotope techniques were developed which allowed more accurate measurement of body fat turnover. In addition, it was demonstrated that different foods could alter the amounts of body fat, and that body fat could also be affected by certain responsive glands – the adrenal, thyroid and pituitary glands – even when energy intake was constant.

The flaws exposed

The fact that high-energy diets are more effective for reducing weight has proved very difficult for dieticians and doctors to accept, because of what looks like a challenge to the laws of thermodynamics. However, there are flaws in this theory. To grasp them, we need to go over some basic facts.

The calorie is a unit of heat. The way the energy content of a food is determined is by burning it in a device called a 'bomb calorimeter' and measuring the amount of heat it gives off.

One gram of carbohydrate, burnt in this way gives an energy value of 4.2 calories, or more correctly kilocalories (kcal). A gram of protein gives 5.25 kcal. This time, however, one calorie is deducted because a gram of protein does not oxidise readily, it gives rise to urea and other products which must be subtracted. That gives a final figure for protein of 4.25 kcal. Burning a gram of fat in the bomb calorimeter gives 9.2 kcal.

These figures are then rounded to the nearest whole number – 4, 4 and 9 respectively – and are used in calorie charts to indicate the energy values of foodstuffs and, thus, to allow dieters to measure their food intake.

However, there are four basic flaws in using these figures to determine the amounts of food we should eat.

The first flaw

The most obvious flaw in the argument is that our bodies do not burn foods in the same way that they are burned in a bomb calorimeter. If they did, we would glow in the dark. Our digestive process is also inefficient. The chemical process whereby blood sugar is oxidised to provide energy produces carbon dioxide. About half is exhaled as carbon dioxide, the other half is excreted in sweat, urine and faeces as energy-containing molecules, the energy values of which must be deducted from the original food intake. All of these vary. For example, eating a lot of fat forms ketones, which can be found in urine. The value of a gram of ketones derived from fat is roughly four calories. So, in this case, nearly half the energy from the fat is lost.

The second flaw

The second and more important flaw in the argument is that the body does not use all its food to provide energy. The primary function of dietary proteins, for example, is body cell manufacture and repair: making skin, blood, hair, fingernails and toenails, etc. The amount of protein needed for this purpose is generally accepted to be about one gram per kilogram of lean body weight. As meats contain approximately 23 grams of protein per 100 grams, a person weighing, say, 70 kg (11 stone) needs to eat about 300 g (11 oz) of meat, or its equivalent, every day just to supply his basic protein needs. Even eating this volume of lean chicken would provide some 465 calories. These calories are not used to supply energy, they contribute nothing to the body's calorie needs and so must be deducted if you are counting calories.

Much of the fat we eat is also used to provide materials used by the body in processes other than the production of energy: the manufacture of bile acids and hormones, the essential fatty acids for the brain and nervous system, and so on. All these must be deducted as well. Thus trying to determine, from food intake and energy expenditure alone, how much excess energy your body will store as fat will give a completely wrong answer. However, these other factors cannot be measured. Therefore, calorie-counting, which is the foundation of practically every modern slimming diet, is a complete waste of time.

The third flaw

When 'experts' say that 'a calorie is a calorie', what they mean is that it is impossible for two diets containing exactly the same number of calories to lead to different weight losses. Yet, over the last century a spate of dietary studies has shown that, calorie for calorie, low-carbohydrate diets are much better at reducing weight than the traditional low-fat diets. 'Experts' have heavily criticised these studies saying that the data could not be right because that would violate the laws of thermodynamics, but they don't. It is important to realise that there is more than one law of thermodynamics. The narrow view that 'a calorie is a calorie' might comply with the First Law, but it violates the Second Law of Thermodynamics.

The point is that there is no doubt at all that low-carb, high-fat diets *do* have a metabolic advantage when it comes to weight loss, whatever the 'experts' say.[7] And this metabolic advantage complies fully with the second Law of Thermodynamics – and, incidentally, with the First Law as well.

The First Law, as mentioned above, is a *conservation* law. The Second Law is a *dissipation* law. It is this Second Law which governs the chemical reactions in our bodies.

Let me use an analogy. The energy in the petrol that fuels your car makes the car go along, but it also produces heat, through friction, and noise, which we really don't need. The Second Law is all about efficiency – how much of the energy we put in does useful work and how much is wasted. Thus, although all of the energy in the petrol is accounted for and complies with the First Law, the actual moving of the car, if the waste products (heat and noise) are removed from the equation, does not. The Second Law was developed in this context, and it applies equally when we look at the efficiency of our bodies and how different foods affect our bodies. The Second Law says that no machine is completely efficient: some of the available energy is lost as heat or in the internal rearrangement of chemical compounds and other changes. As different foods use different metabolic pathways, with different levels of efficiency, variations in efficiency must be expected. For this reason, the dogma that a 'calorie is a calorie' violates the second law of thermodynamics as a matter of principle.

It is the differences in chemical changes within our bodies that make low-carb diets better than low-fat, calorie-controlled ones easier to lose weight on. What the diet dictocrats fail to take into consideration when considering the laws of thermodynamics are the energy losses incurred in the different chemical changes within our bodies. When these are taken into consideration, neither law of thermodynamics is violated.

The fourth flaw – Part 1: fats

The last flaw in the argument is that our bodies don't digest or metabolise different foods equally and they are not all equally available. This is demonstrated in the Table below, where the calculated energy value for fats of 9 kcal/gram was compared to the actual value found.

Table 12.1   Calculated energy value of selected fats vs. actual availability in humans[8]

Type of fat or oil	Caloric availability (kcal/gram)
Cocoa butter	6.8
Beef fat	7.3
Coconut oil	7.8
Lard (pork fat)	8.3
Corn oil	8.5

The Table shows clearly that no fats or oils actually provide as many calories as we are told they do, but you will also notice another thing: not all fats are equal. Saturated fats provide less energy than unsaturated fats and oils. It has long been known that people tend to find it easier to lose weight eating animal fats. Well, here is the reason: animal fats, which are normally saturated, contain less available energy. (In the Table, the reason that the energy availability from lard (pork fat) is high is that farmed pigs are fed a more polyunsaturated diet. The oils in this are then incorporated in their body fat, making it more like a vegetable oil than an animal fat.)

The fourth flaw – Part 2: carbs

The same is true of carbs as not all of them give a value of 4 kcal. Chemically, dietary fibre is a carbohydrate but, as it is indigestible, it is excluded from calorie tables. Fibre is listed on foods in different ways in the UK and USA: in the UK, 'fibre' is listed separately from 'carbs'; in the USA, the fibre is included in the total carbs, then listed separately so that it can be deducted when assessing the calorific value of a product. But even these measures do not give a true picture. While fibre is counted as having no calories, it actually supplies between none and 2 kcal/gram depending on the type of fibre it is.[9] Digestible carbs also are not the same: sugar provides 3.9 kcal and starch gives us 4.2 kcal.[10] The difference might look small, but it is a difference of 8% and, when talking in terms of a 2000 calorie diet, that's a difference of 160 kcal.

So practically all the figures used for calorie counting are wrong. To make life easy, the usually accepted calorie figures are used in this book, but these discrepancies and the other flaws make a nonsense of actually counting calories.

The correct way to lose weight

The truth is that it's well nigh impossible to lose weight permanently simply by restricting calories. Eating less and losing excess body fat do not automatically go hand in hand. Certainly enforced starvation will make you lose weight – World War II concentration camps proved that. However, low-fat, low-calorie, diets (which are essentially the same thing as starving) generate a series of biochemical signals in your body that will take you out of balance, making it more difficult to access stored body fat for energy. In a similar way, diets based on calorie limits invariably fail in the long term – you simply cannot stay on them. People on restrictive diets get tired of feeling hungry and deprived. They go off their diets, put the weight back on – primarily as increased body fat – and then feel bad about themselves for not having enough will power, discipline, or motivation. Feeling bad about things tends to make you want to comfort yourself with yet more carbohydrates in the form of sweets or chocolate, thus adding to the problem. However, you shouldn't need willpower – no other animal does; all you really need is the right information.

If you change what you eat to a more natural way of eating – a way of eating more like our pre-agricultural ancestors – you won't have to be overly concerned about how much you eat at all and be continually counting calories. Your body will do that for you, the way it is genetically programmed to do.

Don't lose muscle

There is more to the question about which is the better way to lose weight than mere weight loss. I asked in the first chapter what it was you wanted to lose, and suggested that it was fat. All weight loss diets will reduce your weight, but not all of them do it by reducing body fat.

With all low-fat, calorie controlled diets, weight is lost from muscles. This is because, deprived of its necessary supply from carbs and conditioned to using glucose as a fuel, the calorie-controlled dieter's body uses its alternative source: *gluconeogenesis*. This is where proteins from lean muscle tissue are cannibalised to produce glucose, and that weakens you.

So this is another area where low carbohydrate diets win over the low-calorie ones: by changing the dieter's body to using fats, they preserve muscle mass and favour fat loss. This effect was ably demonstrated in the small study done by Dr Charlotte Young in the early 1970s.[11] Her overweight patients all consumed 1800 kcal per day and they all consumed 115 g of protein per day. Only the fat and carb content was varied. Those eating the most fat (133 g/day) and least carb (30 g) lost more body fat and less muscle mass than those getting more carb (104 g/day) and less fat (103 g/day).

When we are talking of overweight, these findings are tremendously important. Muscles use more energy than fat. This means that, if muscle mass is lost, this lowers the rate at which your body uses energy. Weight loss that involves a significant loss of muscle mass is much more likely to result in rebound weight gain, so that's another good reason to lower your intake of carbs not fats.

Set point weight

Anyone who has followed any diet for a while – especially if they have a lot of weight to lose – has probably experienced the frustration and utter exasperation when after a couple of weeks of rapid weight loss, it stops. It's called a 'stall'. It normally happens when, after two weeks of success, the third week sees that weight loss stop, seemingly for ever. Why? What's gone wrong?

The cause lies, as you might suspect, in our genes. Over the years, our bodies learn how much energy they need to store. They learn this from the periods of starvation they have to endure. This tends to set a point where your weight will stabilise. It's called your 'set point weight'. The set point is a natural weight, specific to you, which your body will try to maintain at all costs.

There was a survival advantage in this. Regularly, throughout human history, food has been in short supply – during the winter months and in the Ice Ages, for example. During our evolution we developed the ability to store energy against hard times. Those who stored the most had the best chance of surviving. We still have that ability, but we now live in a time when there is anything but a food shortage.

Dr Xavier Pi-Sunyer, Director of the Obesity Research Center, St Luke's Roosevelt Hospital, New York, is convinced that a person's set point works only one way: upward. He explains that the body tends to allow weight gain without adjustment, but if a person's weight remains at the higher weight for a while, the new higher weight becomes the set point and the body will do its utmost to maintain it.[12]

It has been found that if lean people are forced to overeat so that they put on weight, as soon as they return to a normal eating pattern, their weight goes down to where it started – their set point. Similarly when overweight people go on a low-calorie diet, their bodies try desperately to maintain the higher, set point weight. For this reason, as soon as the diet finishes, their bodies use the opportunity to put weight back on – to return to the set point weight. If you are continually low-calorie dieting, you will be much fatter than if you don't for the simple reason that your body recognises that you are starving and stores more fat in the expectation of more starvation in the future. This is another reason that low-calorie dieting is doomed to failure, and so are diets that start with a very rapid weight loss.

While every low-calorie, low-fat diet will tend to increase your set point weight, they don't always involve stalls, but low-carb diets that start with a rapid weight loss often do. This is another reason why it is better to start slowly, then you avoid the frustration and the deep sense of disappointment that low-carb is another diet that doesn't work.

So don't be in too much of a hurry. If your weight stops going down, and you are still overweight and doing everything right, then continue. You just have to wait for your body to get used to the idea that it isn't going to be starved again and decide to move on. Don't worry, your weight *will* start to fall again.

Energy regulation systems

Eat only as many calories as your body uses, dieticians tell us. How can this be done? It is impossible to measure by mental arithmetic your energy input to the nearest calorie and tailor your workload to use up exactly the same amount as you put in. However, while you can't measure this accurately, your body can – if you let it.

The systems which regulate food input and energy output are complex but completely self-regulating and extremely accurate. Your body knows exactly how much of any particular nutrient it needs and, if you are aware of it, it will tell you.

The control systems may be divided into two: those which regulate energy input and those which regulate energy output, the two working together to achieve a balance.

Energy intake controls

On the energy intake side, the controls are hunger and appetite. Through appetite the body tells you what combination of proteins, fats, carbohydrates and other nutrients to eat. Without hunger you would not know when to eat and without appetite you would not know what and how much to eat. These are the signals with which your body communicates with you. They measure and time your body's needs very precisely. If these signals are not heeded, those needs are not met and permanent damage can result.

As food is eaten, sensors in the upper gut assess its nutritional appropriateness and set up a chain of electro-chemical reactions involving the gut opiates, chemical messengers that are similar to morphine in their properties but much stronger.[13] Most are in the intestinal nerve cells, others in the hypothalamus. The opiates control hunger and appetite. As each nutrient is supplied, the appetite for it diminishes until, eventually, the appetite for it is satisfied and 'switches off'. When all our energy needs are met, we no longer feel hungry and we (should) stop eating.

The opiates work extremely efficiently with fats and proteins, but they hardly appear to work at all with carbohydrates. You will find that you cannot eat too much fat. You may like butter or cream but try to eat a lot of either and you will soon develop an aversion to it. Try a little experiment with two items of food that you like, one a sweet carbohydrate food such as toffees, the other one of fat, such as butter. You will find that you will be able to eat the toffees until they 'come out of your ears'. Try the same with butter, however, and you probably won't get beyond the second teaspoon before you begin to go off it. Your body is telling you it has had enough. Disregard this signal and you will probably be sick. On the other hand, it is all too easy to eat too many sweets and other refined carbohydrates such as bread and pasta.

It is possible, however, to fool the body to some extent. Andrew Prentice and Susan Jebb of the Medical Research Council's Dunn Clinical Nutrition Centre suggest that adding sugar to fatty foods can allow you to eat more fat by disguising it and making the fat more palatable.[14] They point out that studies have already been done which showed a reciprocal relation between fat and sugar intake. This is particularly true when fat is combined with sugar and starch in such confections as cakes and chocolates. These are the mixtures that are fattening. The foods which are the major natural contributors to fat intake – meat, fat spreads and oils, dairy products, eggs and fish – are not combined to any great extent with sugar, and are not fattening.

Brown fat cells

The body's use of energy, the output side of the body's energy balance, is controlled by our brown fat. Although mainly located in the upper back, there are clusters of brown fat cells in many parts of the body. Their job is to regulate the amount of energy the body uses. Brown fat is a special fat that is fundamentally different from ordinary white fat both in composition and function. White fat is mainly an energy storage system where excess calories are deposited and stored for future use. Brown fat, on the other hand, is an energy-using material that is stimulated by the nervous system to burn up calories. Thus brown fat reduces the amount of white fat. Brown fat's primary task is to regulate and maintain our body temperature. As it uses energy much faster than other body cells, it is used to produce warmth in cold weather. When this warmth is not required it is dissipated. Brown fat also plays an important part in weight control by burning off excess calories.[15]

White fat cells

The white fat cells that are used to store fat in the body are called adipocytes. Even a lean person has between twenty and forty billion adipocytes. These are not simply inert storage vessels, they are active living cells. As they store fat, adipocytes swell, but they can only double in size, so there should be a limit to how much fat we can carry. Unfortunately for people who eat the wrong foods, Nature has thoughtfully provided us with a vast reserve of extremely small cells called preadipocytes of which we are completely unaware – until they mutate into adipocytes. After adipocytes have been used to store fat to their limit, preadipocytes are converted for use. Insulin, the hormone produced as a response to excessively high blood sugar levels, triggers this mutation. Once this happens you have the extra adipocytes for life: these fat cells can get smaller, but never fewer, a fact that has serious implications for successful weight-loss programmes.

The earlier in your life that you convert more preadipocytes into fat cells, the more difficult it will be to retain a normal weight. Not surprisingly, therefore, the most difficult form of obesity to correct is childhood onset obesity. People who were obese as children have a very hard time trying to lose weight and are much more likely to regain lost weight quickly.

The rhythm method of girth control

Using the controls outlined above, the healthy body can regulate very precisely the rate at which it uses fuel in conjunction with the amount ingested – if it is given the right materials to work with, and in the right proportions.

When you eat less than your appetite says you need, the first effect is that your appetite is not satisfied. This is abnormal and unnatural. If you continue, your appetite becomes blunted until eventually it no longer works correctly. At the same time, if your energy intake is insufficient, you start to use up your energy stores and lose weight, but if your energy intake continues to be less than you need, the brown fat recognises that you are starving and reduces its activity. It conserves energy by slowing down the rate at which your body uses it. Other metabolic processes are also run more energy-efficiently. This is one reason why weight loss may be high at the start of a diet but then becomes progressively less, and also why when you resume a 'normal' eating pattern, after the period of low-calorie dieting, your body takes the opportunity to store extra energy, in the form of fat: it's in case of more hard times to come.

This is the way to put weight on. A recent survey by European obesity experts showed that repeated dieting was a greater cause of obesity than lack of will power, inactivity or depression leading to overeating. Yo-yo dieting is probably the surest way to become overweight in later life.

The long-term effects of yo-yo dieting were studied in a cohort of 1772 former elite male athletes and 651 healthy age-matched non-athletes who acted as controls. The athletes included 273 men engaged in power sports that forced them to yo-yo diet.[16]

By 1985 the yo-yo dieting power athletes had put on much more weight than either the other athletes or the controls, and there were three times as many cases of clinical obesity in the yo-yo group as among the other athletes and twice as many as among the controls.

Similarly, a 1986 Dutch study showed that men who had experienced several weight changes within a short space of time put weight on.[17] A year later this excess weight had disappeared in all subgroups except one: a group who had resorted to low-calorie dieting to lose their excess weight – they had put on even more weight!

This is why most people who diet get progressively fatter over the years. The process leads to ever more stringent diets, the brown fat is damaged, it atrophies and stops working.

Changing from one diet to another and alternating periods of dieting and normal eating weaken your weight-regulating mechanisms, making it necessary for you to undertake ever more stringent diets to achieve the same weight loss. This effect was demonstrated in a trial using subjects who had never dieted before. The first time they dieted they lost an average 1.5 kg (3½ lb) a week, but they lost only 1 kg (2½ lb) a week during their second period of dieting.

Persistent low-calorie dieting can damage any of the control systems. Many people crave food all day. In them there may be damage to the 'switch-off' opiates, their appetite becomes defective and they are never satisfied. These are the people who cannot help nibbling between meals. There are others who get fat and yet eat very little (and have great difficulty in convincing their doctors of this). Here it is the activation of their brown fat that may be at fault. Eventually, both the opiate and the brown fat systems may become flawed.

Low-calorie dietary regimes invariably fail. More importantly, they damage your health, engender a feeling of disillusion and failure, lower morale and increase mental as well as physical stress.

Normalisation of controls

For the natural controls to work correctly they must be normalised. Appetite and hunger are natural and vital signals – and both must be satisfied. Therefore, you should undertake no dietary regime that is harmful to the body. Any diet should follow a pattern that is normal and natural.

Modern low-calorie diets, whether they are obviously faddy – relying on a very restricted range of nutrient-poor foods – or requiring a more subtle reduction of calorific intake, are abnormal. They all encourage hunger but do not satisfy it. Neither, usually, do they satisfy the appetite.

Insulin is the main storage hormone in the body. In the presence of large amounts of insulin, produced by eating carbohydrates, typically simple sugars and starches, the body is primed to store energy as fat. When insulin levels are lower, as is common on a low-carb, higher-fat diet, your body is reluctant to store energy in your fat stores, and more likely to burn that fat.

The most important prerequisite of any diet, then, is to get your body's systems working normally again. If you are comparatively new to dieting, this should not be too big a problem. It may take a little longer, however, if you have been low-calorie dieting for many years. Nevertheless, it is never too late to begin eating properly.

So, what should we eat?

We now know that it is simplistic to claim that people get fat simply because they eat too much, although if you become overweight it is because you have consumed more energy than you have used. To understand obesity, you first need some knowledge of what happens to food and how the body metabolises and regulates energy.

Your body gets its energy from the foods – carbohydrates, proteins and fats – that you eat. Digestion breaks up foods into their constituent compounds. These are then utilised as they are or rebuilt to be used in all your body's processes.

To keep your heart beating, your body warm, your muscles working, and all the other processes going on requires a constant supply of energy (calories). As you cannot eat continuously 24 hours a day, your body ensures that energy is available at all times by storing it in several forms: as glucose in the blood, which is the most readily available; as glycogen, a form of starch, stored in muscles and liver; as lean tissue; and as fat.

Muscles burn both carbohydrate, in the form of glucose, and fat for energy; the heart uses only fat. If you use up more energy than you take in, your store of glycogen is used first and when that is exhausted body fat and lean tissue are cannibalised to provide the energy required. We have discussed carbohydrates already, so let's consider the other two macronutrients: proteins and fats.

Proteins

Proteins are essential to the body, providing the material from which body cells are made and repaired. Proteins are composed of chains of amino acids. There are hundreds of these in nature. Our bodies use around 20, which can be arranged in an almost infinite number of ways. Amino acids are usually split into two groups: *essential* and *non-essential*. The essential amino acids are those that the body cannot make for itself and which must be present in food. There are eight of them. If a protein contains the eight essential amino acids, in the correct proportions, it is called a *complete protein*; if it does not, it is said to be an *incomplete protein*.

Complete proteins are found in meat, fish, eggs, and dairy products. Animal proteins, which are complete, have a high biological value for man. As we are part of the animal kingdom and composed of similar material to other animals, we can use animal proteins with the minimum of waste.

Sources of *incomplete proteins* are cereals, nuts, seeds and legumes. Proportions of amino acids in any one of these types of vegetable food differ markedly from those we need. Maize is deficient in tryptophan, wheat is low in lysine and legumes are low in methionine. Proteins from these vegetable sources are said to be 'of low biological value'. It is necessary, therefore, to combine several vegetable protein sources, fairly accurately, to ensure that the body receives the right amino acid mixture.

In practical terms, it is not too difficult to combine vegetables to meet our bodies' protein requirements. In these circumstances, the real advantage of meat over the vegetables is their associated nutrients: vitamin B, vitamin D, iron, calcium and the more complex fatty acids.

As far as weight loss is concerned there is one other advantage to getting your proteins from animal sources: combining the various sources of incomplete proteins to supply all the essential amino-acids on a vegetarian diet could lead to a high intake of carbohydrates.

Your body needs proteins continually, but it cannot store them in any quantity. Therefore you should eat proteins regularly on a daily basis, and at the same meal, in quantities proportional to your size, but they must be complete proteins: if only one of the essential amino acids is missing, the cell rebuilding process will abort.

Daily protein requirements

Your body needs complete proteins every day, and with proteins come calories. The average woman could realistically get her protein needs from the foods in the table opposite. (Although I do not advocate a low-fat diet, I have deliberately made this example typical of the kinds of foods dieters are advised to eat to illustrate realistically the extent of the danger of malnutrition if you cut calories too much.)

Table 12.2 Example of how to obtain your minimum daily protein requirements

	Protein (grams)	Calories
125 grams lean meat	30	250
1 egg	6	75
570 ml (1 pint) semi-skimmed milk	19	275
50 grams cottage cheese	12	185
2 slices bread	7	120
Total	**74**	**905**

Men by contrast need about 25 to 50 grams more meat or another egg. Your body also needs a certain amount of fat: if only to supply the essential fatty acids needed for proper brain function, you must eat at least 15 grams of these per day. That adds another 135 calories, but as the foods in the examples above all contain these fats, the calories they contain are already included.

It is clear that a 1000-calorie diet, for instance, must be composed almost exclusively of foods which are very high in protein and fats if you are to take in the minimum amount of these nutrients to be healthy. Therefore a crash diet supplying less than, say, 1000 calories a day is almost certainly harmful to health; and the low-fat, high-carbohydrate slimming diets advocated today cannot help but be dangerously deficient in protein.

The importance of fat

The science of nutrition is highly complex and, even today, little is known about the vital part that fat plays in our health and well-being. Nutrients interact: a deficiency of one can have a profound effect on the metabolism of others. Today, a lack of dietary fat probably causes a wider range of abnormalities than deficiencies of any other single nutrient.

Fat provides more energy than carbohydrate. But it does much more: it contains lipids used in the brain and nervous system, without which we become irritable and aggressive; sterols, precursors of a number of hormones (including the sex hormones); and it is essential if we are to use the fat-soluble vitamins A, D, E and K. These vitamins can be found in other foods, but without the presence of dietary fat, the body cannot metabolise them.

Fat has a high calorific value, which is why all modern low-calorie diets restrict fats, but this can be dangerous and self-defeating. Restriction of dietary fat causes a range of problems including dry skin and eczema, damage to ovaries in females, infertility in males, kidney damage, and weight gain through water retention in the body. When there is little or no fat in the gut, there is nothing to stimulate the production of bile, the gallbladder is not emptied and the bile is held in reserve. This leads to the formation of gallstones. If a fat-free diet is continued for a long time, the gallbladder – a necessary part of the digestive system – may atrophy.

Malabsorption of the fat-soluble vitamins A, D, E and K has consequences for yet more nutrients. If vitamin D and fat are not present in the intestine, for example, calcium is not absorbed. For a woman, whose chance of suffering from osteoporosis is high, this is an important consideration. Dieters are usually told to drink skimmed milk. This has the advantage, they are told, that it contains more calcium than full-cream milk. This is true, but skimmed milk does not contain fat. As a consequence, only about 5% of the calcium in skimmed milk is absorbed, compared to around 50% from full-cream milk. This small absorption of calcium is reduced still further if the skimmed milk is eaten with a bran-laden breakfast cereal. Calcium-enriched milk sold in supermarkets may seem worth the extra expense but it is invariably calcium-enriched *skimmed* milk and, without the cream, most of that extra calcium is simply excreted.

Fat is best

- All body cells require a continuous supply of various fatty acids. If insufficient quantities are supplied from food, the body tries to make them from sugar. This causes blood sugar levels to fall, you feel very hungry and eat more, generally of the wrong things – and gain weight.
- Fat also has a satiety value: it takes longer to digest and stops you feeling hungry. Eat 100 calories less fat at a meal and you will probably feel hungry so quickly that you will eat three times as many calories – in the form of sugary or starchy foods, because they are convenient.
- It seems that the gut's nutrient-measuring system works so well with fat that it is difficult, if not impossible, to eat too much of it. Try, and you will make yourself sick, but for the same reason eating fat stops you eating too much in total. If your body needs 10 grams of fat, your appetite will not be satisfied until you have consumed those 10 grams of fat. If you eat those 10 grams as 25 grams (1 oz) of

Cheddar cheese, you will take in about 125 calories. If you eat them as wholemeal bread thinly spread with a very low-fat spread, you will need to eat eight slices – a total of about 200 calories!

Conclusion

If the global problem of overweight and obesity, as well the 'epidemics' of other related diseases is to be conquered, it is essential that our bodies' regulatory systems are retuned to a state of normality; that they are allowed to work as Nature intended. For this to happen, it will take a paradigm shift by the establishment. We must reduce carb intake and increase fats.

However, it is important that you eat the right – the healthy – fats. As this is where much of the confusion about fats is found today, these are discussed in the next chapters.

References

1. Sigal RJ, El-Hashimy M, Martin BC, et al. Acute postchallenge hyperinsulinemia predicts weight gain: a prospective study. *Diabetes* 1997; 46:1025–1029.
2. Odeleye OE, de Courten M, Pettitt DJ, Ravussin E. Fasting hyperinsulinemia is a predictor of increased body weight gain and obesity in Pima Indian children. *Diabetes* 1997; 46: 1341–1345.
3. Meijssen S, Cabezas MC, Ballieux CG, et al. Insulin mediated inhibition of hormone sensitive lipase activity in vivo in relation to endogenous catecholamines in healthy subjects. *J Clin Endocrinol Metab* 2001; 86: 4193–4197.
4. Bruning JC, Gautam D, Burks DJ, et al. Role of brain insulin receptor in control of body weight and reproduction. *Science* 2000; 289: 2122–2125.
5. Heini AF, Weinsier RL. Divergent trends in obesity and fat intake patterns: the American paradox. *Am J Med* 1997; 102: 259–264.
6. Kekwick A. The metabolism of fat. *J R Coll Gen Pract* 1967; 13 (Suppl 7): 95.
7. Feinman RD, Fine EJ. Thermodynamics and metabolic advantage of weight loss diets. *Metabol Syndr Relat Disord* 2003; 1: 209–219.
8. Finley JW, Leveille GA, Klemman LP, et al. Growth method for estimating the caloric availability of fats and oils. *J Agric Food Chem* 1994; 42: 489–494.
9. Livesy G. A perspective on food energy standards for nutrition labelling. *Br J Nutr* 2001; 85:271–287.
10. Ottoboni A, Ottoboni F. *The Modern Nutritional Diseases: heart disease, stroke, type-2 diabetes, obesity, cancer, and how to prevent them.* Vincente Books, Sparks, Nevada. 2002.

11. Young C. Weight loss on 1800 kcal diets varying in carbohydrate content. *Am J Clin Nutr* 1971; 290–296.

12. Pi-Sunyer, F.X. A review of long-term studies evaluating the efficacy of weight loss in ameliorating disorders associated with obesity. *Clin Therapeut* 1996; 18: 1006–1035.

13. Shimomura Y, et al. Opiate receptors, food intake and obesity. *Physiol Behav* 1982; 28: 441.

14. Prentice AM, Jebb SA, Black AE. Extrinsic sugar as a vehicle for dietary fat. *Lancet* 1995; 346: 695.

15. a. Himms-Hagen J. Obesity may be due to a malfunctioning of brown fat. *Can Med Assn J* 1979; 121: 1361.

     b. Thyroid hormones and thermogenesis. In: Girardier L, NI Stock, eds. *Mammalian Thermogenesis*. Chapman and Hall, London, 1983.

     c. Rothwell NJ, Stock NJ. A role for brown adipose tissue in diet-induced thermogenesis. *Nature* 1979; 281: 31.

     d. Schutz Y, et al. Diet-induced thermogenesis measured over a whole day in obese and non-obese women. *Am J Clin Nutr* 1984; 40: 542.

16. Rissanen A, Kaprio J, Sarna S, Koshenvuo M. Department of Public Health, University of Helsinki, 5th European Congress on Obesity, 10–12 June 1992.

17. Rookus MA, Burema J, Frijters JE. Changes in body mass index in young adults in relation to number of life events experienced. *Int J Obes* 1988; 12: 29–39.

Chapter Thirteen

Why blame cholesterol?

Reluctance to admit that any aspect of health may be better elsewhere than in the United States is an obstacle to proper evaluation of the problem of prevention of ischemic heart disease.

Dr Ancel Keys

Of all our nutritional mantras, the one most widely and emphatically proclaimed is the relationship between saturated fats and coronary artery disease. You would think a 'fact' so ingrained in our social psyche would be supported by mountains of evidence. It isn't.

For many years I have been concerned with the way in which saturated fats have been cited as a cause of heart disease, despite the complete lack of evidence that they do. Animal fats are referred to as saturated fats – but they only contain *some* saturated fatty acids; all saturated fatty acids are lumped together as though they all function in an identical manner; and while we are told that higher HDL levels are a good thing, saturated fatty acids that raise HDL levels are ignored. People were advised to switch from butter to margarine and now, despite the fact that the dangers of *trans*-fatty acids that these margarines contain have been recognised for over a decade, no agency that promoted their consumption is willing to risk losing face by admitting 'oops, sorry, we made a mistake'. It seems they would rather risk your health.

The current 'healthy' dietary experiment aimed at reducing heart disease – and it is only an experiment – is a disaster not just because it has so dramatically increased the numbers of cases of obesity and diabetes, but because it has also increased the numbers of people suffering from the very disease against which it was aimed!

The reality is that the data to support the 'diet–heart' hypothesis lies somewhere between flimsy and non-existent. In an extensive review of the literature, a Swedish professor, Uffe Ravnskov, who specialises in this field of medicine, came to the conclusion that:

> 'Few observations agree with the diet–heart idea, but a large number have been falsified most effectively. Man's diet possibly includes factors of importance to the vessels or the heart, but there is little evidence that saturated fatty acids as a group are harmful or that polyunsaturated fatty acids as a group are beneficial.'[1]

In a similar review, Dr Mary Enig, Consulting Editor to the *Journal of the American College of Nutrition*, and a world-renowned expert on fats and oils, was also unable to find any causal relationship between saturated fats and heart disease. Dr Enig says:

> 'The idea that saturated fats cause heart disease is completely wrong, but the statement has been "published" so many times over the last three or more decades that it is very difficult to convince people otherwise unless they are willing to take the time to read and learn what . . . produced the anti-saturated fat agenda.'[2]

Dr Enig came to the conclusion that the causative factor was much more likely to be the inordinate increase in *trans*-fatty acid consumption from vegetable margarines and cooking oils. These are the so-called 'healthy' ones.

Conventional wisdom tells us that high levels of blood cholesterol are to blame for the alarming incidence of heart disease throughout the industrialised world, and that animal fats are the cause of that elevated cholesterol. There is now such a strong 'cholesterolphobia' engendered by establishment propaganda in the population over the past several decades that 'fat', once called 'the most valuable food known to Man', by the late Dr John Yudkin, Professor of Nutrition and Dietetics at London

University, has now been turned into a 'four letter word'. We have all been brainwashed into believing that eating foods with any type of fat is a heart attack on a plate, despite the fact that saturated and mono-unsaturated fats have *never* been shown to cause heart disease, but have been shown to protect against this and many other serious diseases.

'Protein-Rich Diets May Reduce Heart Disease Risk': This was the headline in the August 3, 1999 edition of *The Medical Tribune*. It was reporting findings from the Nurses' Health Study, a study which began in 1976 to evaluate lifestyle factors and health among more than 120,000 female nurses aged 30 to 55.[3]

The researchers, led by Dr Frank Hu, said that this study 'strongly rejects' the theory that high-protein diets may promote heart disease. In fact, the researchers at Harvard Medical School discovered that women with the highest protein intakes were 26% less likely than those who ate the least protein to develop coronary heart disease. The study also found that a menu rich in animal and vegetable proteins may actually cut heart disease risk, and it didn't matter how much fat they ate.

Meat and dairy products, as well as certain vegetable oils such as coconut and palm oils, are the main sources of dietary saturated fats. Because saturated fats were thought to raise blood levels of cholesterol, it was thought that diets rich in animal products might promote heart disease. Therefore, we were taught to reduce our fat intake, especially from animal fats, and replace these with carbohydrates, but the Nurses' Health Study and other studies showed that this approach is wrong.

The British should eat more fat

Throughout our history a healthy diet was one which was based mainly on foods of animal origin and high in fat. Where the major health problems occurred in Britain, it was not among people who ate a lot of fat, but in those who did not get enough. The comparatively wealthy, who ate meat and dairy produce regularly, had average lifespans which were comparable with or better than those of today. It was the poor who could not afford such foods who suffered high levels of infant mortality, poor growth and shorter, less healthy lives.

In the 1920s, Sir John Boyd Orr conducted a number of studies which compared growth rates of children in public schools with those in the state-run schools.[4] He found that those from wealthier backgrounds were significantly taller than their poorer peers. After examining their relative diets and changing the constituents, Boyd Orr proved conclusively that children of the socially deprived, who lived on a largely carbohydrate diet of bread and potatoes, benefited from a diet supplemented with full-cream milk.

Boyd Orr's studies found confirmation in observations among the peoples of India made by Sir Robert McCarrison, a colonial medical officer. He compared the southern Indians, who ate very little in the way of dairy produce and who were of stunted growth and prone to disease, with their neighbours to the north, the Sikhs who drank a great deal of milk and were fit and healthy.[5] Similar research in Africa contrasted the tall, slender and healthy Maasai, who lived almost exclusively on blood and milk, with their unhealthy vegetarian neighbours, the Kikuyu.[6] That added to the weight of evidence.

Boyd Orr concluded that the food intake of half the British population was seriously deficient in a number of what he called 'protective constituents' which were necessary for good health. In the late 1930s he proposed that the British people should drink more milk, and eat more dairy produce and meat. The British government of the time recommended that milk consumption should be doubled and introduced free school milk. The British Medical Association, giving specific amounts, advised that the population should consume 80% more milk, 55% percent more eggs, 40% more butter and 30% more meat. Later, with the advent of television advertising, the government sponsored its own 'go to work on an egg' campaign.

Except for the period of food rationing during the 1940s and early 1950s, Boyd Orr's recommended diet was the standard British fare. We ate breakfasts of eggs and fatty bacon fried in lard; dripping, the fat from the Sunday roast, was saved to have on bread and toast; we drank full-cream milk and ate butter. Only the poor ate margarine; and only the poor had high levels of disease. The recommendations to eat a relatively high-fat, high-animal protein diet led to a spectacular decrease in diseases: rickets, called the 'English Disease' because it was so widespread, together with other deficiency diseases largely disappeared from our lives; child deaths from diphtheria, measles, scarlet fever and whooping cough also fell dramatically well before the introduction of antibiotics and widespread immunisation. Although other factors helped, most important was the higher resistance of children to disease that followed from better nutrition. That dietary advice, given to the people of Britain in 1938 remained the basis of our diet for nearly 50 years, during which time our mean life expectancy increased from 60 years in 1930 to 70 years by 1960 and by 1990 it had reached 75 years.

Cholesterol and heart disease

However, a dramatic change was to come. In the 1920s a new disease – which we now call coronary heart disease (CHD) – suddenly took off all over the Western industrialised world. By the 1940s it had become a major cause of premature death – and nobody knew why. Doctors were both puzzled as to the cause and worried by it. Heart attacks occur when an insufficient supply of blood and oxygen reaches the heart. It was known that this could be due to the build-up of fatty deposits in the arteries which supply the heart. The problem was that there are no symptoms associated with the partial blockage of the coronary arteries, so how could doctors tell, without a direct examination of those arteries, who was in danger? They had to find what was different in those with the disease and those free of it. Cutting people open wasn't an option; it was a problem that seemed to have no solution.

In 1950 a team of American doctors led by Dr John Gofman, hypothesised that blood cholesterol was to blame.[7] Quickly, trials were conducted on rabbits to verify the truth of this hypothesis and, sure enough, those rabbits fed a high-cholesterol diet developed blockages in their arteries. However, the rabbit is a herbivore; such a diet is quite alien to the creature and several scientists pointed out that the results were more likely to be an allergic reaction to the unnatural diet.

Another American doctor, Ancel Keys, pointed out the error of this approach when he wrote in 1956:

> 'For many years there was argument as to whether cholesterol in the diet promotes atherosclerosis in man. One cause of the disagreement resided in the persistent error in attributing to man the same responses seen in rabbits and chicks fed large amounts of cholesterol. The other major source of confusion was the fact that most human high-cholesterol diets are also high-fat diets. *It is now clear that dietary cholesterol per se, which is contained in almost all foods of animal origin, has little or no effect on the serum cholesterol concentration in man*'.[8] (emphasis added)

Nevertheless, based on this one study and despite the lack of evidence from human studies, Gofman and colleagues said 'Preliminary evidence indicates that exogenous cholesterol in the human as well as in the rabbit is a factor . . .'

Is cholesterol really to blame?

What Gofman's group had missed was that blood cholesterol had already been considered as a possible cause of heart disease 14 years earlier – and ruled out.

A study to look at the effects of blood cholesterol on the coronary arteries was published in 1936 by Drs Kurt Landé and Warren Sperry of New York University's Department of Forensic Medicine.[9] They measured the amounts of cholesterol in a large number of accident victims' blood and, by dissecting their arteries, measured their degree of atherosclerosis (furring up of the arteries). Landé and Sperry fully expected to find that the two were related. What they found, to their surprise, was

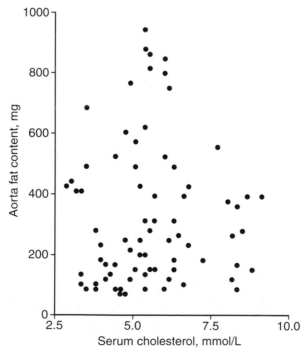

Figure 4   Blood cholesterol and atherosclerosis[9]

that there was absolutely no relation between the amount of cholesterol in the blood and the degree of atherosclerosis (see Fig. 4). Landé and Sperry were very cautious, thorough and methodical; their study was well conducted. If those who later promoted the idea that blood cholesterol were to blame for CHD had read this paper before they began their research, they might well have dropped the idea right there.

Dietary fat

It was Ancel Keys who in 1953 suggested that a fatty diet might play a part as a cause of CHD.[10] Using data from just six countries, Keys compared the death rates from CHD and the amounts of fats eaten in those countries to demonstrate, he said, that heart disease mortality was higher in the countries that consumed more fat than it was in those countries that consumed less. As Figure 5 shows, there is an almost perfect fit, and so the 'diet/heart' hypothesis was born.

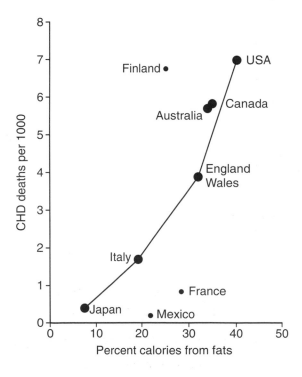

Figure 5   Heart deaths and fat intake[10]

However, at that time, data from another 16 countries were available. If they are added the picture is a lot less clear. For example, Finland near the top has seven times as many deaths as France, yet Finns eat less fat.

Despite its faults, some of which didn't become apparent until later, Keys had what looked like a plausible hypothesis to explain the high levels of heart disease in some countries. However, anyone can have an idea; what you have to do then is prove it. In medicine, the usual way is to select two groups of people, as identical for sex, age, and lifestyle as possible. One group, called the *intervention group*, tries the new diet, drug or whatever, while the other, called the *control group*, carries on as normal. After a suitable time, the two groups are compared and differences noted.

Keys' 'fatty diet causes heart disease' hypothesis was persuasive. To test it, many large-scale, long-term, human intervention studies were set up in many parts of the world. These involved hundreds of thousands of subjects and hundreds of doctors and scientists and cost billions of dollars in an attempt to prove that a fatty diet caused heart disease.

The longest running and most respected is the Framingham Heart Study. This study was set up in the town of Framingham, Massachusetts, by Harvard University Medical School in 1948 and is still going on today. It was this study that gave rise to many of the other 'risk factors' with which we all are so familiar today: smoking, lack of exercise and so on. The Framingham researchers thought that they knew exactly why some people had more cholesterol in their blood than others – they ate more in their diet. To prove the link, they measured cholesterol intake and compared it with blood cholesterol. As Table 13.1 shows, although subjects consumed cholesterol over a wide range, there was little or no difference in the levels of cholesterol in their blood and, thus, no relationship between the amount of cholesterol eaten and levels of blood cholesterol was found.

Table 13.1 Cholesterol intake – The Framingham Heart Study

	Cholesterol intake (mg/day)	**Blood cholesterol in those below median intake (mmol/L)**	**Blood cholesterol in those above median intake (mmol/L)**
Men	704 ± 220.9	6.16	6.16
Women	492 ± 170.0	6.37	6.26

Next, the scientists studied intakes of saturated fats but again they could find no relation. There was still no relation when they studied total calorie intake. The researchers then considered the possibility that something was masking the effects of diet, but no other factor made the slightest difference. After 22 years of research, the researchers concluded:

> 'There is, in short, no suggestion of any relation between diet and the subsequent development of CHD in the study group.'[11]

That was in 1970, and no finding since has changed that view.

The other studies also show little convincing correlation between either the amount of fat eaten and heart disease or the type of fat eaten and heart disease. Professor Uffe Ravnskov, a heart specialist from Lund University, Sweden, published a review in 1992 of studies published to that date. He concluded:

> 'Lowering serum cholesterol concentrations does not reduce mortality and is unlikely to prevent coronary heart disease. Claims of the opposite are based on preferential citation of supportive trials.'[12]

One that did seem to support the 'healthy' recommendations was a Finnish trial involving 1222 men published in 1985.[13] Men in the intervention group were seen regularly and advised about diet, physical activity and smoking. If they had high blood pressure or high cholesterol levels, it was treated with drugs. The predicted risks for CHD were halved during the trial and, even though there were more non-fatal coronary events and more cardiac deaths in the intervention group, it was hailed as a success because 'The program markedly improved the risk factor status.' In December 1991, the results of a 15-year follow-up to that trial were published.[14] During this period the intervention group continued to be instructed on diet, smoking and exercise and treated for high blood pressure and cholesterol when present. Were they healthier? Did they live longer? The results are shown in Table 13.2.

Table 13.2 Deaths during 15-year follow-up

	Intervention group	Control group
Total deaths	67	46
Heart disease deaths	34	14

Not only do these figures show that those people who continued to follow the carefully controlled, cholesterol-lowering diet had more deaths in total, they were more than twice as likely to die of heart disease as those who didn't – some success!

   Dr Michael Oliver, Professor of Cardiology at Edinburgh University's Cardiovascular Research Unit, commenting on these results in the *British Medical Journal*, wrote:[15]

> 'As multiple intervention against risk factors for coronary heart disease in middle aged men at only moderate risk seem to have failed to reduce both morbidity and mortality such interventions become increasingly difficult to justify. This runs counter to the recommendations of many national and international advisory bodies which must now take the recent findings from Finland into consideration. Not to do so may be ethically unacceptable. . . We must now face the fact that the evidence from large, well conducted trials gives little support to hopes that altering the lifestyle of the community at large, when started in middle age, will reduce cardiac deaths or total mortality.'

Saturated fats are healthier than polyunsaturated

In his 1956 paper, Ancel Keys had noted:

> 'It has been reported that patients on a formula diet providing a very high percentage [up to 85%] of corn oil, which is highly unsaturated, and no other fats and no carbohydrates, show substantial declines in the serum cholesterol concentration. This might mean either that great quantities of corn oil specifically depress the serum cholesterol or that some factor in the fats in ordinary diets maintains the serum level at higher levels.'

This led to the assertion that polyunsaturated vegetable fats would be healthier. No one took any notice when the Tecumseh Study found that blood cholesterol levels were the same no matter what type of fats were eaten.[16]

   What they also missed was that Keys had also written 'and no carbohydrates'. Having decided, without any corroborating evidence, that fats were to blame, they completely overlooked the fact that the people who didn't have heart disease were also on diets that contained low levels of carbohydrate.

In view of the results of the Tecumseh Study, it seems that type of fat probably doesn't matter as far as heart disease is concerned. The significant factor is carbohydrate intake, but not one of the many intervention studies conducted around the world at that time even considered carbs; they were concerned only with fats.

This is a good example of where, if you don't ask the right questions, you won't get the right answers. The right answers are essential in this case because, while polyunsaturated fats might lower cholesterol, that's not much use if they also increase the risk of a heart attack.

Scientists at the Wynn Institute for Metabolic Research, London, UK, compared the fatty-acid composition of artery blockages. What they found was a high proportion of both omega-3 and omega-6 polyunsaturated fatty acids; what they did *not* find was saturated fatty acids. In their conclusions they say: 'These findings imply a direct influence of dietary polyunsaturated fatty acids . . . and suggest that current trends favouring increased intake of polyunsaturated fatty acids should be reconsidered.'[17]

The animal fats called 'saturated' by the ignorant, are actually mostly *un*saturated. For example, pork fat (lard) is 57% unsaturated, eggs are 65% unsaturated, as is chicken fat; even beef fat is 55% unsaturated. The most saturated fat in Nature is coconut oil, which is over 90% saturated. Yet, until they started to eat Western foods, Pacific islanders, who call the coconut the 'tree of life' and eat coconuts in large amounts, had no history of heart disease – or any other chronic degenerative disease.

Cholesterol and women

Women seem to worry more about their cholesterol levels than men. Yet, for women, research has demonstrated that a high cholesterol level is healthier than a low one. In 1992 a report of 19 major studies published over the previous 20 years suggested that public policy for reducing blood cholesterol should be reviewed. The report's author, Dr Stephen Hulley, published figures showing the relative risk of death from all causes associated with levels of blood cholesterol in men and women. As can be seen in Figure 6, it is clear that risk increases as blood cholesterol levels fall.[18] Dr Hulley states:

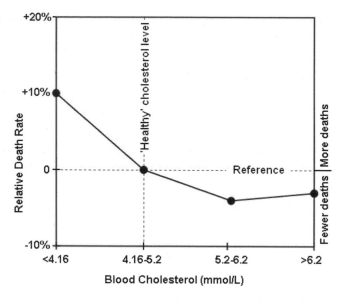

Figure 6   Blood cholesterol and total mortality

'We are coming to realise that the resulting cardiovascular research, which represents the great majority of the effort so far, may not apply to women.'

This confirmed a study published three years earlier in which Dr Bernard Forette and a team of researchers in Paris found that elderly women with very high cholesterol levels lived the longest. They also showed that the death rate for women who had very low levels of cholesterol in their blood was more than five times higher.[19] In their report, the French doctors warned against lowering cholesterol in elderly women, but they could just as well have warned against cholesterol lowering in women at any age.

What about people who have already had a heart attack?

People who have had one heart attack are obviously in the high-risk group. They are invariably told by their doctors to cut out butter and use polyunsaturated margarines instead, but is there evidence that this will prolong their lives? No! In fact the opposite is shown. As long ago as 1965 survival rates were studied in patients eating different fats and oils.[20] In this study, patients who had already had a heart attack were assigned to one of three groups. These were given polyunsaturated corn oil, mono-unsaturated olive oil or saturated animal fats respectively. Blood cholesterol levels were lowered by an average of 30% in the polyunsaturated group, while there was no change in the other two groups. At first sight, therefore, it seemed that men in the polyunsaturated group had the best chance of survival. However, at the end of the trial only 52% of the polyunsaturated group were still alive and free of a second heart attack. Those in the mono-unsaturated group fared little better: 57% survived and had no further attack. But the saturated animal fats group fared the best with 75% surviving and without a further attack. So yet again, saturated fat turns out to be the healthiest.

So why are we still trying to lower cholesterol?

Good question. The Framingham Heart study's first pronouncement wasn't until 1970. But people were dying of heart disease and the arguments for fat being a cause were compelling. In 1968, Dr J.B. Hickie from Melbourne, Australia, suggested that the situation was too urgent to wait for convincing evidence from organised trials.[21] He estimated that by changing diet and taking more exercise, mortality from heart disease would drop by 40% in men over 40 years of age. Many other doctors had similar faith.

However, the only evidence published to that date had come from useless animal trials. Landé and Sperry's study was in the archives so, by now, probably none of the proponents had even heard of it. By the time the large human intervention studies were published in the 1970s and 1980s, doctors had been telling people to cut down on fats to prevent heart disease for so long that they couldn't reverse their advice without risking losing face and credibility.

In 1983 Dr Michael Oliver reminded doctors:

> 'Oliver Cromwell wrote in 1650 . . . "I beseech you, in the bowels of Christ, think it possible you may be mistaken." This admonition might now be appropriately addressed to some of the epidemiologists and the many over-enthusiastic health educators concerned with the prevention of coronary heart disease, for the evidence against substantial benefit to the community from multiple risk factor intervention is increasing.'[22]

You won't be surprised to learn that Professor Oliver went unheeded. The juggernaut had already started to roll the previous year when the American Heart Association published its dietary guidelines which recommended a reduction of fat intake and a change to polyunsaturated oils.[23] Britain followed immediately when in 1983, the National Advisory Committee on Nutrition Education (NACNE) published a discussion paper which suggested cutting fat intake,[24] and the following year the Committee on Medical Aspects of Food Policy (COMA) published official guidelines for dietary policy.[25] All three were remarkably similar.

In 1986 Professor Oliver pointed out that:

> 'Cardiologists and physicians throughout the world are being persuaded by health educationalists . . . that the only way to prevent CHD is to endorse and promulgate changes in lifestyle by the public at large. Such is the force of the juggernaut set forth . . . that little credence is given to genuine scientific scepticism. One result is that there are increasing numbers in the medical-scientific community who regard those of their number who dare to question whether health education has or is likely to reduce the incidence of CHD as irresponsible. Much of the faith in the value of changing lifestyles is little more than wishful thinking.'

But by now the 'fatty diet causes heart disease' dogma was official. Nothing would be allowed to stop it.

Low cholesterol is bad for the young and old alike

In 1991 the US National Cholesterol Education Programme recommended that children over two years old should adopt a low-fat, low-cholesterol diet to prevent CHD in later life. A Table showing a good correlation between fat and cholesterol intakes and blood cholesterol in seven to nine-year-old boys from six countries was published to support this advice. What it did not show, however, was the strong correlation between blood cholesterol and childhood deaths in those countries.[26] As is clearly demonstrated in Table 13.3, the death rate rises dramatically as blood cholesterol levels fall.

Table 13.3 Blood cholesterol and mortality in under-5s in six countries

	Blood cholesterol (mmol/L)	Childhood deaths (per 1000)
Finland	4.9	7
Netherlands	4.5	9
USA	4.3	12
Italy	4.1	12
Philippines	3.8	72
Ghana	3.3	145

Two studies, which considered total blood cholesterol levels and mortality in the elderly, were published in the *Lancet* almost simultaneously in 1997. In the first, scientists working at Leiden University's Medical Centre found that 'each 1 mmol/L increase in total cholesterol corresponded to a 15% decrease in mortality'.[27] Similarly, doctors at Reykjavik Hospital and Heart Preventive Clinic in Iceland noted that the major studies had not included the elderly. They too studied total mortality and blood cholesterol in men over 80 to show that those with blood cholesterol levels over 6.5 mmol/L had less than half the death rate (48%) of those whose cholesterol level was a 'healthy' 5.2 mmol/L.[28]

Studies in Japan added even more weight to this argument. Japan is reported to have low levels of death from coronary heart disease but Okinawa has the lowest of all. Blood cholesterol levels are generally low in Japan, but Okinawan levels are much higher – similar to those in Scotland. In 1992, a paper examined the relationship of nutritional status to further life expectancy and health in the Japanese elderly based on three population studies.[29] It found that Japanese who lived to the age of 100 were those who got their protein from meat rather than from rice and pulses. The centenarians also had higher intakes of animal foods such as eggs, milk, meat and fish; significantly, their carbohydrate intake was lower than that of their fellow countrymen who died younger.

These comparisons are important, as Japan might not actually have the low levels of heart disease deaths that have been attributed to it. Although heart disease deaths are reportedly low, deaths from stroke and cerebral haemorrhage are very high. Keys attributed the lowest levels of heart deaths to Japan in his studies. These findings have been used to support recommendations that we should adopt Japanese eating patterns based on fish and rice, but vital statistics from death certificates are too unreliable for scientific use. One of the recognised facts about Japanese statistics is that at the time of the Keys Study the cause of many deaths was not certified by a qualified doctor. Another is that coronary heart disease was regarded as an undesirable cause of death; stroke was a more desirable one as it was thought to be indicative of intelligence in the family. More recent autopsies have revealed that stroke is not as common as once believed and that heart disease is much more common than original figures suggested.[30] This is a typical example of why vital statistics used by Keys and others may be unreliable.

However, if we lump deaths from all causes together, we get a figure that cannot be fudged. Comparing average age at death from all causes and food intake, we find that the Japanese who live longest are the ones who eat the most animal products and the least carbs.

What is cholesterol?

Having discussed cholesterol and heart disease, you might like to know just what cholesterol is and what it does. The first thing to note is that cholesterol is not a fat: chemically it is an alcohol. Cholesterol is one of a number of 'sterols' widely distributed in plants and animals (although cholesterol is found only in animals). Cholesterol is ingested in animal products; the richest sources being brain, fish roe, eggs, liver, hard cheese and butter.

Because of the propaganda, you can be forgiven for thinking that cholesterol is a harmful, alien substance which should be avoided at all costs, but nothing could be further from the truth. Cholesterol is an essential component for many body processes:

- It is a major building block from which body cells are continually being made and repaired.
- It is found in all body cells, particularly in the brain and nerve cells, where it is essential for nerve transmission and for brain function.
- Its importance for brain function is so great that the brain has the ability to make its own supply of cholesterol.
- It is vital for keeping cell membranes throughout the body intact and permeable so that nutrients can pass into the cells, and waste products can leave them.

- If you radically restrict your cholesterol intake to the point that there is not enough cholesterol to repair and build tissue, cell growth is disrupted.
- It is used to maintain normal hormone production including the sex hormones in both men and women.
- It is essential for the proper functioning of the immune system.
- It is crucial for the manufacture of the important anti-stress factor, cortisol.
- It is used, in conjunction with sun on the skin, to make vitamin D3.
- It is so important that almost every body cell has the ability to make it.

'Good' and 'bad' cholesterol

At this point, let me scotch another myth: there is no such thing as 'good' and 'bad' cholesterol. Cholesterol is only one chemical compound and all cholesterol is exactly the same. Talking of 'LDL' and 'HDL' as if they were two different types of cholesterol is quite misleading.

Cholesterol is not water-soluble, so it cannot travel freely in the bloodstream to where it is needed. It has to be transported in conjunction with other materials, notably fats and proteins. LDL stands for 'low-density lipoprotein' and HDL is 'high-density lipoprotein'. Lipoprotein is a contraction of the words 'lipid', which encompasses cholesterol and all fats and waxes, and 'protein'. Neither LDL nor HDL is cholesterol; they are merely the carriers of cholesterol. So, when your doctor measures your cholesterol level, he is not making a definitive measurement but an informed guess.

LDL carries cholesterol made in the liver out around the body to where it is needed for cell repair, et cetera, and as the body abhors waste and is a great recycler, HDL carries 'second-hand' cholesterol from cells being replaced back to the liver for re-use. Neither HDL nor LDL is 'bad'; both are essential.

Eat as much cholesterol as you like

Your body can absorb only about 300 mg of cholesterol per day from the foods you eat and, as your body needs many times that amount, it then makes up the difference. Although the major proportion – up to 3000 mg a day – is manufactured in the liver, almost all body cells can manufacture cholesterol. For this reason, if you cut down on the amount of cholesterol you eat, all that happens is that your body makes more. You can eat as much as five times the usual 300 mg without it having any effect on the amount of cholesterol in your blood, so it really doesn't matter how much cholesterol you eat; whatever that amount is, it will certainly be less than your body needs.

Conclusion

In the 1990s a new class of cholesterol-lowering drugs, called statins, were developed to lower cholesterol. And they were remarkably successful in doing so. Professor Oliver told me that in the light of such advances in medical research, he would not now make the statement he made earlier. However, I think we should bear in mind that heart disease is not caused by a deficiency of a drug, but an incorrect lifestyle, as is evidenced by the many populations who take no drugs and among whom heart disease is unknown.

Although the media and food companies still warn against cholesterol in your diet, it has been repeatedly demonstrated that the amount of cholesterol you eat has little or no effect on the level of cholesterol in your blood.

This book does not have the scope to discuss all the trials and studies in detail. However, what it all boils down to is this:

- High cholesterol is said to be dangerous for Americans and Britons but not for Canadians, Stockholmers, Russians, Japanese or Maori.
- High cholesterol is said to be dangerous for men, but not for women.
- High cholesterol is said to be dangerous for healthy men, but not for coronary patients.
- High cholesterol is said to be dangerous for men of 30, but not for those older than 47.
- High cholesterol is beneficial for older people of both sexes.

'Such discrepancies', says Dr Ravnskov, 'indicate that the association between high cholesterol and CHD is not due to simple cause and effect. The most likely interpretation is that high cholesterol is not dangerous in itself, but that it is a marker for something else.'

What has become quite clear is that blood cholesterol is a relatively poor predictor of who will have a heart attack. It is also clear now that the hypothesis that a fried breakfast is a 'heart attack on a plate' is based more on myth and wishful thinking than on any coherent body of supportive evidence.

This is the shaky basis for an enormous 'health' industry which is proving to be such an unmitigated disaster as, since 'healthy eating' was introduced two decades ago, the numbers of cases of obesity, diabetes and the other diseases listed in Appendix A have all risen. This is not a coincidence; it is a classic case of cause and effect.

Incidentally, you will be pleased to know that Dr Broda Barnes of Colorado State University, in a paper entitled *A Practical Diet For Weight Reduction*, noted that:

'No heart attacks have occurred during the use of diets rich in saturated fats for over 25 years.'[31]

References

1. Ravnskov U. The Questionable Role of Saturated and Polyunsaturated Fatty Acids in Cardiovascular Disease. *J Clin Epidemiol* 1998; 51:443–460.
2. Enig M. Diet, serum cholesterol and coronary heart disease. In: Mann G, ed. *Coronary Heart Disease*. Janus Publishing, London, 1993.
3. Hu FB, Stampfer MJ, Manson JE, et al. Dietary protein and risk of ischemic heart disease in women. *Am J Clin Nutr* 1999; 70: 221–227.
4. Orr J B. *Food, Health and Income*. Macmillan, London, 1936.
5. McCarrison R. Nutrition in health and disease. *BMJ* 1936; 26 September: p.611.
6. Orr JB, Gilks JL. *Studies of Nutrition: The Physique and Health of Two African Tribes*. HMSO, London, 1931.
7. Gofman JW, et al. The role of lipids and lipoproteins in atherosclerosis. *Science* 1950; 111: 166.
8. Keys A. The diet and the development of coronary heart disease. *J Chron Dis* 1956; 4: 364–380.
9. Landé KE, Sperry WM. Human atherosclerosis in relation to the cholesterol content of the blood serum. *Arch Path* 1936; 22: 301–312.
10. Keys A. Atherosclerosis: a problem in newer public health. *J Mt Sinai Hosp* 1953; 20: 118.
11. Kannel WB and Gordon T. *The Framingham Diet Study: diet and the regulations of serum cholesterol*, (Sect 24). Washington DC, Department of Health, Education and Welfare, 1970.
12. Ravnskov U. Cholesterol lowering trials in coronary heart disease: frequency of citation and outcome. *BMJ* 1992; 305: 15–19.
13. Miettinen TA, et al. Multifactorial primary prevention of cardiovascular diseases in middle-aged men. *JAMA* 1985; 254: 2097–2102.
14. Strandberg TE, Salomaa VV, Naukkarinen VA, et al. Long term mortality after 5-year multifactorial primary prevention of cardiovascular diseases in middle-aged men. *JAMA* 1991; 266: 1225–1229.

15. Oliver MF. Doubts about preventing coronary heart disease. *BMJ* 1992; 304: 393–394.
16. Nichols AB, et al. Daily nutritional intake and serum lipid levels: The Tecumseh Study. *Am J Clin Nutr* 1976; 29: 1384.
17. Felton CV, Crook D, Davies MJ, Oliver MF. Dietary polyunsaturated fatty acids and composition of human aortic plaques. *Lancet* 1994; 344:1195–1196.
18. Hulley S. Editorial on Conference on low blood cholesterol. *Circulation* 1992; 86 (3): 1026–1029.
19. Forette B, Tortrat D, Wolmark Y. Cholesterol as a risk factor for mortality in elderly women. *Lancet* 1989; I: 868–870.
20. Rose GA, et al. Corn oil in treatment of ischaemic heart disease. *BMJ* 1965; 1: 1531–1533.
21. Hickie JB. The prevention of coronary heart disease. *Med J Aust* 1968; 1: 159–166.
22. Oliver MF. Should we not forget about mass control of coronary risk factors? *Lancet* 1983; ii: 37–38.
23. Grundy SM, Bilheimer D, Blackburn H, et al. Rationale of the diet heart statement of the American Heart Association, report of the Nutrition Committee. *Circulation* 1982; 65: 839A–854A.
24. National Advisory Committee on Nutrition Education. *A Discussion Paper on Proposals for Nutritional Guidelines for Health Education in Britain.* HEC, 1983.
25. Committee on Medical Aspects of Food. *Diet and Cardiovascular Disease.* DHSS, London, 1984.
26. Child mortality under age 5 per 1000. *1992 Britannia Book of the Year.* Encyclopaedia Britannica, Chicago.
27. Weverling-Rijnsburger AWE, et al. Total cholesterol and risk of mortality in the oldest old. *Lancet* 1997; 350: 1119–1123.
28. Jonsson A, Sigvaldason H, Sigfusson N. Total cholesterol and mortality after age 80 years. *Lancet* 1997; 350: 1778–1779.
29. Shibata H, et al. Nutrition for the Japanese elderly. *Nutr Health* 1992; 8(2–3): 165–175.
30. Stehbens WE. *The Lipid Hypothesis of Atherogenesis.* RG Landes Co, Austin, Texas, 1993.
31. Barnes BO. A Practical Diet for Weight Reduction. *Federation Proceedings* 1965; 24: 314.

Note: There have been many, more recent studies confirming what is referenced here but the references above show how long helpful evidence has been available if only we were prepared to listen.

Chapter Fourteen

Why healthy eating isn't

> The tragedy of science is the slaying of a beautiful hypothesis by an ugly fact.
>
> *T.H. Huxley*

So the only basis for 'healthy eating' – that it may reduce the rates of heart disease – is a sham. That raises the questions of whether 'healthy eating' would be of benefit anyway; and whether it could be harmful. This chapter looks at this issue.

The main pillars of a 'healthy' diet are:

- **Eat five portions of fruit and vegetables a day.**
- **Base meals on starchy foods** such as bread, pasta, breakfast cereals and root vegetables.
- **Increase dietary fibre intake.**
- **Eat less fat**, particularly saturated fats from animal sources.
- **Change to polyunsaturated fats.** These fats, from vegetable sources, are claimed to lower cholesterol levels.

Eat five portions of fruit and vegetables a day

Some time ago I was making a documentary video. The then-current craze for low-carb diets, sparked by a sudden upsurge in the Atkins diet, was causing all kinds of confusion. The idea of the documentary was to sort out the truth from the hype and, hopefully, give some useful advice. I was the interviewer on the documentary as well as its nutrition consultant.

To get an all-round picture, we interviewed many dieters, medical practitioners and nutritionists/dieticians.

One of the dieticians, I'll call her Jane, came directly from the headquarters of a national nutrition organisation. During the interview, I asked Jane why her institution recommended five portions of fruit and vegetables a day. 'Because that's healthy eating,' she replied. 'Yes,' I said, 'but what is the evidence that recommendation is based on?' Jane told me that it was government advice. 'But,' I persisted, 'that isn't evidence.' I asked again which study or studies had shown that 'five portions' was necessary?' 'It's healthy eating', she replied. We continued in this vein for a few minutes but it was obvious that she had no idea why she recommended five portions.

I decided on another tack. The BDA and American Dietetic Association base their recommendations on The Framingham Heart Study. I knew that this study had been misrepresented so I decided to ask for her comments on the various pronouncements from Framingham that did not agree with the BDA's recommendations. I started by asking her: Would she agree that the Framingham Study was the world's most influential and respected study into the dietary causes of heart disease?

'What's the Framingham Study?' she asked. That stopped me in my tracks and, although I did ask further questions, it effectively finished the interview.

Jane was paid her fee and left. A week later her cheque was returned with a letter from her solicitor warning us that action would be taken if we used any part of her interview in the programme.

Jane's was not an isolated case. In the end, although we used material from all the doctors, we couldn't, in all conscience, use any material from any of the nutritionists/dieticians we interviewed without compromising their careers. It was obvious even to our camera crew that none of them knew their subject.

So what is the evidence for '5 portions a day'?

This is a question I found I could not answer until recently as there didn't seem to be any answer, but there is now, and it doesn't support the recommendations.

Fruit and vegetables are recommended to prevent heart disease and cancer because of their antioxidant properties – they are supposed to prevent the creation of harmful free radicals.

In 2002, scientists at the University of Helsinki studied the effects of high and low intakes of vegetables, berries, and apples on oxidation in subjects consuming diets high in the unsaturated fatty acids, linoleic or oleic acid, both of which are subject to oxidation.[1] What they found was that 'there were no significant differences between the diets'.

In 2003 the prestigious CARDIO2000 study published its results.[2] This study was looking specifically at intakes of fruit and vegetables with relation to heart disease. They found that fruit and vegetables did reduce the risk of heart disease, but significantly, it didn't need five portions a day for this effect. In their conclusions the researchers say 'Consumption of two or more servings per week is associated with about 70% reduction in relative risk.' There was no more benefit after that.

The Daily Mail reported this study and interviewed Professor Sir Charles George, medical director of the British Heart Foundation, about this obvious conflict with the '5-a-day' guidelines. Professor Sir Charles George answered 'There is some argument about how much you need. I think five may be an arbitrary figure.' By so doing, he admitted that this was another example of dietary advice which was based on nothing more than guesswork or wishful thinking.

So we don't need to eat anything like 5 a day to derive benefits in terms of heart disease, but is there a benefit in terms of other chronic diseases such as cancer? This, too, was considered in another study, published in 2004, of over 100,000 people. Conducted by the Harvard School of Public Health, it showed that, 'Increased fruit and vegetable consumption was associated with a modest *although not statistically significant* reduction in the development of major chronic disease' (emphasis added). The 'major chronic disease' they were talking about was heart disease. They continued: 'The benefits appeared to be primarily for cardiovascular disease and not for cancer.'[3] Their conclusions were: 'Consumption of five or more servings of fruits and vegetables has been recommended . . . but the protective effect of fruit and vegetable intake may have been overstated.'

Not surprisingly, supporters of the '5-a-day' campaign were outraged by the findings, repeating their mantra that eating the recommended number of fruits and vegetables has numerous health benefits – without saying what those benefits might be.

You can eat too much fruit and veges

Animals in their natural habitat don't catch infectious diseases unless they eat infected food or are wounded; neither do 'primitive' humans, despite the fact that they do not have the 'benefits' of our sterilised lifestyle. This is because Nature endowed us with a very effective immune system. The evidence suggests that at least part of our loss of immunity to infectious disease lies in our unnatural diet. The good news is that we can regain our immunity quite easily.

Sugars lower our immunity to infectious diseases

As part of our immune system we have white blood cells called *leukocytes* which circulate in our blood streams and mop up any bacteria, viruses or other foreign bodies they come across. This process is called *phagocytosis*. The measure of how many organisms one leukocyte can eat in an hour is called its '*leukocytic index*' (LI). It is a simple measure: if a leukocyte eats ten organisms in an hour, its LI is 10.

Forty years ago researchers carried out a series of studies that examined how the sugar we eat weakens the ability of leukocytes to destroy bacteria.[4] When no sugar was eaten, a leukocyte could mop up 14 bacteria; 12 teaspoons reduced the number to 5.5 and 24 teaspoons just about wiped out the leukocytes' effectiveness altogether. To put that in context, it means that just two cans of a popular fizzy drink can wipe out your immune system altogether for a while.

However, white granulated sugar (sucrose) is only one form of 'sugar' that we eat. In 1973 another study tested the effects of several forms of sugar. In this study, subjects were fed 100 grams of a specific carbohydrate – a sugar or starch.[5] Table 14.1 shows

Table 14.1　Reduction in immune function with different carbohydrates

	Fasting LI	Lowest point LI	Decline (%)	Time before returning to normal
Fructose	15.5	8.5	45.1	more than 5 hours
Sucrose	15.2	8.6	44.0	more than 5 hours
Orange juice	16.6	9.6	42.1	more than 5 hours
Glucose	16.2	9.6	40.5	more than 5 hours
Honey	15.9	9.7	39.0	more than 5 hours
Starch	15.7	13.6	13.4	more than 5 hours

that all forms of carbohydrate – starch as well as sugars – reduced leukocytes' ability to destroy bacteria and other micro-organisms, in the case of the sugars by almost half.

A third study found that 24 fluid ounces of sugar sweetened Cola reduced immune function by 50%.[6] Based on these studies, any person who eats the recommended 'healthy' diet could lose up to half their immunity to disease for the whole of the waking day.

It is important to note that the worst sugar in Table 14.1 is fructose. Fructose is another name for fruit sugar – and modern fruits, selectively bred for sweetness, are today little more than sugared water. So if you are fed up with catching colds or if you want to reduce the risk of MRSA in hospital 'five portions of fruit' may not be such a good idea, even if veges are.

Cancers are sugar junkies

Seventy years ago Otto Warburg, PhD won the Nobel Prize in medicine for discovering that cancer cells don't like oxygen. The significance of his finding is that, unlike normal healthy cells, cancers cells cannot use ketone bodies and fats for energy as they need oxygen for their metabolism, they can only use glucose (blood sugar) for growth. Most cells have a requirement for glucose, but cancer cells consume as much as four or five times more than normal cells. In fact, cancer cells seem to have great difficulty surviving at all without glucose.

A study carried out by Johns Hopkins researchers found that some cancer cells will self-destruct when deprived of glucose.[7] 'The change when we took away glucose was dramatic,' said Dr Chi Van Dang, director of haematology. 'By the next day we knew very quickly that the cells we had altered to resemble cancers were dying off in large numbers.' He continued: 'Scientists have long suspected that the cancer cells' heavy reliance on glucose (sugar) – its main source of strength and vitality – could also be one of its great weaknesses.'

If cancers cannot survive without glucose, then it follows that a low-carb diet is likely to prevent a cancer starting in the first place. Just that piece of knowledge could stop all the heartbreak, pain and misery that cancer causes. I say low-carb, not low-sugar, because *all* carbs become the blood sugar, glucose.

Don't take 'healthy' advice

We are told to 'Base meals on starchy foods, reduce fats'. Starchy foods – or complex carbohydrates as they are also called – have been shown to have all sorts of adverse effects. The most obvious is the subject of this book: overweight and obesity. There are many others. As an increase in carbs and a decrease in fats go together, I will treat the two aspects together.

Obesity

We have known since the days of Banting that carbs are fattening. Modern trials confirm this: The *American Journal of Medicine* reported in 1997:[8]

> 'Reduced fat and calorie intake and frequent use of low-calorie food products have been associated with a paradoxical increase in the prevalence of obesity.'

'Healthy diet' increases heart disease risk for diabetics, post-menopausal women, and in fact everyone!

Obese people often do go on to suffer type-2 diabetes, and diabetics are more prone to heart disease. For this reason diabetics are counselled to eat a 'healthy' low-fat, high-carb diet, but as a paper in the medical journal, *Diabetes Care*, pointed out:

> 'In general, study has demonstrated that multiple risk factors for coronary heart disease are worsened for diabetics who consume the low-fat, high-carbohydrate diet so often recommended to reduce these risks.'[9]

In June 1999 the 81st Annual Meeting of The Endocrine Society was told:

> 'A very high-fat, low-carbohydrate diet has been shown to have astounding effects in helping type 2 diabetics lose weight and improve their blood lipid profiles. The thing many diabetics coming into the office don't realise is that other forms of carbohydrates will increase their sugar, too. Dieticians will point toward complex carbohydrates . . . oatmeal and whole wheat bread, but we have to deliver the message that these are carbohydrates that increase blood sugars, too.'[10]

In 1997 it was discovered that 'Low-fat, high-carbohydrate diets [15% protein, 60% carbohydrate, 25% fat] increase the risk of heart disease in post-menopausal women.'[11]

A 2000 study compared a low-fat, high-carbohydrate diet with a high-fat, low-carbohydrate diet on blood fats and cholesterol. They found their subjects on the 'healthy' high-carbohydrate, low-fat diet, both after fasting and after breakfast and lunch had much worse blood profiles than those on the high-fat diet. The authors conclude:

> 'Given the atherogenic potential of these changes in lipoprotein metabolism, it seems appropriate to question the wisdom of recommending that all Americans should replace dietary saturated fat with [carbohydrate]'.[12]

Back in 1992, the Framingham study had already noted that: 'In Framingham, Mass, the more saturated fat one ate, the more cholesterol one ate, the more calories one ate, the lower the person's serum cholesterol'.[13]

Could carbs cause heart disease?

The popular belief that a fatty diet causes heart disease is untenable because the process that creates atherosclerotic plaques is not fatty formations in the arteries themselves, as we are led to believe, but the intrusion of LDL particles into the walls of the arteries. Yet there is no way LDL can get through the lining of artery walls of an otherwise healthy person. Artery walls are a barrier to LDL. Let's face it; arteries wouldn't be much use if they leaked.

The only way LDL can get through the lining and into the artery wall is if that lining is damaged in some way. What is attributed to cholesterol is really a combination of damage to the artery followed by the formation of a clot (thrombus) which contains cholesterol over the area of damage. This inflammatory/healing process causes plaques to grow. They continue inside the artery wall until, eventually, they rupture, causing a blockage in an artery.

A cut or similar damage is unlikely in the coronary arteries as they are buried too deep in the body, but how about a bacterial or viral attack which damages the artery, for example? A large number of studies have reported associations between heart disease and certain persistent bacterial and viral infections.[14]

Could carbohydrates, particularly sugars and fruit juices allow this damage to occur by reducing the body's ability to fight infection, as well as making blood more likely to clot? These two factors could be a deadly combination. So is it merely coincidence that diseases for which carbohydrates are implicated have risen so dramatically since we have eaten more carbohydrates?

'Healthy' diet increases breast cancer risk

Lastly, the largest and most comprehensive study on diet and breast cancer to date found that women with the *highest* intake of starch also had a significantly *higher* incidence of breast cancer.[15]

Get off the bran wagon

Bran is another name for cereal fibre. It was first advocated to reduce colon cancer and, later, heart disease, but neither of these conditions has been found to be helped by bran. Bran's other supposed benefits aren't apparent in the literature either. For example, bran has been a popular way to treat irritable bowel syndrome (IBS) for many years, but a test at St Bartholomew's Hospital showed that far from helping IBS patients, it was the bran that caused it.[16] The authors say:

> 'The results of this study suggest that the use of bran in IBS should be reconsidered. The study also raises the possibility that excessive consumption of bran in the community may actually be creating patients with IBS by exacerbating mild, non-complaining cases.'

Tests into the supposed benefits of dietary fibre soon showed that there could be other harmful side effects. All the nutrients in food are absorbed through the gut wall and this takes time. By speeding food through the gut faster, fewer nutrients are absorbed. More importantly, phytic acid, a chemical found in cereal fibre (bran) binds with calcium, iron and zinc to form indigestible phytates, which in turn causes malabsorption. One study, for example, showed that subjects absorbed more iron from white bread than from wholemeal bread even though their intakes of iron were 50% higher with the wholemeal bread. Bran has also been shown to deplete the body of calcium, iron, zinc, phosphorus, nitrogen, fats, fatty acids and sterols.

These findings are a cause for concern in several sections of the population who are at considerable risk from eating too much fibre – and bran fibre in particular:[17]

- The incidence of osteoporosis (brittle bone disease) is increasing and now affects one in two post-menopausal women. Osteoporosis is also increasingly affecting men. Bran both inhibits the absorption of calcium from food and depletes the body of the calcium it has. Moreover, zinc, which bones need to heal, is another mineral whose absorption is adversely affected by bran.[18]
- Infants may suffer brain damage if fed soy-based baby milk as this too has a high phytate content.[19]
- Vitamin deficiency diseases such as rickets that were common in Britain until a diet high in dairy products and meat was advocated are on the increase again. The situation is getting so bad that doctors suggest that vegetarian-based fad diets should be classified as a form of child abuse.[20]
- In the UK, USA, Canada and South Africa the intake of dietary fibre that impairs the absorption of iron, accompanied by a low intake of meat (another result of the 'healthy' recommendations), is producing a real risk of iron deficiency anaemia.[21]
- Depression, anorexia, low birth weight, slow growth, mental retardation, and amenorrhoea are associated with deficiencies of zinc and the first five of these are also associated with a deficiency of iron.[22]
- Lastly, excess fibre affects the onset of menstruation, retards uterine growth and, later, is associated with menstrual dysfunction.[23]

Because of the phytate, Professor David Southgate, arguably the world's leading authority on the effects of fibre, concluded that infants, children, young adolescents and pregnant women whose mineral needs are greater should be protected from excessive consumption of fibre.[24] And, writing of the colon cancer risk, Drs H.S. Wasan and R.A. Goodlad of the Imperial Cancer Research Fund stated in 1996:

> 'Until individual constituents of fibre have been shown to have, at the very least, a non-detrimental effect in prospective human trials, we urge that restraint should be shown in adding fibre supplements to foods, and that unsubstantiated health claims be restricted.'. . . 'Specific dietary fibre supplements, embraced as nutriceuticals or functional foods, are an unknown and potentially damaging way to influence modern dietary habits of the general population.'[25]

The results of the largest, long-term trial to date of 88,757 women studied for 16 years, also suggests that a high-fibre intake does not protect against cancer.[26] The authors say:

> 'no significant association between fiber intake and the risk of colorectal adenoma was found'. They conclude: 'Our data do not support the existence of an important protective effect of dietary fiber against colorectal cancer or adenoma'.

This was reinforced still further in 2005 by a huge review of 17 studies involving over three-quarters of a million people.[27] This study found that 'high dietary fiber intake was not associated with a reduced risk of colorectal cancer.'

Constipation

In the event your colon does need a little help, the best way to increase the fibre content of your diet is with salads and raw vegetables.

Understanding fats

Fat is the principal form in which the body stores energy; it is used as an insulating material both just beneath the skin and around some of the internal organs. As part of a meal, fats slow down absorption so you can go longer without feeling hungry. But fat does much more:

- Fat is essential in the diet to supply an adequate amount of essential fatty acids.
- It is necessary for the absorption of minerals and the fat-soluble vitamins A, D, E and K.
- Dietary fats are needed for the conversion of carotene to vitamin A.
- Fat used to make many hormones and similar substances.

All fats contain a mixture of different fatty acids, both saturated and unsaturated. The fatty acid contents of some typical foods are shown in Table 14.2. The total percentages are less than 100% because of the glycerol and other compounds that are present. Note that, although animal fats are generally thought of as being saturated fats, most are less than 50% saturated.

Table 14.2   Fatty acid content of typical foods

	% Fat	Percentage of fat Sat	Mono	Poly
Milk, cow's	3.9	64	28	3
Milk, human	4.1	50	39	9
Cheese, Cheddar	33.5	63	27	4
Eggs	10.9	31	39	11
Beef	27.4	41	47	4
Pork	25.5	35	42	15
Chicken	12.8	30	45	20
Liver, lamb's	6.2	28	29	15
Mackerel	22.9	20	49	20
Butter	76.9	50	34	3
Lard	95.5	39	45	11
Margarine, hard	81.0	39	47	10
Margarine, polyunsaturated	81.0	17	27	52
Blended cooking oil	99.9	13	25	58
Peanuts, roasted	49.0	12	38	37
Chocolate, milk	30.3	58	33	4

Why change to polyunsaturated fats?

Nutritionists tell us that it is the saturated fats that cause cancer and heart disease; that's why we should change to polyunsaturated oils. This advice has resulted in fundamental changes in the Western diet. However, the truth is that saturated fats are healthy and it is the polyunsaturates that cause so much ill-health.[28]

Before the 20th century, most of the fatty acids in the diet were either saturated or mono-unsaturated, primarily from animal fats such as butter, lard, and beef and mutton dripping. In those days, fewer than one in 27 people got cancer, and heart disease was so rare that very few doctors had even heard of it, let alone seen a case. At the beginning of the 21st century, most of the fats in the diet are polyunsaturated from vegetable oils, and cancer now affects nearly one person in two and cardiovascular disease is the major killer.

The reason that polyunsaturates cause so many health problems is that they are easily attacked by oxygen. Just like iron left out in the rain, fats oxidise ('rust'). Oxygen can only attack fats because of their 'double bonds'. Saturated fats have no double bonds and don't oxidise but mono-unsaturated fats have one double bond and polyunsaturates have two or more. And the more double bonds a fatty acid has, the more it oxidises and the more 'free radicals' it creates. These free radicals are highly destructive to the body. This is why polyunsaturated margarines must be kept in the fridge. Polyunsaturates oxidise even faster when subjected to heat. The last thing you should do with polyunsaturated cooking oil is cook with it.

Cancer

Probably the greatest danger from eating too much polyunsaturated margarine and cooking oil lies in the increased risk of cancer. There are three ways in which something can increase the risk of cancer:

- It can suppress the body's immune system so that we lose our protection from disease.
- It can cause a cancer to start.
- It can promote or encourage a cancer's growth.

Certain fats have been shown to do all three. These are the ones to avoid.

Polyunsaturated fats compromise the immune system

In the early days of kidney transplantation, doctors first encountered the problem of tissue rejection as their patients' bodies destroyed the alien transplanted kidneys. If transplantation were to be a success, they had to find a way to suppress the immune system, and they found one: they fed their patients linoleic acid, the major fatty acid in all polyunsaturated margarines and cooking oils.[29] Then they noticed an increase of cancers in the linoleic treated patients – and the practice was stopped.

Heart trials using diets that were high in polyunsaturated fats (PUFs) also reported an excess of cancer deaths from as early as 1971.[30] The *British Medical Journal* carried an editorial in its 6 October 1973 issue which concluded that PUFs were carcinogenic. Despite these findings, by the early 1980s, we were being exhorted by doctors and nutritionists to eat more PUFs because they were 'good for us'.

Carcinogens continually attack us all. Normally, the immune system deals with any small focus of cancer cells so formed and that is the end of it. However, with a high intake of polyunsaturates, a small focus of cancer cells may grow too rapidly for the weakened immune system to cope, thus increasing the risk of a cancer developing.

Polyunsaturated fats cause cancer

No matter how many birthdays you have had, very little of your body is more than about eight years old. This is because of a process of programmed cell death and renewal that goes on throughout our lives. In this process of cell division to make new cells, the DNA, the genetic blueprint in the nucleus of the cell, which is in the form of a double helix, 'unzips' itself, dividing into two strands, each with half of the original genetic code. Then each of these strands reconstructs the original other half. This 'replication' process allows the one cell to produce two genetically identical daughter cells. In this way is the body first made, grown during childhood and repaired throughout adult life. It is here that free radicals are particularly dangerous. Free radicals cannot exist for long in nature. They immediately latch onto another atom. If a polyunsaturated fat creates free radicals when a cell's DNA is replicating, these could disrupt or change the genetic code and lead to mutations and the deregulation we call cancer.

The increase of polyunsaturated fats has been blamed for the alarming increase in malignant melanoma (skin cancer) in Australia.[31] Dr Bruce Mackie on Australia's sunshine coast found in patients of his, that those who developed skin cancers were those who had reduced considerably their intakes of saturated fat and replaced it with polyunsaturated fat. Polyunsaturated oils are oxidised readily by ultra-violet radiation from the sun.

That the sun is not to blame is confirmed by other findings:

- Melanoma occurs ten times as often in Orkney and Shetland as it does on Mediterranean islands.
- It also occurs more frequently on areas of the body that are *not* exposed to the sun – the ovaries, for example.
- In Scotland there are five times as many melanomas on the feet as on the hands.
- In Japan, 40% of melanomas on feet are on the soles of the feet.[32]

Polyunsaturated fats promote cancer

Many laboratories have shown that diets high in polyunsaturated fatty acids promote tumours. Cancer promotion is not the same as causing cancer; promoters are substances that help to speed up reproduction of existing cancer cells.

It has been known since the early 1970s that it is linoleic acid that is the major culprit. As Professor Raymond Kearney of Sydney University put it: 'Many laboratories have shown that a greater proportion of polyunsaturated fats are superior to diets rich in saturated fats in promoting the yield of experimental mammary tumours. In such studies, omega-6 linoleic acid appeared to be the crucial fatty acid . . .' He stated categorically 'Vegetable oils (e.g. corn oil and sunflower oil) which are rich in linoleic acid are potent promoters of tumour growth.'[33]

Polyunsaturated fats increase breast cancer risk

Over the past 15 years, there have been many studies into breast cancer and fat intakes.[34] They have demonstrated that it is polyunsaturated fats that increase the risk, but don't cut down on all fats because, interestingly, the studies also showed that women who had the highest intakes of the right types of fats had less breast cancer: mono-unsaturated fats reduced the risk of breast cancer, and saturated fats were neutral.

Animal fats are almost half mono-unsaturated, and almost half saturated, with a little polyunsaturated, which is about as safe as it gets.

Animal fat prevents cancer, but animal fats get the blame anyway

Linoleic acid is one of the essential fatty acids that our bodies need but cannot synthesise. Fortunately there is one form of linoleic acid that is beneficial. *Conjugated* linoleic acid (CLA) differs from the normal form of linoleic acid only in the position of one of the bonds that join its atoms, but this small difference has been shown to give it powerful anti-cancer properties.[35,36] Even at concentrations of less than one per cent, CLA in the diet is protective against several cancers including breast cancer, colorectal cancer and malignant melanoma. CLA has one other difference from the usual form – it is not found in vegetables but in the fat of ruminant animals. The best sources are dairy products and the fat on red meat, principally beef.[37]

As well as CLA, the saturated fatty acids lauric acid and capric acid found in animal fat also have anti-cancer properties.[38]

It has been suggested that the consumption of red meat increases the risk of colon cancer, yet in Britain there is no evidence to support this.[39] It may be significant that all the evidence implicating red meat in cancer comes from the USA – where they cut the fat off.

But beware: there are two forms of CLA. The one found in animal fat that helps to prevent cancer has double bonds at positions 9 and 11. The one sold in healthfood shops is made from vegetable oils. It has double bonds at positions 10 and 12 – and not only does it not work, it is toxic.

An American study of 90,655 women aged 26 to 46, conducted by the Harvard Medical School published in 2003 came up with different findings. This study was reported in the American press with the headline: **'Animal Fats Linked to Increased Breast Cancer Risk, Study Finds.'** It reported that a diet high in animal fat raised the risk by as much as 54%. But that's not what the figures showed.[40]

The women were divided into five 'quintiles' depending on their fat intakes: the first quintile eating the least fat and the fifth quintile the most. The study's abstract read: '... the [relative risks] for the increasing quintiles of animal fat intake were 1.00 (referent), 1.28, 1.37, 1.54, and 1.33'. It's that 1.54 for the fourth quintile that provides the 54% figure.

But there are no absolute risk figures. Without these, the findings are misleading. However we can work out the numbers of women who did *not* get breast cancer from the study's data for each quintile: 99.3, 99.2, 99.2, 99.1, 99.3. The number of women who did *not* get cancer is 99.3% in both the first and the fifth quintiles. Thus there is no trend of increasing cancer as fats increase.

If eating animal fat increased the risk of breast cancer, you would expect that the more animal fat is eaten, the more breast cancer there would be. That was not the case in this study, and it's not the case in world populations. Note, the dramatic sounding '54%' increased risk is actually a 0.2% increase. But relative risks are so much better for headlines.

Another thing that is suspect about this study is that the authors had published another paper only four months earlier in which they were unable to find a breast cancer risk for red meat intake.[41] In that study, they 'found no evidence that intake of meat or fish during mid-life and later was associated with risk of breast cancer.' It refutes their other study. Interestingly this study isn't even referred to in their later study.

All polyunsaturated margarines, from the brand leader to shops' own brands are 39% linoleic acid. Cooking oils, that is sunflower, safflower, soya and corn oils, are between 50% and 78% linoleic acid. I am sure this is dangerously high. Butter, on the other hand, has a mere 2%, and lard is around 9% linoleic acid.

There are some polyunsaturated fatty acids which are essential to the body, but we don't need much: about 2% of calories in the form of omega-6, linoleic acid. With a 2000-calorie intake, that is about a teaspoonful. We also need about half that amount of omega-3, alpha-linolenic acid and/or EPA. These amounts are readily available from animal fats and fish oils with this way of eating unless the enzyme needed to convert them into a usable form is compromised in some way.

Saturated fats are beneficial

Saturated fats and animal fats are usually blamed for all manner of diseases in Western society, but what all the work in the last half century demonstrated was that they are not the cause of our modern diseases. In fact, they play many important roles in our bodies:

- Saturated fatty acids constitute at least fifty per cent of body cell membranes. They are what gives our cells necessary stiffness and integrity.
- For calcium to be effectively incorporated into our bones, at least fifty per cent of our dietary fats should be saturated.[42]
- Saturated fats lower Lp(a), a substance in the blood that indicates proneness to heart disease.[43]
- They protect the liver from alcohol and other toxins.[44]
- They enhance the immune system.[45]
- The essential fatty acids are polyunsaturated, but our body's use of them is enhanced by saturated fatty acids.[46]
- Saturated fatty acids are the preferred energy source for the heart, which is why the fat around the heart muscle is highly saturated.[47]
- Saturated fats enhance the immune system – short-chain saturated fatty acids kill viruses and bacteria.

The scientific evidence does not support the idea that saturated fats cause heart disease.[48] Most of the fats found in clogged arteries are polyunsaturated.

One last thought: our bodies store energy as fat, and what sort of fat is that? It's a fat similar to any other animal fat, NOT vegetable oil. Since our bodies are not in the habit of making substances that harm themselves, surely the form of fat our bodies make is exactly the type of fat that is healthiest for them?

Conclusion

Research over the last half century has demonstrated no evidence whatsoever of a need to endure an unpalatable, fatless, bran-laden diet. Apart from being less pleasurable to eat, it is now abundantly clear that 'healthy eating' is not so healthy after all.

References

1. Freese R, Alfthan G, Jauhiainen M, et al. High intakes of vegetables, berries, and apples combined with a high intake of linoleic or oleic acid only slightly affect markers of lipid peroxidation and lipoprotein metabolism in healthy subjects. *Am J Clin Nutr* 2002; 76: 950–960.
2. Panagiotakos DB, Pitsavos C, Kokkinos P, et al. Consumption of fruits and vegetables in relation to the risk of developing acute coronary syndromes; the CARDIO2000 case-control study. *Nutr J* 2003; 2: 2.
3. Hung H-C, Joshipura KJ, Jiang R, et al. Fruit and vegetable intake and risk of major chronic disease. *J Natl Canc Inst* 2004; 96: 1577–1584.
4. Kijak E, Foust G, Steinman RR. Relationship of blood sugar level and leukocytic phagocytosis. *South Calif Dent Assn* 1964; 32: 349–351.
5. Sanchez A, et al. Role of sugars in human neutrophilic phagocytosis. *Am J Clin Nutr* 1973; 26: 1180–1184.
6. Ringsdorf WM Jr, Cheraskin E, Ramsey RR Jr. Sucrose, neutrophilic phagocytosis, and resistance to disease. *Dent Surv* 1976; 52: 46–48.
7. *Proceedings of the National Academy of Sciences USA*, 1998; 95: 1511–1516.
8. Heini AF, Weinsier RL. Divergent trends in obesity and fat intake patterns: the American paradox. *Am J Med* 1997; 102: 259–264.
9. Chen YD, et al. Why do low-fat, high-carbohydrate diets accentuate postprandial lipemia in patients with NIDDM? *Diabetes Care* 1995; 18: 10–16.
10. Hays J. *Diabetics improve health with very high-fat, low carb diet*. Paper presented to the 81st Annual Meeting of the Endocrine Society, 15 June 1999.
11. Jeppeson J, et al. Effects of low-fat, high-carbohydrate diets on risk factors for ischemic heart disease in postmenopausal women. *Am J Clin Nutr* 1997; 65: 1027–1033.
12. Abbasi F, et al. High carbohydrate diets, triglyceride-rich lipoproteins and coronary heart disease risk. *Am J Cardiol* 2000; 85: 45–48.
13. Castelli WP. *Arch Int Med* 1992; 152: 1371–1372.

14. Patel P, Mendall MA, Carrington D, et al. Association of *Helicobacter pylori* and *Chlamydia pneumoniae* infections with coronary heart disease and cardiovascular risk factors. *BMJ* 1995; 311: 711–714.

15. Franceschi S, et al. Intake of macronutrients and risk of breast cancer. *Lancet* 1996; 347: 1351–1356.

16. Francis CY, Whorwell PJ. Bran and irritable bowel syndrome: time for reappraisal. *Lancet* 1994; 344: 39.

17. Kelsay JL. A review of research on effect of fibre intake on man. *Am J Clin Nutr* 1978; 31: 142–159.

18. a. Editorial. The Bran Wagon. *Lancet* 1987; i: 782–783.
    b. Suri YP. The Bran Wagon. *Lancet* 1987; ii: 42–43.

19. Bishop N, et al. Aluminium in infant formulas. *Lancet* 1989; i: 490.

20. Roberts IF, West RJ, Ogilvie D, Dillon MJ. Malnutrition in infants receiving cult diets: a form of child abuse. *BMJ* 1979; 1: 296–268.

21. Bindra GS, Gibson RS. Iron status of predominantly lacto-ovo-vegetarian East Indian immigrants to Canada: a model approach. *Am J Clin Nutr* 1986; 44: 643.

22. a. Hambidge M. The role of zinc and other trace metals in paediatric nutrition and health. *Paediat Clin N Am* 1977; 24: 95.
    b. Bryce-Smith D, Simpson R. Anorexia, depression and zinc deficiency. *Lancet* 1984; ii: 1162.
    c. Fonesca V, Harvard C. Electrolyte disturbances and cardiac failure with hypomagnesaemia in anorexia nervosa. *BMJ* 1985; 291: 1680.
    d. Meadows N, et al. Zinc and small babies. *Lancet* 1981; ii: 1135.
    e. Bryce-Smith D. Environmental chemical influences on behaviour and mentation. John Jeyes lecture. *Chem Soc Rev* 1986; 15: 93.
    f. McMichael A, et al. A prospective study of serial maternal zinc levels and pregnancy outcome. *Early Human Development*. 1982; 7: 59, Elsevier, Edinburgh.

23. a. Hughes RE. A new look at dietary fibre. *Hum Nutr Clin Nutr* 1986; 40c: 81.
    b. Hughes RE, Johns E. Apparent relation between dietary fibre and reproductive function in the female. *Ann Hum Biol* 1985; 12: 325.
    c. Lloyd T, et al. Inter-relationships of diet, athletic activity, menstrual status and bone density in collegiate women. *Am J Clin Nutr* 1987; 46: 681.

24. Southgate DAT. Minerals, trace elements and potential hazards. *Am J Clin Nutr* 1987; 45: 1256.

25. Wasan HS, Goodlad RA. Fiber-supplemented foods may damage your health. *Lancet* 1996; 348: 319–320.

26. Fuchs CS, et al. Dietary fiber and the risk of colorectal cancer and adenoma in women. *New Engl J Med* 1999; 340: 169–176, 223–224.

27. Park Y, Hunter DJ, Spiegelman D, et al. Dietary fiber intake and risk of colorectal cancer: a pooled analysis of prospective cohort studies. *JAMA* 2005; 294(22): 2849–2857.

28. a. Pinckney ER, Pinckney C. *The Cholesterol Controversy.* Sherbourne Press, Los Angeles, 1973, pp.127–131.

    b. Felton CV, et al. Dietary polyunsaturated fatty acids and composition of human aortic plaques. *Lancet* 1994; 344: 1195–1196.

29. Uldall PR, Wilkinson R, McHugh MI, et al. Unsaturated fatty acids and renal transplantation. *Lancet* 1974; 2: 514.

30. Pearce ML, Dayton S. Incidence of cancer in men on a diet high in polyunsaturated fat. *Lancet* 1971; i: 464.

31. Mackie BS. Do polyunsaturated fats predispose to malignant melanoma? *Med J Austr* 1974; 1: 810.

32. Karnauchow PN. Melanoma and sun exposure. *Lancet* 1995; 346: 915.

33. Kearney R. Promotion and prevention of tumour growth – effects of endotoxin, inflammation and dietary lipids. *Int Clin Nutr Rev* 1987; 7: 157.

34. a. Carroll KK. Dietary fats and cancer. *Am J Clin Nutr* 1991; 53: 1064S.

    b. France T, Brown P. Test-tube cancers raise doubts over fats. *New Sci*, 7 December 1991, p.12.

    c. Franceschi S, et al. Intake of macronutrients and risk of breast cancer. *Lancet* 1996; 347: 1351–1356.

    d. Holmes MD, et al. Association of dietary intake of fat and fatty acids with risk of breast cancer. *JAMA* 1999; 281: 914.

    e. Wolk A, et al. A prospective study of association of monounsaturated fat and other types of fat with risk of breast cancer. *Arch Intern Med* 1998; 158: 41–45.

35. Ip C, Scimeca JA, Thompson HJ. Conjugated linoleic acid: a powerful anticarcinogen from animal fat sources. *Cancer* 1994; 74(3 Suppl): 1050–1054.

36. Shultz TD, et al. Inhibitory effect of conjugated dienoic derivatives of linoleic acid and beta-carotene on the in vitro growth of human cancer cells. *Cancer Lett* 1992; 63: 125–133.

37. Lin H, et al. Survey of the conjugated linoleic acid contents of dairy products. *J Dairy Sci* 1995; 78: 2358–2365.

38. Cohen LA, et al. Dietary fat and mammary cancer. II. Modulation of serum and tumor lipid composition and tumor prostaglandins by different dietary fats: association with tumor incidence patterns. *J Natl Cancer Inst* 1986; 77: 43.

39. Cox BD, Whichelow MJ. Frequent consumption of red meat is not a risk factor for cancer. *BMJ* 1997; 315: 1018.

40. Cho E, Spiegelman D, Hunter DJ, et al. Premenopausal fat intake and risk of breast cancer. *J Natl Cancer Inst* 2003; 95: 1079–1085.

41. Holmes MD, Colditz GA, Hunter DJ, et al. Meat, fish and egg intake and risk of breast cancer. *Int J Cancer* 2003; 104: 221–227.

42. a. Watkins BA, et al. Importance of vitamin E in bone formation and in chrondrocyte function. *AOCS Proceedings*, 1996.

b. Watkins BA, Seifert MF. Food lipids and bone health. In: McDonald RE, Min DB, eds. *Food Lipids and Health*. Marcel Dekker, New York, NY, 1996, p.101.

43. a. Dahlen GH, et al. The importance of serum lipoprotein (a) as an independent risk factor for premature coronary artery disease in middle-aged black and white women from the United States. *J Intern Med* 1998; 244: 417–424.

b. Khosla P, Hayes KC. Dietary trans-monounsaturated fatty acids negatively impact plasma lipids in humans: critical review of the evidence. *J Am Coll Nutr* 1996; 15: 325–339.

c. Clevidence BA, et al. Plasma lipoprotein (a) levels in men and women consuming diets enriched in saturated, cis-, or trans-monounsaturated fatty acids. *Arterioscler Thromb Vasc Biol* 1997; 17:1657–1661.

44. a. Nanji AA, et al. Dietary saturated fatty acids: a novel treatment for alcoholic liver disease. *Gastroenterology* 1995; 109: 547–54.

b. Cha YS, Sachan DS. Opposite effects of dietary saturated and unsaturated fatty acids on ethanol-pharmacokinetics, triglycerides and carnitines. *J Am Coll Nutr* 1994; 13: 338–343.

c. Hargrove HL, et al. *FASEB J*, Meeting Abstracts, Mar 1999, #204.1, p.A222.

45. a. Kabara JJ. *The Pharmacological Effects of Lipids*. The American Oil Chemists Society, Champaign, IL, 1978, 1–14.

b. Cohen LA, et al. Dietary fat and mammary cancer. II. Modulation of serum and tumor lipid composition and tumor prostaglandins by different dietary fats: association with tumor incidence patterns. *J Natl Cancer Inst* 1986; 77: 43–51.

46. Garg ML, et al. *FASEB J*, 1988; 2: 4:A852; Oliart Ros RM, et al. Meeting Abstracts, *AOCS Proceedings*, May 1998, 7, Chicago, IL.

47. a. Lawson LD, Kummerow F. beta-Oxidation of the coenzyme A esters of vaccenic, elaidic, and petroselaidic acids by rat heart mitochondria. *Lipids* 1979; 14: 501–503.

b. Garg ML. Dietary saturated fat level alters the competition between alpha-linolenic and linoleic acid. *Lipids* 1989; 24: 334–339.

48. Ravnskov U. The questionable role of saturated and polyunsaturated fatty acids in cardiovascular disease. *J Clin Epidemiol* 1998; 51: 443–460.

Chapter Fifteen

Why your low-carb diet must be high-fat, not high-protein

Fat is the most valuable food known to Man.

Professor John Yudkin

Introduction

We now know that we should eat a diet that is low in carbohydrates, particularly avoiding those with a high GI. However, a plethora of books published in the last decade have been 'low-carb, high-protein', or 'low-carb, high-fat', or 'low-carb, high-'good'-fats', or all sorts of other mixtures. In other words, the real confusion lies in what we should replace the carbohydrates with: for example, should it be protein or fats? And if fats, what sort of fats?

All the evidence suggests that carbs should be replaced with fats, and those fats should be mainly from animal sources.

ATP: our bodies' fuel

Our bodies' energy comes either from glucose, which is supplied mainly from the carbs we eat, or from fatty acids which, in turn, are derived either from the food we eat or by breaking down fats already stored in our bodies.

If you are eating the so-called 'healthy' way, most of your energy will come from dietary carbs. When you cut down on carbs, the energy your body needs has to come from somewhere else. There are only two choices: protein or fat.

The fuel that body cells use for energy is actually neither glucose nor fat; it is a chemical called *adenosine triphosphate* (ATP). A typical human cell may contain nearly one billion molecules of ATP at any one moment, and those may be used and re-supplied every three minutes.[1] This huge demand for ATP, and our evolutionary history, has resulted in our bodies' developing several different pathways for its manufacture.

Oxygen and mitochondria

Living organisms have two means to produce the energy they need to live. The first is fermentation, a primitive process that doesn't require the presence of oxygen. This is the way that *anaerobic* (meaning 'without oxygen') bacteria break down glucose to produce energy. Our body cells can use this method.

The second, *aerobic* (meaning 'using oxygen'), method began after the Earth began to cool down and its atmosphere became rich in oxygen. After this event, a new type of cell – a *eukaryotic* cell – evolved to use it. Today all organisms more complex than bacteria use this property and all animal life requires oxygen to function. When we breathe in, our lungs extract the oxygen in air and pass it to the bloodstream for transport through the body. In our bodies, it is little power plants called *mitochondria* in our body's cells that use this oxygen to produce most of the energy our bodies need. The process is called 'respiration'. This process takes the basic fuel source and oxidises it to produce ATP. The numbers of mitochondria in each cell vary, but as much as half of the total cell volume can be mitochondria. The important point to note is that mitochondria are primarily designed to use fats.

Which source of base material is best?

The question now, in this era of dietary plenty, is: which source is best? There are three possible choices:

- Glucose, which comes mainly from carbohydrates, although protein can also be utilised as a glucose source by the body if necessary.
- Fatty acids, both from the diet and from stored body fats.
- Ketones, which are derived from the metabolism of fats.

Not all cells in our bodies use the same base material. Cells that can employ fatty acids are those that contain many mitochondria, such as heart muscle cells, for example. These cells can make energy from fatty acids or glucose or ketones, but given a choice, they much prefer to use fats. The second type of cells are those that cannot use fats but can use either glucose or ketones. These cells which also contain mitochondria will shift to preferentially using ketones. We also have cells that contain few or no mitochondria. Examples of cells with few mitochondria are white blood cells, testes and inner parts of the kidneys; and cells which contain no mitochondria are red blood cells, and the retina, lens and cornea in the eyes. These are entirely dependent on glucose and must still be sustained by glucose.

To understand how a low carb diet works, we need to look at how we eat. This process is one of eating, digestion, hunger and eating again. During our evolution, we also must have experienced long periods when food was in short supply and we starved. This is a pattern our bodies are adapted to; they have developed mechanisms to cope with a wide range of circumstances.

First, the human body must contain adequate levels of energy to sustain the essential body parts that rely on glucose. The brain and central nervous system may be a particular case as, although the brain represents only a small percentage of body weight, it uses around a quarter of all the resting energy used by the body.[2] Fortunately the brain can also use ketone bodies derived from fats. During fasting in humans, and when we are short of food, blood glucose levels are maintained by the breakdown of glycogen in liver and muscle and by the production of glucose primarily from the breakdown of muscle proteins in a process called *gluconeogenesis*, which literally means 'glucose new birth'.[3]

However, we don't want to use lean muscle tissue in this way: it weakens us. We want to get the glucose our bodies need from what we eat. Some of that will come from carbs, the rest from dietary proteins. Our bodies need a constant supply of protein to sustain a healthy structure. This requires a fairly minimal amount of protein: about 1 to 1.5 grams per kilogram of lean body weight per day is all that is necessary to preserve muscle mass.[4] Any protein over and above this amount can be used as a source of glucose.

Dietary proteins are converted to glucose at about 58% efficiency, so approximately 100 g of protein can produce 58 g of glucose via gluconeogenesis.[5] Body fats are stored as triglycerides, molecules that contain three fatty acids combined with glycerol. The fatty acids are used directly as a fuel, with the glycerol stripped off. This is not wasted. As the glycerol is nearly 10% of triglyceride by weight and two molecules of glycerol combine to form one molecule of glucose, this also supplies a source of glucose. During prolonged fasting, glycerol released from the breakdown of triglycerides in body fat may account for nearly 20% of gluconeogenesis.[6]

The case for getting energy from fat and ketones

When most people think of eating a low-carb diet, they tend to think of it as being a protein-based one. This is false. All traditional carnivorous diets, whether eaten by animals or humans, are always preferred with a ratio of about 80% of calories from fat and 20% of calories from protein.

Similarly, the main fuel produced by a modern low-carb diet should also be fatty acids derived from dietary fat and body fat. We find in practice that free fatty acids are higher in the bloodstream on a low-carb diet compared with a conventional diet.[7,8]

Fats also produce an important secondary fuel called 'ketone bodies'. Ketones were first discovered in the urine of diabetic patients in the mid-19th century; for almost 50 years thereafter, they were thought to be abnormal and undesirable by-products of incomplete fat oxidation. In the early 20th century, however, they were recognised as normal circulating metabolites produced by the liver and readily utilised by body tissues. Ketones are the preferred energy source for highly active tissues such as heart and muscle tissues.[9]

Ketones are an important substitute for glucose. During prolonged periods of starvation, fatty acids are made from the breakdown of stored triglycerides in body fat.[10] Free fatty acids are converted to ketones by the liver. They then provide energy to all cells with mitochondria. Within a cell, ketones are used to generate ATP. And where glucose needs the intervention of bacterial fermentation to convert it for energy use, ketones can be used directly.

Reduction of carbohydrate intake stimulates the synthesis of ketones from body fat.[11] This is one reason why reducing carbs is important. Another is that reducing carbohydrate and protein intake also leads to a lower insulin level in the blood. This, in turn, reduces the risks associated with insulin resistance: diseases such as diabetes and heart disease.

Ketone formation and a shift to using more fatty acids also reduce the body's overall need for glucose. Even during high-energy demand from exercise, a low-carb diet has what is called a 'glucoprotective' effect. What this all means is that ketosis arising from a low-carb diet is capable of accommodating a wide range of metabolic demands to sustain body functions and health while not using, and thus sparing, firstly the stored glycogen, and secondly, protein from lean muscle tissue.

All this means that more glucose is available for essential tissues which are dependent on glucose.

The case against getting energy from protein

We know, then, that dietary fats can produce all the energy the body needs, either directly as fatty acids or as ketone bodies, but as there is still some debate about the health implications of using fats, why not play safe and eat more protein?

There is one simple reason why not: while the body can use protein as an energy source in an emergency, it is not at all healthy to use this method in the long term. All carbs are made up of just three elements: carbon, hydrogen and oxygen. Fats are also made of the same three elements. Proteins, however, also contain nitrogen and other elements. When proteins are used to provide energy, these must be got rid of in some way. This is not only wasteful, it can put a strain on the body, particularly on the liver and kidneys.

Excess intake of protein and its use for energy leads in a short space of time to *hyperammonaemia*, which is a build up of ammonia in the bloodstream. This is toxic to the brain. Protein also requires vitamin A – a fat-soluble vitamin – for its metabolism. A diet too high in protein without adequate fat rapidly depletes vitamin A stores, leading to serious consequences such as heart arrhythmias, kidney problems, autoimmune disease and thyroid disorders. While protein does not raise glucose, it does raise insulin. For this reason, high-protein diets that reduce both carbs *and* fats, are not as healthy as they could be. Fats raise neither glucose nor insulin.

Many human cultures survive on a purely animal diet, but *only* if it is high in fat.[12,13] All primitive peoples avoid protein-rich, low-fat diets. These can lead to nausea in as few as three days, you develop symptoms of starvation in a week to ten days, severe debilitation in 12 days and possibly death in just a few weeks. A high-fat diet, however, is completely healthy for a lifetime.

Perhaps one of the best documented studies is that of the Arctic explorer,

Vilhjalmur Stefansson and a colleague, Dr Karsten Andersen.[14] They ate an animal meat diet for more than a year to see whether such a diet could be healthy. Everything was fine until they were asked to eat only lean meat. Dr Walter S. McClelland, the lead scientist, wrote:

> 'At our request [Stefansson] began eating lean meat only, although he had previously noted, in the North, that very lean meat sometimes produced digestive disturbances. On the third day nausea and diarrhea developed. When fat meat was added to the diet, a full recovery was made in two days.'

This was a hospital-based clinical study, but Stefansson had already lived for nearly 20 years on an all-meat diet with the Canadian Inuit. He and his team suffered no ill effects whatsoever unless only lean meat was available. They then found that they developed what they called 'rabbit hunger' within a couple of days and had to find fat to cure the condition.

So don't be tempted to add protein powders to up the protein content without adding calories at the same time. The result could well be a low-carb, low-fat diet which is unnaturally high in protein. That is probably the unhealthiest diet of all.

Low-carb, high-fat diet and weight loss

There is just one other consideration. If you want to lose weight, the actual material you want to rid your body of is fat, but to do that you have to change your body from using glucose as a fuel to using fat – including your own body fat. This is another reason not to use protein as a substitute for carbs, because protein is also converted to glucose.

If you think about it, Nature stores excess energy in our bodies as fat, not as protein. It makes much more sense, therefore, to use what we are designed by Nature to use.

Which fats are best?

Now that we know that fats are the most efficient basic raw material for energy production, the next question to answer is: which ones are best, particularly in terms of our health.

When we listen to news items and read press health articles, they normally talk about 'fats' as if all fats are the same. This is quite wrong. Some fats are essential, some are not; some fats are beneficial, others are not. Lumping all fats together gives quite the wrong message. They really should be classified by their other properties: degree of saturation and length.

Saturation

Saturated fatty acids. A fatty acid is saturated when all its carbon bonds are occupied by a hydrogen atom. Because of this, saturated fats are highly stable. This means that they do not normally go rancid, even when heated. This in turn means that they do not create free radicals.

Figure 7 shows the structure of stearic acid. It has 18 carbon atoms and no double bonds, and is therefore designated 18:0. Because all the carbon atoms are surrounded by hydrogen atoms, it is called *saturated*. As the hydrogen atoms are all symmetrical, stearic acid and other long saturates can pack together neatly like toothpicks. This makes them difficult molecules to bend when cold. It is this resistance to bending that makes most saturated fats solid at room temperature. However, in their liquid form, in the body of a warm animal, they bend every which way.

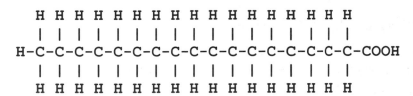

Figure 7 Structure of stearic acid

Mono-unsaturated fatty acids are fatty acids with one double bond (shown as =).

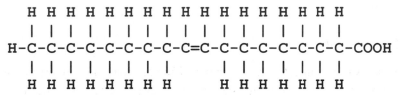

Figure 8 Structure of oleic acid

Oleic acid is another 18 carbon fatty acid but with one *double bond* in the middle. Fatty acids with one double bond are called *mono*-unsaturated. It is designated by the term 18:1. C=C bonds and the nearest carbons are held rigid C–C=C–C with a 120° angle between the triplet of carbon atoms. The inability of oleic acid to pack well with other molecules makes its melting point lower than that of 18:0, and it is liquid at room temperature. Oleic acid is the major fatty acid in olive oil and also the most abundant fatty acid in all animal fats including human fat. Because the double break is after the ninth carbon atom it is an omega-9 fatty acid. The shorthand for oleic acid is 18:,n-9.

Poly-unsaturated fatty acids are those with two or more double bonds.

Figure 9 shows linoleic acid, the most abundant fatty acid in vegetable seed oils such as sunflower, safflower, soya and corn oils. This has two double bonds, the first after the sixth carbon atom. This makes it an **omega-6** fatty acid. The shorthand for linoleic acid is 18:2,n-6. If the first double bond follows the third carbon atom, the fatty acid is an **omega-3** fatty acid.

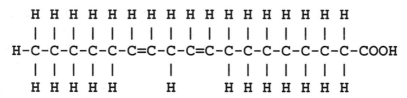

Figure 9   Structure of linoleic acid

Some fatty acids come in two configurations: omega-3 and omega-6. **Linolenic acid**, an 18-carbon molecule with three double bonds, is an example of this. **Alpha-linolenic acid** is **omega-3**, while **gamma-linolenic acid** is **omega-6**.

All polyunsaturated fatty acids are liquid at room temperature.

Lengths of fatty acids

As well as degree of saturation, scientists also classify fatty acids by their length.

Short-chain fatty acids, which are always saturated (in animal fats and tropical oils only), have four to six carbon atoms. Bile is not needed for their digestion and they are directly absorbed for quick energy. For this reason, they are less likely to cause weight gain than olive oil or commercial vegetable oils.[15] But they also have other important properties. They are anti-microbial, meaning that they protect the body from viruses, bacteria and yeasts in the gut. They also contribute to the health of the immune system.[16] Four-carbon *butyric acid* is found mostly in butterfat from cows, and six-carbon *capric acid* is found mostly in butterfat from goats.

Medium-chain fatty acids, which again are all saturated, have eight to twelve carbon atoms. These fatty acids have the same health benefits as short-chain fatty acids. They are found mostly in butterfat and coconut and palm oils.

Long-chain fatty acids have fourteen or more carbon atoms. These can be saturated, mono-unsaturated or polyunsaturated. *Stearic acid* is an 18-carbon saturated fatty acid found chiefly in beef and lamb fats. An important mono-unsaturated fatty acid found almost exclusively in animal fats is 16-carbon *palmitoleic acid* which has strong anti-microbial properties. *Oleic acid* is an 18-carbon mono-unsaturated fatty acid which is the chief component of olive oil and also the major fatty acid in animal fats. The two essential fatty acids, omega-6 *linoleic acid* (LA), and omega-3 *alpha-linolenic acid* (ALA), are also 18 carbons in length. LA is the major fatty acid in seed oils such as sunflower, safflower, soya and corn oils, where it forms 55–70% of their fatty acid content. It is these which are used for the manufacture of 'high-in-polyunsaturates' margarines and as cooking oils. Human fats contain very little linoleic acid. ALA comes mostly from animal fats and some genetically modified seed oils.

Very-long-chain fatty acids with 20 to 24 carbon atoms are highly unsaturated, with four, five or six double bonds. Most people's bodies can manufacture these from the essential fatty acids, but some people lack the necessary enzymes. These people must obtain these important fats by eating animal foods such as fish oils, organ meats, egg yolks, and butter (although, having said that, there is still some debate about whether 'essential fatty acids' really are essential). The two most important very-long-chain fatty acids are *eicosapentaenoic acid* (EPA) with 20 carbons and five double bonds; and *docosahexaenoic acid* (DHA) with 22 carbons and six double bonds. Very-long-chain fatty acids are used in the production of tissue hormones that govern many processes in the cells and are important to the proper growth and functioning of the brain and nervous system.[17]

Cis and trans bonds

Generally, in Nature, fatty acids' double bonds are as shown above with the single hydrogen atoms at a double bond on the same side of the molecule. This is called a *cis* configuration. However, in the process of margarine manufacture, liquid oils are not much good. They have to be made more solid. The process which does this is called hydrogenation. During hydrogenation, some of the double bonds are twisted so that the hydrogen atoms lie on opposite sides, as in Figure 10. This configuration is called ***trans***.

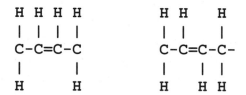

Figure 10 Examples of *cis* and *trans* bonds

In the diagram above, the first double is shown *cis*, the second is shown *trans*.

These *trans* fats are artificially hardened to resemble saturated fats such as butter. It is only these 'saturated' fats that have been shown to be toxic. Natural saturated fats are healthy. However, when the media and many scientists talk of good and bad fats, they invariably lump *trans* fats together with saturated fats. This is how natural saturated fats have acquired their undeserved notoriety.

The significance of temperature

Have you ever wondered why polyunsaturated margarine has to be kept in a fridge, yet coconut oil can be kept out at room temperature for a year or more without any untoward effects?

All fats and oils in Nature are a mixture of saturated, mono-unsaturated and polyunsaturated fatty acids. The only difference between them is the proportions of each. Whether they are in plant or animal tissues, this is governed by the temperature at which the different fats and oils are designed to operate. This point, which is often neglected when discussing the healthiness or otherwise of fats and oils, is actually the most important consideration. The degree of saturation or unsaturation determines not only a fat's melting point, but also its chemical stability and its likelihood of auto-oxidising and creating harmful free radicals. The higher the proportion of saturated fatty acids a fat is, the less likely it is to go rancid; the more polyunsaturated fatty acids it contains, the more difficult it is to stop it going bad.

In plants, oils are usually found in their seeds. The degree of saturation of plant oils and fats is entirely dependent on the temperature in which they are grown. These oils provide a store of energy for the seeds' germination, usually in early spring when the weather is cool. For this reason, the energy contained in the oils must be accessible when the temperatures are low. Unsaturated oils melt at lower temperatures, and the more unsaturated they are, the lower the temperature at which they are viable. So we find oils that are highly saturated, such as coconut oil which is over 95% saturated, in the tropics; palm oil, which grows further from the equator, is less saturated; mono-unsaturated oils are found in olives grown in Mediterranean regions; and polyunsaturated oils in the seeds of plants grown in cooler climates. It has also been shown that the same plant species grown in a warm climate will be more saturated than if grown in a cooler region.[18]

The same is true of animals. Pigs dressed in sweaters were also found to have more saturated fat than unclothed pigs.[19] Animals must have body fats which are liquid, otherwise they would be too stiff to move. This is why cold-blooded animals such as fish, which also live in cold water, contain highly polyunsaturated fatty acids with many double bonds (the EPA and DHA of cod liver oil have five and six double bonds respectively). As body or environmental temperatures rise, so we find fats tending to become more saturated. The fats of all warm-blooded animals contain mixtures of saturated and unsaturated fatty acids, but the degree of saturation is still quite high. Human fat is naturally about 40% saturated, 56% mono-unsaturated and only 4% polyunsaturated.

The temperature at which a fat is used is highly relevant because, as the temperature rises, the more likely unsaturated fats are to auto-oxidise. Fat must be stable at the temperature at which it is going to be used. If it is attacked by oxygen and goes rancid, as polyunsaturated margarines do if they are not refrigerated, then they become unfit for consumption if they are outside the body, and extremely harmful if they are inside it.

All polyunsaturated fatty acids will auto-oxidise at body temperature unless they are protected in some way. Let's look at how Nature makes sure it doesn't happen.

Coconuts are found in equatorial regions where the ambient temperature is well over 40°C (104°F). Coconut oil contains a small percentage of polyunsaturated fatty acids – but significantly, coconut oil doesn't go rancid at this temperature as a polyunsaturated margarine very quickly would. This is because the polyunsaturated fatty acids in coconut oil are protected by the high percentage of saturated fatty acids.

Our body temperature at 37°C (98.6°F) is not much lower than the coconut's environment. Our fat must also be liquid at this temperature but it must also be stable. So it, too, contains a high proportion of saturated fat and only a small amount of polyunsaturated fat. Just like the coconut, the saturated fatty acids in our bodies protect the polyunsaturated fatty acids from oxidation. However, if we eat a diet that contains high levels of polyunsaturated fats, as 'healthy eating' tells us we should, those fats will be incorporated in our body cells. And that, as we will see later, makes them a recipe for disaster.

Fish, whether in the cold Arctic or in warmer waters, contain a higher proportion of polyunsaturated fats than do warm blooded animals. In the tropics, where diets tend to include lots of fish, coconut oil is also eaten in plenty. Human cultures in the tropics eat high levels of saturated coconut oil and they don't suffer heart disease. South Pacific islanders are protected from the harmful effects of the polyunsaturated fats in the fish by the saturated fats in the coconuts.

We in cooler climates have the same body temperatures as Pacific islanders and we eat animals such as cattle, pigs and sheep. The natural fat of those food animals is very similar to our own fat. If the animals are allowed to feed naturally, the saturated fatty acids in animal fat protect the polyunsaturated element in our diet. This makes these fats entirely healthy for both them and us. There is one caveat, however: nowadays, the establishment is trying to make fats 'healthier' by feeding animals with commercially produced foodstuffs that contain high levels of polyunsaturated seed oils, notably from soya and maize (corn).

In Table 15.1, the figures for food animals are based on animals eating their natural diet (as they did when these values were determined). Today, however, many food animals are fed on foods such as soya bean whose fats are mostly polyunsaturated – and the figures can be very different. For example, pork fat which should be about 8% polyunsaturated, can now be well over 30%.[20] And as many of our intensively farmed food animals are now fed large amounts of grains and soya, it is no longer accurate to speak of their fats as 'animal fats' – in many cases they are more akin to vegetable oils. In the same way that these are taken up by the animals we eat, they are also incorporated in our body cells. That turns what should be a

Table 15.1   Fatty acid composition of selected fats

Fat or oil	Saturated (%)	Mono-unsaturated (%)	Polyunsaturated (%)
Coconut	91	6	3
Palm kernel	83	16	1
Butter	60	34	6
Human milk	54	39	8
Lamb	53	41	5
Beef	45	51	5
Pork	43	48	8
Human (body fat)	40	57	3
Hen's egg	39	47	14
Chicken	35	48	16
Cod	26	16	59
Margarine (polyunsaturated)	24	21	55
Soya oil	18	24	58
Olive oil	17	74	9
Corn oil	13	24	59
Sunflower oil	10	20	66
Safflower oil	9	12	75

healthy fatty acid profile into a decidedly unhealthy one, with serious implications not only for those animals, but for our health as well.

So what levels of carbs, fats and proteins are required?

We now know that the animal fats we are advised not to eat are really very much healthier then the polyunsaturated vegetable margarines and cooking oils we are told we should eat. That just leaves the question of how much carb, protein and fat we should eat.

Clinical experience and studies into low-carb diets over the last century suggest that everybody has a threshold level of dietary carbohydrate intake where the changeover from glucose-burning to fat and ketone burning takes place. This varies between about 65 and 180 grams of carbs per day.[21] If your carb intake is below this threshold, then your body fat will be broken down to generate ketones to supply your brain and other cells that would normally use glucose.

In the early trials for the treatment of obesity mentioned in Chapter 8, carb levels were very much reduced to supply only about 10% of calories. This works out at around 50 or 60 grams of carb (see Appendix E) for a 2000 calorie daily intake.

For diabetics, the level may need to be lower to counteract insulin resistance. Typical levels of carb intake for a type-2 diabetic are around 50 grams per day; the level should be lower still at about 30 grams a day for a type-1 diabetic.

A Polish doctor, Jan Kwaśniewski, who has used a low-carb diet to treat patients with a wide range of medical conditions for over 30 years, recommends a ratio of one part carb to two parts protein to between three and four parts fat, by weight. I see no reason to disagree with this. What it means in practice is that on a 2000 calorie per day diet, we should get:

- 10–15% of calories from carbs.
- 20–30% of calories from protein.
- 60–70% of calories from fats.

Or put another way, as it is difficult to work out percentages in this way, with a common dietary intake of around 2000 calories, 50–75 grams of carbs, mostly from vegetables, and the rest from meat, fish, eggs, cheese, with their natural fats.

Traditional fats are better for weight loss

There is one other aspect as far as weight is concerned. No matter how careful you are, it is always possible to eat too much and put a bit of weight on. However, scientists at the Faculty of Medicine, University of Geneva in Switzerland, found that the more saturated a fat was, the less likely it was to put weight on. Similarly, they found that fats which were composed of shorter chain fatty acids, were also less fattening.[22] They say:

> 'The results indicate that for both body fat and protein, the efficiency of deposition was dependent on the dietary fat type. The most striking differences were found (1) between diets rich in n-3 and n-6 polyunsaturated fatty acids (PUFA), with the diet high in fish oil resulting in a greater body fat deposition and lower protein gain than the diet high in safflower oil; and (2) between diets rich in long-chain (LCT) and medium-chain triglycerides (MCT), with the diet high in

lard resulting in a greater gain in both body fat and protein than the diet high in coconut oil. Furthermore, the diet high in olive oil (a mono-unsaturated fat) and the mixed-fat diet (containing all fat types) were found to be similar to the fish oil diet in that the efficiency of fat deposition was greater (and that of protein gain lower) than with the diet high in safflower oil.'

This is because the unsaturated fats are fully digested to give more calories per gram than saturated fats as I mentioned earlier in Chapter 12. As animal fats are a mixture of both saturated and unsaturated fatty acids, a more accurate figure for fats from warm-blooded animals such as cattle and sheep is not 9 kcal, but about 7.5 kcal per gram. In other words, fish oils are the most fattening; vegetable oils and olive oil come next. Less likely to put fat on are animal fats; and least fattening of all is coconut oil. This is another good reason to eat the traditional animal fats and coconut oil, and avoid modern processed vegetable oils.

Potential for other diseases

The traditional Inuit (Eskimo) diet is a no-carb diet. It is notable that the Inuit diet described by Drs Vilhjalmur Stefansson and Hugh Sinclair in the 1950s is very similar in regard to percentages of fat/protein/carb intake to the experimental low-carb diets used in recent obesity studies.[23] The Inuit diet was comprised of seal, whale, salmon, and sometimes a very limited amount of berries and the partially digested contents of animals' stomachs. On this diet, blood cholesterol levels were very high as were free fatty acids, but – and this is much more important – triglycerides were low.[24,25]

It is interesting to note that the Inuit were of great interest to research scientists because they suffered none of the diseases we suffer. They had no obesity, no coronary heart disease, no diabetes and no cancer.[26,27]

A list diseases helped or prevented by this way of eating is at Appendix A.

References

1. Alberts B. *Molecular Biology of the Cell*, 4th edn. Garland Science, New York, 2002, p.93.
2. Cahill GF. Survival in starvation. *Am J Clin Nutr* 1998; 68: 1–2.
3. Exton JH. Gluconeogenesis. *Metabolism* 1972; 21: 945–990.

4. Volek JS, Sharman MJ, Love DM, et al. Body composition and hormonal responses to a carbohydrate-restricted diet. *Metabolism* 2002; 51: 864–870.

5. Krebs HA. The metabolic fate of amino acids. In: Munro HN, Allison JB, eds. *Mammalian Protein Metabolism*, vol 1. Academic Press, New York, 1964, p.164.

6. Vazquez JA, Kazi U. Lipolysis and gluconeogenesis from glycerol during weight reduction with very low calorie diets. *Metabolism* 1994; 43: 1293–1299.

7. Phinney SD, Bistrian BR, Wolfe RR, Blackburn GL. The human metabolic response to chronic ketosis without caloric restriction: physical and biochemical adaptation. *Metabolism* 1983; 32: 757–768.

8. Bisshop PH, Arias AM, Ackermans MT, et al. The effects of carbohydrate variation in isocaloric diets on glycogenolysis and gluconeogenesis in healthy men. *J Clin Endocrinol Metab* 2000; 85: 1963–1967.

9. Neely JR, Morgan HE. Relationship between carbohydrate and lipid metabolism and the energy balance of heart muscle. *Annu Rev Physiol* 1974; 36: 413–459.

10. Cahill GF Jr. Starvation in man. *N Engl J Med* 1970; 19: 668–675.

11. Klein S, Wolfe RR. Carbohydrate restriction regulates the adaptive response to fasting. *Am J Physiol* 1992; 262: E631–E636.

12. Speth JD, Spielmann KA. Energy source, protein metabolism, and hunter-gatherer subsistence strategies. *J Anthropol Archaeol* 1982; 2: 1–31.

13. Noli D, Avery G. Protein poisoning and coastal subsistence. *J Archaeol Sci* 1988; 15: 395–401.

14. McClellan WS, et al. Prolonged meat diets with a study of kidney function and ketosis. *J Biol Chem* 1930–31; 87:651; 87: 669; 93: 419.

15. Portillo MP, et al. Energy restriction with high-fat diet enriched with coconut oil gives higher UCP1 and lower white fat in rats. *Int J Obes Relat Metab Disord* 1998; 22: 947–949.

16. a. Kabara JJ. *The Pharmacological Effects of Lipids*. The American Oil Chemists' Society, Champaign, IL, 1978, 1–14.

    b. Cohen LA, et al. *J Natl Cancer Inst* 1986: 77: 43.

17. a. Guesry P. The role of nutrition in brain development. *Prev Med* 1998; 27: 189–194.

    b. Willatts P, Forsyth J, DiModugno M, et al. Effect of long-chain polyunsaturated fatty acids in infant formula on problem solving at 10 months of age. *Lancet* 1998; 352: 688–691.

18. Wolf RB. Effect of temperature on soybean seed constituents. *J Am Oil Chem Soc* 1982; 59: 230–232.

19. Wolfe R. Chemistry of nutrients and world food. *Univ Oregon Chem* October 16, 1986; 121.

20. McHenry EW, Cornett ML. The role of vitamins in anabolism of fats. *Vit Hormon* 1944; 2: 1–27.

21. Klein S, Wolfe RR. Op cit.

22. Dulloo AG, Mensi N, Seydoux J, Girardier L. Differential effects of high-fat diets varying in fatty acid composition on the efficiency of lean and fat tissue deposition during weight recovery after low food intake. *Metabolism* 1995; 44: 273–279.

23. Stefansson V. *The Fat of the Land*. Macmillan Press, New York, 1957; Sinclair HM. The diet of Canadian Indians and Eskimos. *Proc Nutr Soc* 1952; 12: 69–82.

24. Bang HO, Dyerberg J, Nielsen AB. Plasma lipid and lipoprotein pattern in Greenlandic West-Coast Eskimos. *Lancet* 1971; I: 1143–1146.

25. Feldman SA, Ho KJ, Lewis LA, et al. Lipid and cholesterol metabolism in Alaskan arctic Eskimos. *Arch Pathol* 1972; 94: 42–58.

26. Bjerregaard P, Dyerberg J. Mortality from ischaemic heart disease and cerebrovascular disease in Greenland. *Int J Epidem* 1988; 17: 514–519.

27. Sagild U, Littauer J, Jespersen CS, Andersen S. Epidemiological studies in Greenland 1962–1964. I. Diabetes mellitus in Eskimos. *Acta Med Scand* 1966; 179: 29–39.

Chapter Sixteen

Exercise isn't necessary

You may enjoy exercise; it may be helpful socially; it may make you look and feel better. But all the rest is myth.

Dr Henry Solomon

Introduction

Together with diet, exercise is touted as a cure for obesity and other associated conditions, but does this hypothesis stand up to objective scrutiny? Just how much benefit is there really to undertaking a strenuous exercise regime? And can you have too much? This chapter looks at the evidence for both benefit and adverse effects. It also discusses why low-carb diets are better for sportsmen and fitness.

How much exercise is natural?

If you watch animals in the wild you will see that on the whole, they take as little exercise as possible. The lion, for example, spends most of his day lying down or asleep, yet he doesn't get fat or suffer any other diseases. It is his wife, the lioness, who does the shopping, but she hunts only once every two or three days and even then expends as little energy as possible doing it. Similarly, grazing animals have a slow and steady lifestyle, moving quickly only when threatened by a predator. The same is true of modern hunter-gatherer human tribes. In the wild, nature protects the heart from stress. It's starting to look as if Dr Solomon may have a point.

Think about our hunter-gatherer ancestors. We have a good brain, but not a lot of speed. Did we chase our prey? It's not likely: there wouldn't be much point as they could all run faster than us. No, we crept up on them stealthily until we were close enough to throw something at them, or we ambushed them or set traps.

Animals that run for a living have efficient built-in shock absorbers in their legs; we haven't. With merely the arch of the foot, we simply aren't designed to run. We are designed for stealth and for walking at a slow, deliberate pace which does not send shock waves up our lower limbs. It is not surprising, therefore, that our love affair with exercise has resulted in a huge burden on the NHS from injuries sustained while running and jogging. Today, 20% of hospital orthopaedic beds are filled by exercise fanatics.

Exercise for weight loss

The combination of exercise and thinness is a well-established stereotype. The overweight are frequently criticised for not taking up the more strenuous physical activities enjoyed by slimmer people. Drs Andrew Prentice and Susan Jebb of the Medical Research Council pointed out that between 1980 and 1991 calorie intake in Britain fell by some 20%, while the number of people who were overweight doubled.[1] As we seem to be heeding the current dietary advice to eat less, but are nevertheless getting fatter, Prentice and Jebb conclude that the overweight are lazy. But are they?

Most modern diets advocate the twin strategies of taking in less energy (calorie-counting) while at the same time using more (exercising), and so dieters are urged to take up some form of physical activity to burn up the calories.

But the overriding philosophy – that exercise is the only sure way to lose fat – has always ignored one important fact: it doesn't work! Every single study on exercise to date, regardless of the type of exercise, (aerobic, anaerobic, resistance training, split routines and combo approaches) has shown that exercise almost always fails to alleviate obesity – whether it is combined with a low-calorie and/or low fat diet or not.

A great deal of research has been carried out in the hope of demonstrating that exercise reduces weight in the obese and prevents weight gain. It has been consistently unsuccessful and very few studies have tried to discover why. Here are the results of some of them:

1. In 1976 Dr Per Björntorp and colleagues at the University of Gothenburg, Sweden, studied normal and overweight subjects on a six-month course of physical training.[2] Although those at normal weight did lose weight on this programme, the overweight ones didn't.
2. Two years later Dr Martin Krotkiewski and colleagues conducted a similar study.[3] They found that while mildly obese patients did tend to lose weight; severely obese patients actually put on weight. These findings were not confined to Scandinavia.
3. In 1989 Drs I.E. Yale, L.A. Leiter and E.B. Marliss, at McGill University, Montreal and the University of Toronto, also found that exercise was fattening.[4] Measuring blood insulin levels, they discovered that these remained much higher in obese patients for more than an hour after exercising. This means that their bodies were taking glucose out of the blood and storing it as glycogen and fat.

Studies published in the early 1990s found no causal relationship between low physical activity and obesity in either children or the elderly.[5]

All this is borne out by the following case history which shows that there is no need to exercise to lose weight if you eat the right foods:

E.K. has multiple sclerosis. She was first diagnosed with MS when she was 19. She is now 40. Almost all of that time she has spent in a wheelchair, getting no exercise at all. You won't be surprised to hear that over the early years E.K. put on a lot of weight. Eventually, she decided to adopt the low-carb diet I recommended – and it worked beyond her wildest dreams. E.K. didn't weigh herself; she couldn't, but she did know what she measured. After less that a year, she had gone down three bra sizes and, she told me, 'it is getting expensive!' As I write this, five years after starting the diet, E.K. has maintained a normal weight for over four years.

The truth is that exercise as a means of achieving permanent weight loss simply doesn't work unless it is approached in the right way.

Exercise and energy stores

Your body stores energy in two forms: glycogen, a form of starch to serve as a ready supply of glucose, and body fat or adipose tissue, which is a store of fat. The aim is to lose the fat. This means you have to change your diet to one that is low in carbs or it simply won't work.

If you eat a carb-based, low-fat diet as most dieters do, then your body will be geared to burn glucose, so when you exercise, it will use up the glucose in your bloodstream and then mobilise the glycogen stored in your muscles and liver. When this is getting low, it will look for another source of glucose, and it will convert protein from your muscles into glucose.

You cannot keep on exercising forever without stopping, so as soon as you eat your next carb-rich meal, your glucose and glycogen stores will be replenished. You will then be right back where you started – but weaker. As every ounce of glycogen is stored with about three ounces of water, you can put that weight back on very quickly. On top of this you probably won't have burned up any body fat – which was the whole point of exercise in the first place!

This form of exercising for weight loss is costly, short-term, potentially dangerous and self-defeating. If, when you exercise, you burn up less energy than the amount of easily accessible glycogen stored in the liver and muscles you won't use up any of your body fat – and therefore you won't lose any weight. If you use more energy than is immediately available, any weight lost is at a cost of stress on your body.

The formula is another form of calorie-counting: increasing energy output through exercise is the same as decreasing energy input with a low-calorie diet. The overall effect is the same: you are eating less than you need (starving) and, no matter how long you exercise, as soon as you stop, you will put the weight back on again.

Exercise for weight loss – the right way

To lose weight, you *must* mobilise your fat stores. This means getting your body to burn fat and that, in turn, means making it change from using glucose to using fat. The only way to do that is to deprive your body of the sources of glucose, so it has no choice in the matter.

If you think about it, it really is quite logical: to lose weight, you merely have to change to a low-carb, high-fat diet. Or, of course, you can continue to starve.

Exercise and heart disease

But we are also told to exercise for other reasons. With respect to heart disease, it is suggested that regular exercise will enlarge the arteries thus lessening the likelihood of their becoming blocked and so reducing the risk of coronary heart disease. It was noted that bus drivers have a higher incidence of coronary heart disease than bus conductors and, as the drivers have a less energetic working life, this may be seen to support the argument. It was also noted, however, that dock labourers have higher rates of heart disease than building labourers which tends to defeat the argument as the amounts of exercise associated with their jobs are not likely to differ significantly.[6]

Professor John Yudkin published a graph of the early mortality trends from heart disease correlated with radio and TV licences issued at the time in his book, *Sweet & Dangerous*, which showed a strong linear relationship between the two, and that too may suggest that a lack of exercise could be connected with the rise.

The claim that exercise may help in heart disease arose from the fact that seasoned athletes develop increased cardiovascular capacity. However, the view that exercise necessarily protects against heart disease, a strongly emotive factor in the increasing pressure to indulge in high-intensity exercise regardless of physical status, can be dangerous.

The studies disagree

The results of the major studies published so far have found for the most part that there is no convincing correlation between exercise (or the lack of it) and heart disease. For example, while a study of 16,882 executive grade civil servants aged 40 to 64 from 1968–1972 suggested that heavy work such as swimming or gardening may be beneficial if continued for over 15 minutes, its results were inconclusive.[7]

In the UK Heart Disease Project, a part of the WHO European Study, however, the results were conclusive – and different. The Project studied 18,210 men, again in the 'coronary' age group, from 24 factories. Half were given the conventional advice on exercise and overweight, the other half being given no specific advice. The results of this study, published in 1983 showed that instead of the expected benefits, the group which followed the advice on exercise had significantly *higher* rates of cardiovascular mortality and morbidity than that which did not.[8] These results confirmed others that had been published in the USA a few years earlier.

Data from the United States indicated that richer people tend to adopt health innovations more readily than poorer people, and this was particularly evident in the cases of smoking and exercise. Stern cites as an example:

'A dramatic illustration in the case of exercise is that of the approximately 10,000 persons who participated in the recent New York Marathon, 80% had college degrees and of these fully half held graduate degrees!' He continued, 'Since in our society, whites are generally of higher socio-economic status than either blacks or Mexican-Americans, one might have expected that they would experience the steepest CHD mortality declines. . . The data, however, indicate the reverse has been true'.

The statistics from the period show that while mortality in the USA from CHD declined by over 20% between 1968 and 1976, it seems that exercise increased it.[9]

Exercising faith

In June 1991 the British government published its initial *Health of the Nation* green paper in which exercise was promoted on the grounds that it prevented heart disease. Given that a major national effort is invested in promoting exercise on the grounds that it prevents heart disease, you might think it fair to ask for some evidence to substantiate this claim. The *British Medical Journal* conducted a debate into the merits of the green paper and contested the assertion that exercise was helpful. This led to two contributors to the debate revealing the anti-scientific mentality of the health promotion lobby. In their support of 'the role of exercise', Drs Henry Dargie and S. Grant took on the exercise sceptics by writing:

> 'Some would argue that there is no conclusive evidence from controlled trials that regular exercise reduces the number of deaths from coronary heart disease or substantially prolongs life. To demand such proof is to miss the point about exercise, which is that it is valuable for numerous other health benefits it confers and as a catalyst in the adoption of a healthier lifestyle.'[10]

So it seems there is no evidence after all for the benefits of exercise in heart disease – merely 'numerous *other* health benefits'. No doubt to request evidence for these benefits would also be to miss the point, which is that the health promoters firmly believe that exercise is conducive to a healthier lifestyle. It seems it is faith rather than science that justifies exhortations to change public behaviour, and such faith may place a trusting public at greater danger, for exercise may not always be beneficial.

The dangers of over-exercising

'Fitness' is a billion-pound industry which promotes books, exercise machinery, weights, footwear, clothing, and expensive gyms and clubs. If someone tells you that you need to exercise, you would be wise to question whether there is any commercial bias behind their advice.

Sport and exercise of the right kind can be rewarding both as a social outlet and in making you feel good, it may boost your self-esteem if you treat it as a form of group therapy, and it helps to keep muscles in trim and give your body a better shape. As such it has an important role to play, particularly as leisure time for most of us is increasing, but it can easily be overdone with potentially disastrous consequences.

In women, exercise exhaustive enough to cause weight loss can delay the onset of puberty, cause amenorrhoea (cessation of periods), abnormal menstrual cycles, abnormal sex hormone patterns and impaired reproductive function, and the early development of osteoporosis.[11] Male long-distance runners may suffer reductions in the male sex hormone, testosterone.[12] For anyone contemplating taking up the more strenuous forms of exercise, the advice from the *American Heart Journal* is:

> 'Be tested and have an exercise programme devised after clinical trials and tests on the heart as, although regular exercise will lower the overall risk of cardiovascular disease, there is a statistically significant increase in the risk of sudden death.'[13]

There are real risks if those who are not seasoned athletes attempt to break through the pain barrier, or as Jane Fonda put it, 'go for the burn'. The pain barrier is the body's signal that its limit of toleration has been reached. Disregarding it is foolhardy. While seasoned athletes with their increased oxygenating capacity may be able to prolong their muscular activity before the onset of pain, the average person cannot and should not attempt to emulate them. The risk to health and even life is unacceptably high. Over the past few years there have been reports of significant numbers of cases of sudden death in healthy young men out jogging or playing squash because they disregarded the pain barrier.

Most sudden deaths in sport are caused by cardiovascular conditions, although one regularly hears that the benefits of exercise in terms of CHD are 'well established' and may reduce the risk of such events. Victims are often perceived as very fit but it should be noted that 'extreme forms of conditioning, including marathon running, do not prevent severe atherosclerosis or sudden death.'[14]

There have also been a vast number of cases of broken bones, dislocations, and damage to internal organs, muscles, tendons and ligaments. A study from Japan cited a 25% incidence of injury in those undertaking exhaustive exercise and these figures are confirmed in similar Western studies. The increase of sports-related injuries has been such that, had they been caused by a bacterium, it would have been classed as a serious epidemic.

Exercise-induced allergies – asthma, skin itching and urticaria (nettle rash) – are also on the increase, as are cases of cardiovascular collapse and respiratory obstruction.[15] While some conditions may be minor annoyances, others are definitely life-threatening. They typically affect teenagers and young adults.

In a study of 42 Swedish elite runners, 23 had asthma and 31 had asthma-like symptoms. The prevalence of asthma in elite athletes in Finland whose mean age was 22.9 was similar. Of 103 athletes, 16 had documented asthma and 24 more had allergies. All those with asthma and 14 of those with allergies reported having symptoms like exercise-induced asthma. Twenty-three of the remaining 63 also reported having asthma-like symptoms occasionally. Thus over half of the runners in this study were affected.[16]

The usual trigger for an attack is running, but some patients have collapsed after only a brisk walk. It is not possible to predict an attack even among people with a history of such attacks while running. Even joggers, who have been running for many years without incident, frequently collapse. Jim Fixx, author of *The Complete Book of Running*, invented jogging and advocated it to prevent a heart attack. It is ironic that Fixx himself died of a heart attack while out jogging. Current advice to joggers is: never jog alone.

In spite of the risks, or more probably because they are not made aware of them, many people adopt exercise programmes which involve sudden intensive exertion such as squash or aerobics.

The term aerobics means 'using oxygen' and it is claimed that aerobic exercise is beneficial because it increases the amount of oxygen in the body tissues. In fact, the demand for oxygen may increase to a point where it cannot be met, so that, far from increasing tissue oxygenation, aerobic exercise decreases it. Aerobic exercise has been demonstrated to cause a significant and continuous drop in blood pressure – a sign of cardiac fatigue.[17] It can happen in as little as five minutes – and most aerobic sessions last for an hour!

And there is another consideration, particularly where the overweight are concerned: by definition, people who are overweight are already carrying around extra weight. That fact alone means that they must already use more energy than slim people. There is a limit to how much more exercise someone who is massively overweight can do.

Athletes reach altered states such as 'the runner's high'. It makes them feel better and is a form of reward for their effort. The lower potential of overweight people means that they will be denied this satisfaction even if they do lose some weight.

Too much of a good thing?

The reason we have the potential for rapid movement is that we have evolved to be able to escape from danger and to survive in a wide range of dangerous and adverse circumstances. This ability is built into our bodies' emergency system: the 'fight or flight reflex'. When that is activated by the need to run away from danger or stay and fight, or as a result of strenuous exercise, it causes a number of automatic responses which prepare the body to face the danger to come. Amongst these, the heartbeat is accelerated and minor blood vessels are constricted so that more blood is fed to the brain and muscles, and the lungs take in more oxygen; the amount of cholesterol in the blood is increased; adrenaline is pumped into the bloodstream helping these changes, stopping or slowing the digestive process, and stimulating the conversion of glycogen, a form of sugar stored by the body, into glucose which the body can use more easily as a source of energy.

These changes, in the natural world, are designed to last for a short time: the time of the emergency, after which the body can return to normal. In the case of prolonged physical exertion, however, the body is forced to continue, setting in motion a series of changes called the *General Adaption Syndrome*. A major and important change is the prolonged production of a group of adrenal hormones called *corticosteroids*. An excessive production of corticosteroids has been shown to produce heart disease,[18] hypertension and stomach ulcers,[19] and harm the body's ability to fight infectious diseases and cancer[20]; and the depletion of the corticosteroids may cause rheumatoid arthritis.[21]

Other evidence emerged in 2005 which suggested that exercising may actually shorten your life.[22] Dr Peter Axt and his daughter, Dr Michaela Axt-Gadermann, who are both reformed, long-distance runners, argue that exercising increases the production of harmful free radicals – unstable oxygen molecules believed to speed up the ageing process. They add: 'If you lead a stressful life and exercise excessively, your body produces hormones which lead to high blood pressure and can damage your heart and arteries.'

To sum up, moderate exercise and sport do have a healthy social role. People who are part of a social group tend to have fewer health problems than loners. Members of religious groups, supportive families and clubs are also healthier, slimmer and more relaxed. However, excessive exercise is unnatural and can be dangerous. And don't be misled by the hype – athletes are not known for their longevity.

The correct exercise for health

For health generally all that is necessary is moderate exercise such as walking or gardening. To increase the capacity of your cardiovascular system, you need to work harder, but either way, it's a good idea to avoid repetitive 'bouncing' types of exercise that shock the system. This means that walking, cycling and swimming are good, but running and jogging are not.

Although there is some disagreement among experts, it is generally agreed that pulse rate should be raised to between 60% and 80% of its maximum using the 220-minus-age formula:

The 220-Minus-Age Formula

220 minus your age = your maximum pulse rate
This is the maximum rate your heart can beat and optimally pump blood. Your maximum pulse rate declines with age.

Your maximum pulse rate multiplied by 0.6 = your minimum aerobic pulse rate
This is the minimum pulse rate to confer benefit.

Your maximum pulse rate multiplied by 0.8 = your maximum aerobic pulse rate
This is generally accepted as the maximum pulse rate that confers aerobic benefit.

So, to give an example, if you are 35 years old, your maximum pulse rate will be 185 beats per minute and the aerobic zone will be between 111 and 148 beats per minute. You should maintain a rate between 111 and 148 for the period of your exercise. If you are 60, the figures are lower with the aerobic zone between 96 and 128.

Note that these figures are based on averages. There will be some people who naturally have slower or faster pulse rates. It is a good idea, therefore, to take it easy, particularly at first. Monitoring your breathing can also help determine whether you are overdoing it, or can safely put a bit more 'oomph' into your exercise regime.

Your exercise should make you breathe faster but shouldn't make you gasp for air. You should be able to talk, haltingly, while exercising. If you are unable to carry on a limited conversation, you are overdoing it.

If you work your muscles too hard, they will be starved of oxygen and start to work 'anaerobically', or without oxygen. This will change the fuel they use from fat, which uses oxygen, to glucose, which doesn't, and that is the last thing we want.

So don't go mad at it. You should exercise in a steady and continuous way. The idea isn't to see how many calories you can burn up in the quickest time, but to change the way in which your body works. If you want faster results, then exercise longer, not harder.

Unfortunately, most sports – tennis, badminton, football, hockey, cricket, for example – are not useful exercises. They tend to be 'start/stop' – brief spurts of intense movement between lulls of low intensity. Sports like golf and archery, while they are enjoyable, are also not much use as they are low intensity all the time and don't cause the metabolic changes needed to cause the muscles to burn fat. No, for that you need moderate exercise which must be continuous.

Carbs are not as good as fats for athletes

All carbohydrates – sugars and starches – are converted immediately into glucose which the body can use for energy. That is the reason that athletes are told by their coaches and sports nutritionists that it is a good idea for them drink a goodly supply of carbohydrate-rich, sugary drinks throughout a match or tournament. Food and drinks manufacturers, always ready to make a swift buck, have seen this as an opportunity to provide a range of what are laughingly called 'isotonic drinks'. These are little more than sugared water which do nothing for performance (although they do wonders for the manufacturers' profits).

Athletes, like the rest of us, are also usually told to eat a diet high in carbohydrates and low in fats. This, they are told, will increase their performance. However, this was not confirmed in a dietary study published in 1994.[23] Using three diets: normal, high-fat and high-carbohydrate, the study showed that the high-carbohydrate diet increased performance by an average 10% over a normal mixed diet. Not bad, you might think, but the high-fat diet increased performance by a massive 33%. That's much better. The authors conclude that restriction of dietary fat may be detrimental to endurance performance. So, once again, fat is best.

Conclusion

I hope by writing some of the information above I haven't put you off exercising altogether. That was not my intention. I wrote it because there are two aspects to exercise: one is health, which I have covered; the other is fitness. 'Health' and 'fitness' are not the same thing. There is not a great deal of evidence that exercise plays much part in health – unless you eat an unhealthy 'healthy' diet, in which the exercise may help to counter the diet's unhealthy effects – but exercise of the right kind will keep you fit: that is supple, strong and with stamina.

People with only ten pounds or so to lose may be able to lose it with exercise, but anyone who claims that exercise is the key to solving weight problems in the chronically obese is simply not telling the complete truth about what research on the subject has shown.

Fat is the best fuel for an athlete, carbohydrates are the worst. The same goes for weight loss. It really is as simple as that.

References

1. Prentice AM, Jebb SA. Obesity in Britain: gluttony or sloth? *BMJ* 1995; 311: 437–439.
2. Björntorp P, et al. Physical training in human hyperplasic obesity. IV: Effects on hormonal status. *Metabolism* 1977; 26: 319.
3. Krotkiewski M, et al. Effects of long-term physical training on body fat, metabolism, and blood pressure in obesity. *Metabolism* 1979; 28: 650.
4. Yale J-F, Leiter LA, Marliss EB. Metabolic responses to intense exercise in lean and obese subjects. *J Clin Endocrin Metab* 1989; 68: 438–445.
5. a. Oomura Y, Tarui S, Inoue S, Shimazu T, eds. *Prog Obes Res* 1990; p.563. John Libby, London, 1990.

b. Voorrips LE, et al. History of body weight and physical activity of elderly women differing in current physical activity. *Int J Obes* 1992; 16: 199.

6. Yudkin J. Diet and coronary thrombosis. Hypothesis and fact. *Lancet* 1957; ii: 155.

7. Morris JN, et al. Vigorous exercise in leisure time and the incidence of coronary heart disease. *Lancet* 1973; i: 333.

8. Rose G, Tunstall-Pedoe HD, Heller RF. UK Heart Disease Prevention Project: Incidence and mortality results. *Lancet* 1983; iv: 1062.

9. Stern MP. The recent decline in ischaemic heart disease mortality. *Ann Int Med* 1979; 91: 630.

10. Dargie H, Grant S. The Health of the Nation: The BMJ View. *BMJ* 1992; 305: 156.

11. a. Schwartz B, et al. Exercise associated amenorrhea: a distinct entity? *Am J Obstet Gynecol* 1981; 141: 662.
    b. Cumming DC, et al. Exercise and reproductive function in women. *Prog Clin Biol Res* 1983; 117: 113.
    c. Defects in pulsatile release in normally menstruating runners. *J Clin Endocrin Metab* 1985; 60: 810.
    d. Reid RL, van Vugt DA. Weight-related changes in reproductive function. *Fertil Steril* 1987; 48(6): 905.

12. Editorial. Reduced testosterone and prolactin in male distance runners. *JAMA* 1984; 252: 514.

13. Coplan NL, Gleim GW, Nicholas JA. Exercise and sudden cardiac death. *Am Heart J* 1988; 115: 207–212.

14. Hillis WS, McIntyre PD, Maclean J, Goodwin JF, McKenna WJ. Sudden death in sport. *BMJ* 1994; 309: 657–661.

15. Weinstein CE. Exercise-induced allergic syndromes on the increase. *Cleveland Clin J Med* 1989; 56: 665–666.

16. Tikkanen HO, Helenius I. Asthma in runners. *BMJ* 1994; 309: 1087.

17. Ketelhut R, Losem CJ, Messerli FH. Is a decrease in arterial pressure during long-term exercise caused by a fall in cardiac pump function? *Am Heart J* 1994; 127: 567–571.

18. Sholter DE, Armstrong PW. Adverse effects of corticosteroids on the cardiovascular system. *Can J Cardiol* 2000;16: 505–511.

19. Sawrey WL, Weisz JD. An experimental method of producing gastric ulcers. *J Comp Physio Psychol* 1956; 49: 269.

20. a. Selye H. *The Stress of Life*. McGraw-Hill, New York, 1956;
    b. *Annual Report on Stress*. Acta Inc., Montreal, 1951.

21. Solomon GF. Psychophysiological aspects of rheumatoid arthritis and auto-immune disease. In: Hill OW, ed. *Modern Trends in Psychosomatic Medicine* – 2. Butterworths, London, 1970.

22. Axt P, Axt-Gadermann M. *The Joy of Laziness: How to Slow Down and Live Longer*. Bloomsbury, 2005.

23. Muoio DM, et al. Effect of dietary fat on metabolic adjustments to maximal VO-2 and endurance in runners. *Med Sci Sports Exercise* 1994; 26 (1): 81–88.

Chapter Seventeen

Fat or fashion?

Fashion, though Folly's child, and guide of fools,
Rules e'en the wisest, and in learning rules.

George Crabbe

Being overweight is not a desirable state, at least from a medical standpoint; being excessively overweight puts unnecessary strain on the heart, and back and knee joints. It also makes any surgery more difficult. Apart from that, being obese is generally not socially acceptable.

However, there is another side to this coin: we live in a society that makes a virtue out of being skeletally thin. Models on catwalks, pictures in fashion magazines, and the slimming industry may have convinced you that you should shed a few pounds, but are you really overweight? Fads come and go, fashions change, how can you tell? You really need to know, because before you try to lose weight, you really should be sure that you really do need to do so. You should never try to lose weight if you are not overweight as it is even more unhealthy to be underweight than overweight. So there is one last consideration we need to address: are you really overweight, or are you just bowing to fashion?

Having said that, because this way of eating doesn't involve starvation, it won't allow your weight to go too low. Indeed, if you are underweight, you will put weight on. That is one reason why it is so much healthier than the more usual calorie-controlled diets.

Overweight and obesity defined

There are a number of ways to measure whether you are the right weight for your height: skin-fold thickness, body density measurement, height/weight tables, and so on.

The most used definition of overweight is a weight that is above the acceptable weight for your height, and obesity is defined as being 20% or more above the upper limit of the acceptable weight range. And that said, we have to define 'acceptable' as there are now known to be health risks associated with extreme leanness – it is safer to be overweight than underweight.[1]

The acceptable weight ranges at present are those shown in Appendix B (page 283). Until recently, women's acceptable weights have ranged considerably lower than those for men, and, as there is no reason why they should, weights of the two sexes have now been brought into line.[2] You will notice that the small/medium/large frame sizes have disappeared. This is because these were always artificial: doctors had asked for them and the acceptable ranges were split arbitrarily into three. There is no scientific definition of frame size.

The weight ranges for any particular height may seem very wide as they cover a band of nearly 30 lb (13.6 kg) for a woman of 4 ft 9 in (1.45 m) to 45 lb (20.5 kg) for a tall man. However, there is no evidence that weight at one position within this range is any healthier than at any other position. A weight at the top is as healthy as one in the middle or one at the bottom. As muscle is heavier than fat, a body builder with no excess body fat can weigh the same as a person of similar height with considerably more body fat. Your weight also wanders about constantly over a few pounds and many people worry quite unnecessarily about their weights.

Unfortunately, the old tables are still being used in current diet books and slimming magazines, even though the concept of frame sizes, for example, was abandoned as long ago as 1973. But slimming is a multi-billion-dollar industry. If people are told that they ought not to be so thin after all, the industry could lose some of its business – and that is not what they are in business for.

Other tests whereby you pinch a fold of flesh on the upper arm to gauge the amount of fat are more realistic as they are more individual, but a figure of three-quarters of an inch, generally regarded as the norm, still does not allow for individual physiology.

Body Mass Index (BMI) is the most commonly used measure today. To determine your BMI you divide your weight in kilograms by the square of your height in metres (kg/m^2). If the result is between 20 and 25 you are an acceptable weight, between 25 and 30 is overweight, over 30 is obese and over 40 is morbidly obese. This is the method favoured by clinicians and is the method used to generate the weights in Appendix A.

In Britain the number of adults aged 20–74 years with a body mass index (BMI) greater than 30 kg/m^2 more than doubled between 1980 and 1996 from 6% to 16% in men and from 8 to 17.3% in women.[3]

Another good way to test whether you are overweight is to look at your face. If it is neither bloated around the eyes, which would be an indication of overweight, nor hollowed, an indication of underweight, you are almost certainly within the acceptable weight range. If you do not feel you are overweight, then you are probably not.

Fashions change

In primitive societies it is often fatness that is desired; in the West it is more likely to be slimness. Slimming magazines, women's fashions and the media portray the desirable woman as tall and thin.

We live in a time when slimness is the fashion but it was not always so – fashions change. Centuries ago, celibate early Christian writers were terrified of women's flesh. They were frightened by their own lascivious thoughts – but put the blame on women. In an attempt to make women as sexless as possible, the Church urged women to fast. Travel through time to the 16th and 17th centuries and the fashion had changed dramatically. Rubens' paintings depict women who are considerably cuddlier. At the beginning of the 20th century it was also fashionable to be buxom, but by the 1920s busts were out and it was fashionable to be slim once more. In the 1930s the fashion changed to cuddly again – and back yet again with skinny fashion models in the 1960s. This look has persisted. As the late Duchess of Windsor famously said: 'you can never be too rich or too thin'.

However, we should be less concerned with what is fashionable and concentrate more on what is normal and what is healthy. In reality, the impeccably emaciated women employed in the fashion business today are not normal, they are freaks. The only safe way to look like them is to be born like them, but why would you want to look like them? Ask most men, for example, what shape they desire in a woman, and you will find that they prefer one considerably more rounded. To know what shape a man prefers, look at the centrefold of a man's magazine. The ideal shape, from both a desirability and a health point of view, is nearer to that seen in a Rubens painting than on the catwalk. Indeed the major difference between the sexes is that healthy men tend to be hard and angular and healthy women soft and rounded.

In both sexes, body fat plays an important role: it fills hollows in the skeleton, the eye sockets, joints and neck; it cushions and protects internal organs and provides a reservoir of energy; it is fat that contours the body. When the body loses fat, it sags and shows the signs of ageing. Body fat is synonymous with the looks and actions of youth.

Women have more fat cells than do men. In a woman, up to 24% of body weight should be fat; in men only about 12% should be fat. Curves distinguish women from men. The woman's extra fat is both a natural and a normal phenomenon brought about by sex hormones during puberty. As well as having an aesthetic value, it is of biological importance, preparing women for motherhood. A feminine body is a curvaceous body. Why try to lose it? It is much healthier to be satisfied with what you have rather than continually try to change it.

Heavier may be healthier

The current hysteria over an alleged epidemic of obesity may be overdone – at least to some extent. The abstracts of many papers allegedly showing 'overweight' to be detrimental are at variance with the data presented in these papers.[4]

A standard reference for mortality with respect to height and weight was, for a long time, the extensive data compiled by the Metropolitan Life Insurance Company, which was usually analysed without taking into account the ages of the subjects. When Reuben Andres recalculated these data for 10-year-wide age cohorts, he found that minimal mortality was correlated with *increasing* weight as the ages of the cohorts increased.[6] He also found that the 'ideal' weights were the same for men and women. Thus, if you *don't* gain weight as you age, you may be slipping out of the lowest-mortality weight range.

In *The Obesity Myth*, Paul Campos, a professor of law, pretty much demolishes the case for the existence of an epidemic of obesity.[7] He reckons that the unwarranted concern with 'obesity' has the opposite of the intended effect, since it is very difficult and very uncommon for a person who has lost weight by low-calorie dieting to be able to keep this weight off. This leads to 'yo-yo' weight loss, and he presents horrifying statistics which demonstrate this to be extremely detrimental to health.

Waist/hip ratio

As far as health is concerned, overall weight is not as important as how any excess weight is distributed. There is one very good way of determining whether you need to lose weight for health reasons: if your waist measurement and your hip measurement are such that it's difficult to work out where one stops and the other begins. For women, the distance around your waist should be no more than 80% of that around your hips; for men your waist should measure no more than your hips. In both sexes, upper body fat is more of a risk to health than fat around hips and thighs. Fortunately, fat around the middle is generally easier to lose than fat lower down.

The dangers of low-calorie dieting

Dieting, therefore, is a serious and risky business that should not be embarked upon lightly. How many slimming magazines explain this to their readers? They all give the impression that losing weight is always beneficial.

If you think that you should lose weight, check with your doctor to ensure that it is necessary. This is particularly important if you are only mildly or moderately overweight and thinking of embarking on a crash diet, as you are at increased risk of arrhythmic sudden death on such diets. Then diet in a way that is safe. There is a serious risk of harm on very-low-calorie liquid-protein diets such as the Cambridge Diet even under medical supervision.[8] The 'yo-yo' effect of rapid weight loss, followed inevitably by weight gain, repeated over and over is far more dangerous to health than a high but steady weight.

Unreasonable regimes

Slimming clubs and counsellors are only too aware that the modern slimmer will sacrifice anything to lose weight. They set unreasonably low target weights and encourage unreasonably rapid weight loss. Many dieters find these regimes impossible to resist. Do they work? Only in the short term, and then the weight returns. After losing 140 lb (63 kg) in a year and becoming the British 1980 Weight Watcher of the Year, the recipient of this honour said that the experience had changed his life. Suddenly, he was no longer a loser but a success, but the euphoria did not last for long. As soon as he had reached his target weight, the weight he had lost began to return. After a 12-year struggle, his weight in 1992 was 295 lb (143 kg) – right back where it started. Interviewed on television, he said that the whole weight-loss philosophy was wrong. Dieters' minds are focused and concentrated on food, when food was the last thing they should be thinking about. He went on to say that his mood now was one of depression, disappointment and a loss of self-esteem: feelings all too common in the long-term dieter.

There are many people who are not even slightly overweight, much less obese, who have been influenced by all the publicity to start on an unnecessary slimming program that will ultimately have an adverse effect on their bodies' regulatory systems. Unfortunately, adolescent girls seem to have an exaggerated concern about getting fat regardless of whether they are overweight or not.

Dr Nancy Moses and colleagues of North Shore University Hospital, Manhasset, New York, studied perceptions concerning weight, dieting practices and nutrition of adolescent girls in relation to their body weight.[9] High school girls reported exaggerated concern with obesity regardless of their body weight or nutrition knowledge. As many as 51% of *underweight* girls described themselves as extremely fearful of being overweight and 36% were preoccupied with body fat. Many had a distorted perception of what was an ideal body weight. This was particularly noticeable among underweight girls; normal weight and overweight girls had better concordance between their actual and perceived ideal body weight for height. The team concluded that fear of obesity and inappropriate eating behaviours are pervasive among adolescent girls regardless of body weight or nutrition knowledge. In a society obsessed with body weight, even young girls who are underweight are dieting. Such inappropriate eating patterns are associated with many medical problems and poor growth.

Parents who are dieting also tend to put their young offspring on similar low-calorie diets. This can have devastating results. A growing child needs lots of protein to build body tissue. As a child's stomach is relatively small, he or she must also have a diet that contains lots of energy. Low-fat, low-calorie slimming diets are particularly dangerous to any child prior to puberty.

Conclusion

You should never try to lose weight if you are not overweight. If you are at your correct weight and can maintain it without 'dieting', you have no need to diet.

References

1. Jarrett RJ. Is there an ideal body weight? *BMJ* 1986; ii: 493.
2. Lewin R. Overblown reports distort obesity risks. *Science* 1981; 211: 258.
3. Prescott-Clark P, Primatesta P. *Health Survey for England, 1996.* Stationery Office, London, 1996.
4. Deutsch ME. Obesity and cancer. *New Engl J Med* 2003; 349: 502–504.
5. a. Lee CD, Blair SN, Jackson AS. Cardiorespiratory fitness, body composition, and all-cause and cardiovascular disease mortality in men. *Am J Clin Nutr* 1999; 69: 373–380.
   b. Barlow CE, Kohl HW 3rd, Gibbons LW, Blair SN. Physical fitness, mortality and obesity. *Int J Obes Relat Metab Disord* 1995; 19 Suppl 4: S41–44.
6. Andres R, Elahi D, Tobin JD, et al. Impact of age on weight goals. *Ann Intern Med* 1985; 103: 1030–1033.
7. Campos P. *The Obesity Myth: Why America's Obsession with Weight is Hazardous to your Health.* Gotham Books, New York, 2004.
8. Sours HE, et al. Sudden death associated with very low calorie weight reduction regimes. *Am J Clin Nutr* 1981; 34: 453.
9. Moses N, et al. Fear of obesity among adolescent girls. *Pediatrics* 1989; 83: 393.

Appendix A

Diseases helped or prevented by the *Natural Health and Weight Loss* way of eating

> There are some people that if they don't know, you can't tell 'em.
> *Louis Armstrong*

Many previously rare diseases suddenly 'took off' in the 20th century and new ones also appeared during that period. These then tended to increase dramatically in the last quarter of the last century after we were introduced to the concept of 'healthy eating'. There is a huge body of evidence that this modern carbohydrate-based, low-fat diet may be either a cause of these conditions or a factor in increasing the risk of contracting one or more of them. Unfortunately, detailing this is beyond the scope of this book. Nevertheless, around 70 diseases have been shown to be prevented or successfully treated with the diet recommended in this book. I have listed these below together with the dietary causal component. Note, however, that there may be causal factors other than diet. Note also that this list is not exhaustive.

Acne. *Refined sugar- and starch-rich foods; cereal grains.* In industrialised societies, acne is a universal skin disease. It afflicts 79 to 95% of the adolescent population. Indeed, acne during teenage years is now so widespread it is considered 'normal' in developed nations, but it also continues into adulthood. However, it is noticeable that peoples who do not consume a carbohydrate-rich diet do not suffer the problem.[1]

Allergies. *Incorrect fatty acid balance: too much omega-6 and insufficient omega-3; cereal grains; processed food.* Allergies are caused by too many things to cover here. However, as the numbers of cases have risen dramatically since 'healthy eating' was introduced in 1984, the two are likely to be linked.

Alzheimer's disease. *Bran; cereals; carbohydrate-based 'healthy' diet.* It is said that the recent increase in numbers of people succumbing to Alzheimer's disease is because it is a disease of the elderly and people are living longer, but that theory doesn't stand up as Alzheimer's is increasingly seen in younger people. It is much more prevalent in people with other conditions such as diabetes which is known to be caused by a 'healthy' diet.

Amenorrhoea. *Bran; soya; strict vegetarian diet, low-cal dieting, exercise.* Amenorrhoea is associated with deficiencies of zinc and of iron.[2] Soy and cereal grains inhibit the absorption of both minerals; reduced intake of red meat as part of 'healthy eating' advice also reduces the availability of iron.

Ankylosing spondylitis. *Carbohydrate based 'healthy' diet.* Ankylosing spondylitis is an inflammatory form of back pain. Its cause is not known for sure, but AS is generally thought to be an autoimmune disease. This is similar to several other conditions: coeliac disease or multiple sclerosis for example, so it is not surprising that, in a similar way, taking starch out of the diet has been shown to be highly beneficial.[3] Since 1983, the AS Clinic at the Middlesex Hospital in London has used the low-carb diet in the treatment of AS patients. Over half of these patients have not required any medication and are successfully treated solely by diet.

Anorexia. *Bran; soya; low intake of red meat.* Anorexia is associated with deficiencies of zinc and of iron, whose absorption is inhibited by bran,[4] and the current obsession against red meat.

Antisocial behaviour. *Carbohydrate-based, low-fat diet; low blood cholesterol.* Studies showed that children between 6 and 16 years of age whose cholesterol concentration was below 3.77 mmol/L (145 mg/dL) were almost three times more likely to have been suspended or expelled from schools than their peers with higher cholesterol levels.[5] The conclusion was that low total cholesterol may be a risk factor for aggression or a risk marker for other biologic variables that predispose to aggression.

Arthritis (osteo). *Carbohydrate based 'healthy' diet.* Osteoarthritis tends to accompany osteoporosis.[6] Osteoarthritis is also known to be more prevalent in those who are obese.[7] It's not surprising that joints protest at having to support a heavier body. Studies of ancient peoples and modern clinical trials have also shown that carbohydrates, particularly cereals, in the diet cause arthritis.[8]

Arthritis (rheumatoid). *Carbohydrates; cereals; excess vegetable oils.* Rheumatoid arthritis is never found in animal remains. Neither has it been found in skeletal remains of peoples whose diet is from animal sources, but it has been found in all races and cultures eating wheat, rye and oats. This finding suggests that rheumatoid arthritis is a gluten-induced condition similar to coeliac disease.[9] Incorrect ratios of omega-3 and omega-6 fatty acids is another possible cause as vegetable oils make arthritis worse while eating fish oils and other omega-3 rich oils are of benefit.[10]

Asthma. *High-carbohydrate 'healthy' diet?* Nobody seems quite sure what causes asthma. Too early weaning to cereals is certainly one cause.[11] Being overweight in childhood is another.[12]

Attention deficit hyperactivity disorder (ADHD). *Sugars and refined starches; additives in processed foods.* The most common underlying cause of the behavioural symptoms of ADHD seems to be hypoglycaemia (low blood sugar). When individuals have low blood sugar, the body releases adrenaline to raise it to normal levels. In children, the adrenaline release may cause them to act aggressively. Hypoglycaemia is caused by a high-carb diet. ADHD has also been shown to be caused or exacerbated by a number of chemical food additives. By avoiding the processed and packeted foods that contain carbs, you will not only avoid the excessive carb load, you also avoid the chemicals that are related to ADHD.

Autism. *Cereals and milk casein.* The cause of autism in children is not known. Professor Jean Golding of Bristol University points out that there has been a huge increase in numbers of cases of autism in the last 20 to 30 years. That tells us that the condition cannot be genetic. Some autistic patients have been shown to have increased antibodies to gluten found in wheat, barley, rye and oats, and casein;[13] however, the amelioration of symptoms in response to gluten-free diets was equivocal.[14]

Cancers. *Sugars; high-carbohydrate, fibre-rich, diet; vegetable cooking oils and margarines.* See Chapter 14.

Cataract. *Polyunsaturated vegetable oils; carbohydrates.* Cataract is an eye condition that may be caused by the oxidation of polyunsaturated fats. When damaged proteins gather within one or both lenses, the resulting area becomes cloudy or opaque. This is called cataract. Cataract is the leading cause of blindness worldwide. Cataract is usually attributed to exposure to sunlight while not wearing UV sunglasses,[15] but that happens only while consuming a diet rich in unsaturated fats and their oxidised products.[16] Those who consume a more natural diet do not get cataracts even from lengthy sun exposure.[17] Sugars also increase cataract risk;[18] and a 'healthy' high-carb diet can increase the risk.[19]

Chronic fatigue syndrome. *Vegetarian diet.* CFS is a symptom of slow recycling of ATP. ATP is the body's fuel. CFS manifests as very poor stamina and delayed fatigue. The condition is greatly helped by acetyl l-carnitine, found in meat.[20]

Cirrhosis of the liver (non-alcoholic fatty liver). *High-carbohydrate diet.* Despite its name, fatty liver is not caused by a fatty diet – quite the reverse. The French delicacy, pâté de fois gras, is a perfect example of how a fatty liver develops. The pâté is made from goose livers, but not just any goose livers: they have to be fat ones. To achieve this, the geese whose livers are to be used are force-fed grain which is high in starch for several days. It is this that fattens the liver. The same thing happens in humans who eat a bread, potato and cereal based diet.[21]

Coeliac disease. *Cereal grains.* Coeliac disease is an intestinal disorder in which gliadin, a fraction of gluten – a natural protein commonly found in many grains, including wheat, barley, rye and oats – cannot be tolerated by the body. This causes a malabsorption of food with symptoms of diarrhoea and fatty stools; failure to thrive and grow at normal rates are often the symptoms first noticed in children with coeliac disease. Coeliac disease is one of the most common lifelong disorders in both Europe[22] and the United States.[23]

Cognitive decline. *'Healthy' diet; low blood cholesterol; low red meat intake.* The Framingham Study examined the relationship between total cholesterol and cognitive performance.[24] Cognitive tests measured learning, memory, attention, concentration, abstract reasoning, concept formation, and organisational abilities. The researchers found a significant linear association between blood cholesterol and measures of verbal fluency, attention, concentration, abstract reasoning, and a composite score measuring multiple cognitive domains. Participants with 'desirable' cholesterol levels of less than 5.2 mmol/L (200 mg/dL) performed significantly less well than participants with cholesterol levels higher than 6.25 mmol/L (240 mg/dL). Also, iron is an essential element in maintaining normal brain structure as well as cognitive functions (learning and memory). Red meat is the best supplier of iron.

Constipation. *High-fibre diet; missing breakfast.* See Chapter 2.

Coronary heart disease. *Carbohydrate-based, low-fat, diet.* See Chapter 13.

Crohn's disease. *Carbohydrate-based diet?* Crohn's disease (CD) was first recognised early in the 20th century. Since then the numbers of cases has increased considerably. CD is a chronic condition associated with inflammation and injury of the small intestine. It typically begins to cause symptoms in young adulthood, usually between the ages of 14 and 24. Why it develops is not clear. However, as a diet very low in carbohydrates is an effective treatment,[27] a high-carb diet is the likely cause.

Crowded and misaligned teeth. *High-carb diet – sugars and starches.* This facial malformation, including that of the dental arch, is directly a problem of growth which is determined before birth by what an expectant mother eats. The narrowing of the face and of dental arches were non-existent in primitive races, but have been seen as early as in the first generation of children after their parents adopted the foods of modern white civilisations.[28]

Deep vein thrombosis. *High-carb diet – sugars and starches.* DVT is a condition where clots (thromboses) form in the deep veins of the legs, which may then travel to other parts of the body. If the clot goes to and blocks a major blood vessel – in the lungs or heart, for example – it can have fatal consequences. A high-carb diet which puts high levels of glucose in the blood tends to make the blood stickier, and this makes it clot more readily. The answer to DVT is not necessarily to move about more, do special exercises and wear anti-DVT stockings. These all may reduce the risk, but they don't address the cause: a 'healthy' diet. All one needs to do to prevent DVT is eat less carbohydrate-rich foods.

Dental decay. *High-carb diet – sugars and starches; low intake of dairy products.* Sticky foods like toffee that take a long time to eat are major offenders but starchy foods also present a major risk. Dentists at the Faculty of Odontology, University of Göteborg, Sweden, used a variety of starchy foods: plain potato crisps, sugar-free cheese doodles, and sweetened crackers, and measured acidity levels in the mouth together with how long the foods remained in the mouth.[29] They found that, while sugary foods increased mouth acidity more than starches during the first 30 minutes, all three snack foods were worse than the sugar after that time. Milk and cheese are effective preventatives.

Depression. *Bran; soya; low intake of red meat; sugar.* Depression is also associated with deficiencies of zinc and of iron. (See Amenorrhoea.)

Dermatitis herpeteformis. *Cereal grains.* Dermatitis herpeteformis is caused in a similar way to coeliac disease. It is an autoimmune reaction to a protein in most cereals.

Diabetes (both types). *High-carb diet – sugars and starches.* See Chapter 5.

Diverticular disease. *Fibre-rich cereals.* Diverticulosis and diverticulitis are conditions very common among older adults. In response to pressure, small, balloon-like pouches called *diverticula* may poke outward through the weak spots in the large intestine (colon). At this stage, most people have no symptoms. The trouble starts when a *diverticulum* is filled with faeces which start to ferment. This causes the more serious *diverticulitis* which can infect the colon wall and cause bleeding. Normally, a high-fibre diet is recommended as part of the treatment for this and all conditions affecting the gut. However, it doesn't seem a good idea. The editor the *Lancet* wrote: 'Bran is on the defensive. There is little direct evidence that increasing the intake of fibre by itself has any beneficial effect on health. The notion that people should tolerate the unpalatability of bran and its unpleasant side-effects because it will prevent diseases . . . is founded on shaky evidence.' The answer is to avoid cereal bran and eat the right fibre-rich foods – green leafy vegetables, such as broccoli, cauliflower, celery and lettuce.

Dry eye syndrome. *Excess omega-6 fatty acids from polyunsaturated cooking oils and margarines.* Many millions of people in the industrialised countries, predominantly women, suffer from dry eye syndrome, a painful and debilitating eye disease. Dry eye syndrome is characterised by a decline in the quality or quantity of tears that normally bathe the eye to keep it moist and functioning well. The condition causes symptoms such as pain, irritation, dryness, and a sandy or gritty sensation. If untreated, severe dry eye syndrome can eventually lead to scarring or ulceration of the cornea, and loss of vision. Researchers from Brigham and Women's Hospital and Schepens Eye Research Institute, an affiliate of Harvard University Medical School and the largest independent eye research institute in the world, found that the amount, type and ratio of essential fatty acids in the diet may play a key role in dry eye prevention in women.[30] What they found was that a high intake of omega 6 fatty acids of the type found in many margarines, cooking and salad oils, increased the risk of dry eye syndrome. On the other hand, omega 3 fatty acids found in fish oils and walnuts, reduced the risk.

Eczema. *Various, but cereals are a prime cause.* Eczema follows very closely the same pattern as coeliac disease.

Epilepsy. *Carbohydrate-rich diet; cereals.* Since 1920 a carefully calculated diet, very high in fat, low in protein, and almost carbohydrate free, has proven to be very effective in the treatment of difficult-to-control seizures in children. It was only discontinued for the control of seizures as new medications were developed, although Johns Hopkins Medical Center in the USA has continued to use it with great success.[31] Normally the brain's preferred fuel is glucose derived from dietary carbohydrates. The 'ketogenic diet' as it is called is in stark contrast to the traditional diet in that it forces the brain to use ketone bodies as a fuel source. Ketone bodies are formed when fats are used as fuel rather than carbohydrates. Evidence shows that if cereal-free diets are adopted soon after the onset of epilepsy, seizures can be severely reduced or eliminated.[32] It follows, therefore that such a diet could prevent them.

Fatigue. *High-carb diet – sugars and starches.* The most usual cause of tiredness and fatigue is hypoglycaemia (low-blood sugar). This is cause by a high intake of carbohydrates. These initially raise glucose levels in the blood, but they trigger an insulin dump which lowers glucose again to low levels. The answer is to keep glucose reasonably constant by reducing carb intakes.

Flatulence. *High-fibre diet; bran; soya and other legumes (beans).* Undigested carbohydrates and fibre provide the material from which faecal bacteria produce methane gas.

Gallstones. *Low-fat diet.* Fats are not soluble in water. Before dietary fat can be digested, it has to be emulsified. Bile is used for this purpose. The liver makes bile continuously and stores it in the gallbladder until such time as it is needed. However, if a low-fat diet is eaten, that bile remains in the gallbladder. Gallstones are formed when the gallbladder is not emptied on a regular basis. In people who continually resort to low-fat diets, bile is stored for long periods in the gallbladder – and it stagnates. In time – and it is really quite a short time – if the gallbladder isn't emptied, a 'sludge' begins to form. This then coagulates to form small stones which then become bigger. The speed with which this happens was dramatically demonstrated in a trial at several American University hospitals.[33] After only eight weeks of weight-reduction dieting, more than a quarter of patients had developed gallstones. Where they were fed intravenously, half developed gallbladder sludge after 3 weeks, and *all* had developed sludge by six weeks. Nearly half of those who developed sludge also developed gallstones.

Glaucoma. *'Healthy', high-carb, low-fat diet.* Glaucoma is the second most common cause of blindness in the UK and the USA, affecting around 2% of the population. It is the result of insufficient blood flow due to agglutination (clumping together) of the red blood cells and waste build up in the cells and intercellular fluids. These blood-corpuscle clusters cannot squeeze through the extremely tiny capillaries in the back of the eye, and so they block them, preventing the eyes from getting the nutrients they need. As there is the diabetes connection, this makes a lot more sense and, as it is high levels of glucose in the bloodstream that cause blood to become 'sticky', it should be no surprise that a low-carb diet helps both to treat the condition and prevent it occurring in the first place.

Hearing loss (age related). *High-carb diet – sugars and starches.* Research suggests that diabetes can cause sensorineural hearing loss. Dr Hisaki Fukushima from the International Hearing Foundation, Minneapolis, Minnesota and colleagues examined temporal bones obtained at autopsy from patients with juvenile onset diabetes and compared them with similar bones obtained from normal controls. Diabetics had significant damage to the inner ear. The researchers say 'The findings in our study suggest that the microangiopathy associated with diabetes affects the inner ear vasculature and causes degeneration of inner ear structures.'[34] Diabetes is a condition where blood sugars are high.

Heartburn. *High-carb diet – sugars and starches.* Heartburn risk is much higher among people who are overweight or obese.[35] They also suffer more from diarrhoea. Professor Nicholas Talley, from the Mayo Clinic in Rochester, Minnesota, USA and his team investigated relationships that might exist between body mass index (BMI) and problems with the GI tract, such as heartburn, abdominal pain or stool frequency. Professor Talley and colleagues write: 'Our data suggest that there is a positive independent relationship between increasing BMI and heartburn as well as diarrhoea in the community . . . that obesity *per se* is a risk factor for gastro-esophageal reflux disease.' And obesity is caused by a carbohydrate-rich diet.

Infections, increased susceptibility to. *High-carb diet – sugars and starches.* See Chapter 14.

Infant brain damage. *Soya-based baby formula; low-fat diet.* Infants can suffer brain damage similar to Alzheimer's if fed soya based baby milk. Soya milk has a high phytate content which inhibits the absorption of some minerals, one of which is zinc. Zinc plays a very important part in the developing brain, it is believed that a zinc deficiency caused by soya and other products which contain phytate enhances the uptake and deposition of aluminium in the milk.[36]

Intermittent claudication. *High-carb diet – sugars and starches.* Intermittent claudication is a condition where the small blood vessels in the extremities, particularly the lower leg and foot, become blocked. The major reason for leg amputations, this condition is caused by the raised blood glucose seen in diabetes. Its cause is the same high-carb diet that causes type-2 diabetes.

Iron deficiency anaemia. *Bran; soya; low intake of red meat; vegetarian diet.* If there is a large intake of 'anti-nutrients' such as phytate, dietary fibre and tannins, which impair the absorption of iron,[37] and a low intake of flesh foods (another result of the diet-heart recommendations), there is a real risk of iron deficiency anaemia. Twenty years ago sub-optimal iron intakes were already being found in Britain, USA, Canada and South Africa.[38]

Irritable bowel syndrome. *Bran, wholemeal bread and wholemeal cereals, and the fruit sugar, fructose.* IBS is a common but poorly understood disorder that causes a variety of bowel symptoms including abdominal pain, diarrhoea and/or constipation, bloating, gassiness and cramping. While these symptoms may be caused by a number of different bowel diseases, IBS is usually diagnosed only after your doctor has ruled out the possibility of a more serious problem. Its severity varies from person to person. Fibre has been a popular way to treat IBS for many years, and this despite several studies between 1976 and 1985 showing no evidence of benefit. In 1994, doctors at the University Hospital of South Manchester, looking at the weight of evidence so far, said 'we got the impression that wholemeal wheat and bran products made people with the condition worse rather than better'. So they did a trial – and proved that their impressions were correct. They concluded that their evidence 'suggests that the use of bran in irritable bowel syndrome should be reconsidered' as there was a 'possibility that excessive consumption of bran in the community may actually be creating patients with irritable bowel syndrome by exacerbating mild, non-complaining cases'.[39] A study presented by Young Choi and colleagues from the University of Iowa in Iowa City, USA, also showed that between one third and one half of patients suffering from IBS symptoms were intolerant of the fruit sugar, fructose.[40]

Kidney stones. *Oxalate-rich foods such as spinach, rhubarb, beets, strawberries, wheat bran, nuts and nut butters.* The number of people with kidney stones has been increasing over the past 20 years.[41] And kidney stones strike most typically between the ages of 20 and 40. What change has been made to peoples eating habits in the past 20 years? Oh yes, 'healthy eating' was introduced. And who are the people most likely to follow this message? The 20–40s. But nearly 30 years ago, kidney stones were shown to be associated with high intake of refined carbohydrates.[42]

Learning disabilities. *Bran; soya; low intake of red meat; vegetarian diet.* Learning disabilities are associated with deficiencies of zinc and of iron.[46]

Loss of memory. *High-carbohydrate diet.* Under normal circumstances, the brain uses glucose as its main metabolic energy source. You might expect, therefore, that higher the levels of glucose in your blood would mean that your brain would operate more efficiently. However, this is not necessarily the case, as the rate at which carbohydrates hit the bloodstream is also important. Scientists at the Department of Psychology, University of Wales, measured blood glucose levels for three hours after a 'healthy' carbohydrate-rich, breakfast-like meal in parallel with memory tests. What they found was that a rapid climb in blood glucose had a deleterious effect on cognitive performances such as verbal memory.[43] On the other hand, their subjects performed much better after a meal that did not cause glucose levels to rise quickly.

Low birthweight. *Nutrient poor diet; bran; soya; low intake of red meat; vegetarian diet.* Low birthweight is also associated with deficiencies of zinc and of iron.[44] Nutrient poor vegetable-based diets also make smaller babies more likely.

Macular degeneration. *Vegetable margarines and cooking oils.* Macular degeneration is spreading rapidly throughout Western society like a disease. Affecting millions, macular degeneration is the leading cause of blindness in humans. Researchers at the Massachusetts Eye and Ear Infirmary carried out a study of 349 individuals aged 55 to 80 with MD, and compared their diet to a control group with eye diseases other than MD.[45] Those who consumed foods high in 'healthy' vegetable fat had more than twice the risk of MD of those whose intakes were low. And mono-unsaturated olive oil also carried a 71% higher risk. Diets rich in omega-3 fatty acids, found in fish like tuna and salmon, were protective against MD.

Menstrual dysfunction. *Bran; soya; low intake of red meat; vegetarian diet.* There is an apparent relation between dietary fibre and reproductive function in women. It affects the onset of menstruation and retards uterine growth.[47] Later it is associated with menstrual dysfunction.[48]

Migraine. *High-carbohydrate diet.* Migraines are persistent headaches lasting up to 72 hours, moderate to severe in intensity. There is often throbbing, pain, nausea, vomiting, and sensitivity to light, sound or smell. Analgesics are not usually effective and may worsen the condition over time. It is known that prior to and during a migraine attack there are changes in the blood and scalp arterial blood flow. Tests with low-carbohydrate diets have been shown to be effective.

Multiple sclerosis. *Cereal-based diet; perhaps milk.* MS is an autoimmune disorder, where the body's immune system attacks its own tissue. The condition is similar in many respects to type I diabetes mellitus. Although the two diseases are entirely different clinically, they have nearly identical ethnic and geographic distribution, genetic similarities, and, as is now known, shared environmental risk factors. MS has increased wherever peoples have changed to eating the 'western' way.

Muscle weakness. *Lack of soluble vitamin D; insufficient salt.* The best source of vitamin D is sunlight – but we tend not to get enough of that. The other sources are always found in fats from animals that have been in sunlight. Low-fat diets, therefore, can be harmful.

Myopia (short-sightedness). *High-carb diet – sugars and starches.* Myopia is almost unknown outside western industrialised countries. But there has been a dramatic increase in myopia recently in developed countries. As well as stimulating the production of insulin, diets high in refined starches such as sugar and breads also stimulate production of a related compound called insulin-like growth factor 1 (IGF-1). This stimulates excess growth of the eyeball during its development. This affects the development of the eyeball, making it abnormally long. This is the fundamental defect in myopia.

Nephropathy. *High-carb, low-fat diet. Cereals.* Nephropathy is a common complication of diabetes where the small blood vessels in the kidney become blocked. The condition is caused by the raised blood glucose seen in diabetes. Its cause is the same high-carb diet that causes type-2 diabetes.

Obesity. *High-carb, low-fat diet.*

Osteomalacia. *Bran; cereal fibre; soya; lack of vitamin D.* Osteomalacia is the adult counterpart to rickets. In this disease bones soften due to both insufficient vitamin D because women don't go into the sun enough, and to insufficient calcium in their diet. If not treated soon enough, the condition may be irreversible. Sunlight and the avoidance of bran are effective treatments.

Osteoporosis. *Bran; fibre-rich diet, soya, fizzy drinks; insufficient protein.* Osteoporosis (brittle bone disease) has increased at an alarming rate in the last 20 years. There are now twice as many fractures as there were in the 1950s, and yet there are many cultures in the world where postmenopausal women are fit, active and healthy until the end of their lives. It is also noticeable that the women in these cultures do not suffer from osteoporosis. Fibre-rich diets deplete calcium, while protein promotes stronger bones. Men and women who eat the most animal protein have better bone mass than those who avoid it.[49]

Parkinson's disease. *High-carbohydrate, 'healthy' diet.* Parkinson's disease seems to have similar causes to Alzheimer's disease although it affects only about one-tenth as many people as does Alzheimer's. A low-carb, very high-fat, ketogenic diet has been found effective in treating Parkinson's, so it is likely that such a diet would prevent it.

Psoriasis. *Lack of essential fatty acids; 'healthy' diet.* Although mental stress is a major cause of psoriasis, susceptibility is greatly increased in the overweight.[50] And that, as we know, is caused by a 'healthy' carbohydrate-based diet. Other factors that have an effect on psoriasis activity include the interdependency between inflammation, stress, and insulin resistance, which again is caused by the same diet.

Resistance to authority. *High-carb diet – sugars and starches; low-cholesterol.* Several scientific investigations have linked criminality to diets high in sugar and carbohydrates in adults. Jails are notorious for their problems with defiance of authority and bad behaviour and trials have been conducted into the effects of changing diets on inmates. Usually, these have switched inmates to a low sugar diet with no fizzy drinks. This results in a significant drop in aggressive behaviour. Low blood cholesterol is also associated with aggression and antisocial behaviour. People whose cholesterol was 'healthily' below 5.04 mmol/L were significantly more antisocial compared to others whose cholesterol was above 6.02 mmol/L.[51] Mental patients with blood cholesterol around 7.55 mmol/L were much less regressed and withdrawn than those whose cholesterol levels were around 4.80 mmol/L.

Retinopathy. *High-carbohydrate diet.* Retinopathy is a complication of diabetes where the small blood vessels in the retinas of the eyes become blocked. The condition is caused by the raised blood glucose seen in diabetes. Its cause is the same high-carb diet that causes type-2 diabetes.

Rickets. *Bran; cereal fibre; soya.* Rickets is a disease of children in which the bones do not harden and are malformed. It is caused by a deficiency of calcium and vitamin D. In the archaeological record, rickets is rare or absent in pre-agricultural human skeletons but common in industrialised societies. Early studies showed that rickets was caused by eating wholemeal and other bran-rich breads as phytate in the bran bound calcium.[52] With better nutrition in the 1930s rickets largely disappeared. However, since the advent of 'healthy eating' with its stress on increasing cereal intake, rickets has returned.[53]

Slow childhood growth. *Bran; soya; low intake of red meat; vegetarian diet.* Phytate-rich fibres (cereals and soy) which inhibit the absorption of minerals, are the greatest contributors to growth problems,[54] but any form of nutrient starvation can add to the problem.

Schizophrenia. *'Healthy' carbohydrate-rich diet, particularly cereals containing gluten.* In the 1960s, Dr F. Curtis Dohan noticed that in regions where gluten consumption was common, the rate of schizophrenia was substantially higher than in places where gluten consumption was absent.[55] Between 1966 and 1990 more than 50 articles regarding the role of cereal grains as a cause of schizophrenia were published. Dr Karl Lorenz conducted a meta-analysis of them and concluded: 'In populations eating little or no wheat, rye and barley, the prevalence of schizophrenia is quite low and about the same regardless of type of acculturating influence.'[56]

Stomach ulcers. *High-carb diet – sugars and starches. Gastrin,* a hormone responsible for gastric secretions, is formed when food enters the stomach. This leads to secretion of hydrochloric acid and the enzymes necessary for digestion in the stomach. It is important to note that in cases of hyperacidity, too much *gastrin* is produced. Carbohydrates especially elicit production of gastrin. Both stomach ulcers caused by high acid levels and duodenal ulcers usually heal if carbohydrates are restricted.[57]

Strokes. *Polyunsaturated oils, low-fat diets.* High intakes of animal fats and cholesterol reduce the risk of stroke by almost two-thirds (63%) compared to those with the lowest intakes.[58] Polyunsaturated fats[59] and low-fat diets increase risk.[60]

Suicide and violence. *High-carb diet; low blood cholesterol; vegetarian diet.* The risk of mood disorders, depression, stroke, and violence is increased if cholesterol is low. During trials to lower levels of cholesterol in the blood, it became obvious that there was a tendency towards more suicides and violent deaths in the treatment groups. A study of this trend found that those whose cholesterol was below 4.27 were six times more likely to attempt suicide that those with cholesterol above 5.77.[61] A Medical Research Council study also found that those who committed suicide had low rates of weight gain in infancy. And that could be caused by incorrect diet – one that is carbohydrate rich and nutrient poor.[62]

Ulcerative colitis. *Carbohydrate-based 'healthy' diet.* Ulcerative colitis is a lifelong condition that begins with inflammation of the rectum but can progress to involve much or all of the large intestine. In a similar way to Crohn's disease, ulcerative colitis typically begins to cause symptoms in young adulthood, usually between the ages of 15 and 40. No one knows for sure what triggers the inflammation in ulcerative colitis, but as a low-carb, high-fat diet cures the condition, a carbohydrate-based, low-fat 'healthy' diet is a likely cause.

References

1. Cordain L, et al. Acne vulgaris: a disease of western civilization. *Arch Dermatol* 2002; 138: 1584–1590.

2. a. Reid RL, Van Vugt DA. Weight-related changes in reproductive function. *Fertil Steril* 1987; 48 (6): 905–913.

    b. Lozoff B, et al. Long-term developmental outcome of infants with iron deficiency. *N Eng J Med* 1991; 325: 687–694.

3. Ebringer A, Wilson C. The use of a low starch diet in the treatment of patients suffering from ankylosing spondylitis. *Clin Rheumatol* 1996; 15, Suppl 1: 62–66.

4. Bryce-Smith D, Simpson R. Anorexia, depression and zinc deficiency. *Lancet* 1984; ii: 1162.

5. Zhang J, Muldoon MF, McKeown RE, Cuffe, SP. Association of serum cholesterol and history of school suspension among school-age children and adolescents in the United States. *Am J Epidemiol* 2005; 161: 691–699.

6. Karvonen RL, Miller PR, Nelson DA, et al. Periarticular osteoporosis in osteoarthritis of the knee. *J Rheumatol* 1998; 25: 2187–2194.

7. National Institutes of Health. *Clinical guidelines on the identification, evaluation, and treatment of overweight and obesity in adults: the Evidence Report*. US Department of Health and Human Services, Bethesda, MD, 1998.

8. Darlington LG, Ramsey NW, Mansfield JR. Placebo-controlled, blind study of dietary manipulation therapy in rheumatoid arthritis. *Lancet* 1986; i: 236–238.

9. *Medical World News* December 18, 1964.

10. Hagfors L, Nilsson I, Sköldstam L, Johansson G. Fat intake and composition of fatty acids in serum phospholipids in a randomised, controlled, Mediterranean dietary intervention study on patients with rheumatoid arthritis. *Nutr Metab* 2005; 2: 26.

11. Fomon S. *Infant Nutrition*, 2nd edn. WB Saunders, Philadelphia, 1974, p.455.

12. Mannino DM, Mott J, Ferdinands JM, et al. Boys with high body masses have an increased risk of developing asthma: findings from the National Longitudinal Survey of Youth (NLSY) *Internat J Obes* 2006; 30: 6–13.

13. Reichelt KL, Ekrem J, Scott H. Gluten, milk proteins and autism: dietary intervention effects on behavior and peptide secretion. *J Appl Nutr* 1990; 42: 1–11.

14. Sponheim E. Gluten-free diet in infantile autism: a therapeutic trial. *Tidsskr Norsk Laegeforen* 1991; 111: 704–707.

15. Harmful effects of ultraviolet radiation. *JAMA* 1989; 262: 380–384.

16. Ames BN, Shigenaga MK, Hagen TM. Oxidants, antioxidants, and the degenerative diseases of aging. *Proc Natl Acad Sci USA* 1993; 90: 7915–7922.

17. Leske MC, Chylack LT Jr, He Q, et al. Antioxidant vitamins and nuclear opacities. *Ophthalmology* 1998; 105: 18–36.

18. Rattan SIS, Derventzi A, Clark B. Protein synthesis, post-translational modifications, and aging. *Ann NY Acad Sci* 1992; 663: 48–62.

19. Chiu CJ, Morris MS, Rogers G, et al. Carbohydrate intake and glycemic index in relation to the odds of early cortical and nuclear lens opacities. *Am J Clin Nutr* 2005; 81: 1411–1416.

20. Vermeulen RC, Scholte HR. Exploratory open label, randomized study of acetyl- and propionylcarnitine in chronic fatigue syndrome. *Psychosom Med* 2004; 66: 276–282.

21. Diet for Obese Patient Tied to Liver Inflammation. Reuters Health, 27 October 2003. http://www.reuters.co.uk/newsArticle.jhtml?type=healthNews&storyID=3698408&section=news, accessed 28 October 2003.

22. Catassi C, Fabiani E, Ratsch IM, et al. The coeliac iceberg in Italy: a multicentre antigliadin antibodies screening for coeliac disease in school-age subjects. *Acta Paediatr Suppl* 1996; 412: 29–35.

23. Fasano A, Berti I, Gerarduzzi T, et al. Prevalence of celiac disease in at-risk and not-at-risk groups in the United States: a large multicenter study. *Arch Intern Med* 2003; 163: 286–292.

24. Elias PK, Elias MF, D'Agostino RB, et al. Serum cholesterol and cognitive performance in the Framingham Heart Study. *Psychosom Med* 2005; 67: 24–30.

25. Chassell CF. *Relation between Morality and Intellect*. Columbia, NY, 1935.

26. Burt CL. *Backward Child*. Appleton, New York, 1937.

27. Lutz W. *Dismantling a Myth*. Selecta-Verlag Dr Ildar Idris GmbH & Co, KG Planegg Vor München, 1986, pp.125–180.

28. Weston A. *Nutrition and Physical Degeneration: A Comparison of Primitive and Modern Diets and their Effects*. Paul B. Hoeber, New York, London, 1939.

29. Lingstrom P, Birkhed D. Plaque pH and oral retention after consumption of starchy snack products at normal and low salivary secretion rate. *Acta Odontol Scand* 1993; 51: 379–388.

30. Miljanovic B, Trivedi KA, Reza Dana M, et al. Relation between dietary n-3 and n-6 fatty acids and clinically diagnosed dry eye syndrome in women. *Am J Clin Nutr* 2005; 82: 887–893.

31. http://www.neuro.jhmi.edu/epilepsy/keto.html. Accessed February 2002.

32. Gobbi G, Bouquet F, Greco L, et al. Coeliac disease, epilepsy, and cerebral calcifications: The Italian working group on coeliac disease and epilepsy. *Lancet* 1992; 340: 439–443; Fois A, Vascotto M, DiBartolo RM, Di Marco V. Celiac disease and epilepsy in pediatric patients. *Childs Nerv Syst* 1994; 10: 450–454.

33. Liddle RA, Goldstein RB, Saxton J. Gallstone formation during weight-reduction dieting. *Arch Intern Med* 1989; 149: 1750–1753.

34. Fukushima H, Cureoglu S, Schachern PA, Kusunoki T, Oktay MF, Fukushima N, Paparella MM, Harada T. Cochlear changes in patients with type 1 diabetes mellitus. *Otolaryngol Head Neck Surg* 2005; 133: 100–106.

35. Talley NJ, Quan C, Jones MP, Horowitz M. Association of upper and lower gastrointestinal tract symptoms with body mass index in an Australian cohort. *Neurogastroenterol Motil* 2004; 16: 413–419.

36. Bishop N, McGraw M, Ward N. Aluminium in infant formulas. *Lancet* 1989; i: 490.

37. Addy D. Happiness is: iron. *BMJ* 1986; 292: 969.

38. Bindra GS, Gibson RS. Iron status of predominantly lacto-ovo-vegetarian East Indian immigrants to Canada: a model approach. *Am J Clin Nutr* 1986; 44: 643.

39. Francis CY, Whorwell PJ. Bran and irritable bowel syndrome: time for reappraisal. *Lancet* 1994; 344: 39–40.

40. 68th Annual Scientific Meeting of the American College of Gastroenterology, Baltimore, Maryland, USA, October 2003.

41. http://www.niddk.nih.gov/health/kidney/pubs/stonadul/stonadul.htm, accessed 21 August 2003.

42. Thom JA, et al. The influence of refined carbohydrate on urinary calcium excretion. *Br J Urol* 1978; 50:7, 459–464.

43. Benton D, Ruffin MP, Lassel T, et al. The delivery rate of dietary carbohydrates affects cognitive performance in both rats and humans. *Psychopharmacology* 2003; 166: 86–90.

44. Meadows N, *et al.* Zinc and small babies. *Lancet* 1981; ii: 1135.

45. Seddon JM, Rosner B, Sperduto RD, et al. Dietary fat and risk for advanced age-related macular degeneration. *Arch Ophthalmol* 2001; 119: 1191–1199.

46. a. Lozoff B, Jimenez E, Wolf AW. Long-term developmental outcome of infants with iron deficiency. *N Eng J Med* 1991; 325 (10): 687–694.
    b. Herens MC, Dagnelie PC, Kleber RJ, et al. Nutrition and mental development of 4–5 year old children on macrobiotic diets. *J Hum Nutr Diet* 1992; 5: 1–9.

47. Hughes RE, Johns E. Apparent relation between dietary fibre and reproductive function in the female. *Ann Hum Biol* 1985; 12: 325; Hughes RE. A new look at dietary fibre. *Hum Nutr Clin Nutr* 1986; 40c: 81.

48. Lloyd T, et al. Inter-relationships of diet, athletic activity, menstrual status and bone density in collegiate women. *Am J Clin Nutr* 1987; 46: 681.

49. a. Munger RG, et al. Prospective study of dietary protein intake and risk of hip fracture in postmenopausal women. *Am J Clin Nutr* 1999; 69: 147–152.
    b. Hannan MT, et al. Effect of dietary protein on bone loss in elderly men and women: The Framingham Osteoporosis Study. *J Bone Min Res* 2000; 15: 2504–2512.

50. a. Naldi L. Epidemiology of psoriasis. *Curr Drug Targets Inflamm Allergy* 2004; 3: 121–128.
    b. Wellen KE, Hotamisligil GS. Inflammation, stress, and diabetes. *J Clin Invest* 2005; 115: 1111–1119.

51. Engleberg H. Low serum cholesterol and suicide. *Lancet* 1992; 339: 727–729.

52. McCance R, Widdowson E. Mineral metabolism of healthy adults on white and brown bread dietaries. *J Physiol* 1942; 101: 44–85.

53. a. Clements MR. The problem of rickets in UK Asians. *J Hum Nutr Dietet* 1989; 2: 105–111.
    b. Welch TR, Bergstrom WH, Tsang RC. Vitamin D-deficient rickets: The re-emergence of a once-conquered disease. *J Pediatr* 2000; 137: 143–145.

54. Lifshitz F, et al. Nutritional dwarfing in adolescents. *Semin Adolesc Med* 1987; 3 (4): 255–266.

55. Dohan FC, Grasberger JC. Relapsed schizophrenics: early discharge from the hospital after cereal free, milk free diet. *Am J Psychiatr* 1973; 130: 685–688.

56. Lorenz K. Cereals and schizophrenia. *Adv Cereal Sci Technol* 1990; 10: 435–469.

57. Lutz W. *Dismantling a Myth*. Selecta-Verlag Dr Ildar Idris GmbH & Co, KG Planegg Vor München, 1986, pp.125–180.

58. Sauvaget C, Nagano J, Hayashi M, Yamada M. Animal protein, animal fat, and cholesterol intakes and risk of cerebral infarction mortality in the Adult Health Study. *Stroke* 2004; May 27.

59. Shimamoto T, et al. Trends for coronary heart disease and stroke and their risk factors in Japan. *Circulation* 1989; 79: 503–515.

60. Gillman MW, et al. Inverse association of dietary fat with development of ischemic stroke in men. *JAMA* 1997; 278: 2145–2150.

61. Ellison LF, Morrison HI. Low serum cholesterol concentration and risk of suicide. *Epidemiology* 2001; 12: 168–172.

62. Barker DJP, Osmond C, Rodin I, et al. Low weight gain and suicide in later life. *BMJ* 1995; 311: 1203.

Appendix B

Adult height/weight tables

How much should you weigh?

Age and height are the main factors that determine healthy weight. Within each range, higher weights generally apply to men, who tend to have more muscle and bone. Lower weights generally apply to women. If indoor clothes are worn, their weight should be allowed for. Estimated weights of indoor clothing are: 7–9 lb for men and 4–6 lb for women.

The weight ranges below are based on the Body Mass Index (BMI) scale, widely used to assess weight. Acceptable BMI is normally between 20 and 25. Over 25 means you are overweight and over 30 means clinically obese. BMIs are the ratio of weight to height. In the metric system they are calculated by dividing weight in kilograms by the height in metres squared: i.e. if you are 1.75 m tall and weigh 85.5 kg, your BMI is $85.5 \div 1.75 \div 1.75 = 27.9$. Calculating BMI using imperial measurements is done in a similar way, albeit a bit more complicated: i.e. if you are 5 ft 8 in tall, and weigh 12 st 10 lb, you must first convert your height into inches = 68 (1 ft = 12 in) and your weight into lb = 178 (1 st = 14 lb). The calculation is then done in the same way but the result must be multiplied by 705, so in this case, your BMI is $(178 \div 68 \div 68) \times 705 = 27.1$.

Table B.1 Imperial height and weight table for men and women aged 25–59 years

Height (without shoes) ft in	Weight BMI = 20 st lb	BMI = 25 st lb	BMI = 30 st lb
4 10	6 11	8 7	10 3
4 11	7 1	8 12	10 9
5 0	7 4	9 1	10 12
5 1	7· 8	9 6	11 5
5 2	7 10	9 10	11 9
5 3	8 1	10 1	12 1
5 4	8 5	10 6	12 7
5	8 8	10 10	12 12
5 6	8 12	11 1	13 4
5 7	9 1	11 5	13 9
5 8	9 6	11 11	14 2
5 9	9 9	12 1	14 6
5 10	9 13	12 6	14 13
5 11	10 3	12 10	15 4
6 0	10 7	13 2	15 11
6 1	10 11	13 6	16 2
6 2	11 2	13 13	16 9
6 3	11 7	14 5	17 3

Table B.2 Metric height and weight tables for men and women aged 25–59 years

Height (without shoes) (m)	Weight		
	BMI = 20 (kg)	BMI = 25 (kg)	BMI = 30 (kg)
1.47	43.2	54	64.8
1.49	45	56.3	67.5
1.52	46.2	57.6	69.3
1.55	48.1	60.1	72.1
1.57	49.3	61.6	73.9
1.60	51.2	64	76.8
1.62	53.1	66.4	79.7
1.65	54.5	68.1	81.7
1.67	56.4	70.6	84.7
1.70	57.8	72.3	86.7
1.72	59.9	74.8	89.9
1.75	61.3	76.6	91.9
1.78	63.4	79.2	95.1
1.80	64.8	81	97.2
1.82	67	83.7	100.5
1.85	68.5	85.6	102.7
1.88	70.7	88.4	106.0
1.91	73	91.2	109.4

Appendix C

Glossary

Amino acids are the fundamental constituents of all proteins. There are twenty in the protein foods we eat and our bodies need all of them. Our bodies can manufacture all but eight. These, called the *essential amino acids*, must be obtained from protein in the diet. Not only must all eight be present, they should ideally be in the correct proportions thus:

one part **tryptophan** to
two parts each of **phenylalanine** and **threonine** to
three parts each of **isoleucine, lysine, methionine** and **valine** to
three and a half parts **leucine**.

When all are contained in a food, this is said to be *complete* protein. Egg whites contain all the essential amino acids in the correct proportions. The best sources of the essential amino acids, in approximately the correct proportions, are foods such as liver, eggs, and dairy products. Pulses, cereals and nuts all contain some but not all of the essential amino acids and not in the required proportions. These are called *incomplete* proteins. A strict vegetarian diet must contain a mixture of these foods for all eight essential amino acids to be supplied.

Atheroma is degeneration of artery walls due to the formation in them of fatty plaques and scar tissue. Although atheroma narrows arteries and restricts blood flow, it is usually symptomless. But it can cause complications in later life such as angina, heart attack, stroke and gangrene.

Bioavailability. The bioavailability of a nutrient in a foodstuff is a measure of the proportion of it which can be absorbed into the bloodstream. Bioavailability is affected by a number of factors. For example, no enzyme in the human gut can digest the cellulose from which plant cell walls are made. Therefore, unless those walls are ruptured in some way, the nutrients inside a plant cell will not be available to the digestion. Cooking and chewing, which damage the cell walls, increase bioavailability. Phytic acid which is found in bran, is an 'anti-nutrient'. This substance combines with a number of minerals to form a compound which is indigestible thus reducing their bioavailability.

Calorie. The calorie, or more correctly in dietary terms kilocalorie (kcal), is a unit of heat. It is the amount of heat required to raise the temperature of a kilogram of water by one degree Celsius.

Carbohydrates are one of the three main constituents of food. They are a large group of compounds which include sugars, starches, celluloses and gums. Apart from the indigestible starches (fibre), all carbohydrates are eventually broken down in the body to the simple sugar, glucose. Excess carbohydrate, not immediately needed by the body, is stored in the body: in the liver and muscles as glycogen, a form of starch and as fat. Glycogen is later broken down to glucose to be used as energy.

Cholesterol is a white waxy material. It is not a fat but a form of alcohol called a *lipid alcohol*. In higher animals, it is found in all cells and it is especially abundant in the brain and nervous tissue. In cells, it is used principally as a structural material – cell wall membranes are made of it. In these membranes, its ratio with other lipids has a large impact on the stability and permeability of the membranes. The myelin sheath which is the 'insulation' around nerves has the highest concentration of cholesterol. (Multiple sclerosis is the result of a breakdown of this myelin sheath.)

As well as its structural function cholesterol performs other important functions: it is a precursor for several hormones, including both male and female sex hormones; in the liver it is used to make the bile acids and bile salts which are secreted into the gut as part of the digestive process; and it is used by the body to manufacture vitamin D in conjunction with sunlight.

Cholesterol and other substances in the blood are measured in milli-moles per litre (mmol/L) in Australia and Europe and in milligrams per decilitre (mg/dL) in the United States of America. Normal blood concentration of cholesterol is 3.6–7.8 mmol/L (140–300 mg/dL) but this rises naturally with age: at the age of 50, for example, 9.0 mmol/L (346 mg/dL) would not be abnormal. The normal Western intake of cholesterol from food is 500–1000 mg/day. However, the body uses considerably more than this and the extra required is synthesised from acetate mainly in the liver. Normally the amount of cholesterol in the blood from these two sources is constant because under feedback control, if more is eaten, the liver compensates by making less. On a low-cholesterol diet, the amount synthesised by the liver rises markedly.

Cholesterol is found in equal amounts in both the lean and fat portions of meat.

HDL and LDL cholesterol. Cholesterol is transported around the body by a group of proteins combined with lipids called lipoproteins. The higher the ratio of proteins to lipids, the higher the density of the lipoprotein. Although one normally hears only of high density lipoprotein cholesterol (HDL, the 'good' cholesterol which is believed by some to be protective from heart disease) and low density lipoprotein cholesterol (LDL, the 'bad' cholesterol, which is believed by some to cause heart disease), there are actually several distinct densities: very low density (VLDL), intermediate density, and even HDL is split into HDL2 and HDL3.

Controls. When a medical trial is conducted it is usual to divide the people taking part in the trial into two groups. One group will be given the active treatment while the other will be given none. In this way doctors can assess the effectiveness of the treatment by measuring the differences between the two groups. The group that receives the treatment in called the 'intervention group' and the group that does not receive the treatment is known as the 'control group' or 'controls'.

Cro-Magnon. Our ancestors, whom we call Cro-Magnon, migrated into Europe from the Middle East around 35,000 years ago. They were fully modern men, identical in appearance to the modern European. They apparently had a culture all their own and made better weapons and tools than the Neanderthals. Like the Neanderthals, they occupied caves but in larger groups and on a more permanent basis.

Diabetes is a condition where fasting levels of glucose in the blood are above 7 mmol/L. High levels of glucose cause damage to small blood vessels (microvascular complications) leading in turn to blindness (*retinopathy*), to kidney failure (*nephropathy*) and to nerve damage (*neuropathy*); and damage to the larger arteries (macrovascular complications) leading in turn to damage to the brain (stroke), the heart (coronary heart disease) or to the legs and feet (peripheral vascular disease). It can also lead to difficulties in pregnancy, infection, periodontal disease, and many other conditions. A diagnosis of diabetes should be taken very seriously.

Epidemiology is a branch of science which deals with diseases in population groups. It includes all forms of disease that relate to environmental and lifestyle factors.

Essential fatty acids (EFAs) are a group of three polyunsaturated fatty acids which the body needs but cannot synthesise itself. They are: arachidonic, linoleic and linolenic acid. Although all three are essential, the only one which need be included in the diet is linoleic acid as the body when functioning properly can make the other two from it. Vegetable oils such as sunflower, safflower, soya and corn oils contain large quantities of linoleic acid. Animal fats also contain it but in smaller amounts. Once called vitamin F, the body requires only small quantities of the essential fatty acids.

Fat is a substance which contains one or more fatty acids and is the principal form in which the body stores energy. It is also used as an insulating material both just beneath the skin and around some of the internal organs. Fat is essential in the diet to supply an adequate amount of essential fatty acids and for the absorption of the fat-soluble vitamins: A, D, E and K.

The chemical and physical properties of a fat are determined by the relative amounts of the various fatty acids of which it is composed. Generally, the more saturated the fatty acid content, the harder the fat will be at room temperature; the more unsaturated its content, the runnier it will be.

Fibre, or roughage as it used to be called, is that part of a plant which cannot be digested and absorbed in the human gut. Although, because of its indigestibility it cannot be classed as a food, a certain amount of fibre is believed to be necessary for the correct functioning of the gut and passage of materials through the intestines and bowel. Fibre falls into four groups: celluloses, of which plant cell walls are made; hemicelluloses; lignins, another constituent of cell walls which give a plant stiffness; and pectins. All fruits, vegetables and cereals contain fibre but the types of fibre differ in each.

The major fibre found in fruits is pectin. Not fibrous in texture, it has little effect on the faeces. The major fibre in vegetables is cellulose. In ruminant animals such as cows, cellulose is broken down and used as a food; in Man it passes straight through, as there are no enzymes with which we can digest it. The source of the greatest quantities of fibre are cereals, particularly in bran and wholemeal flours. However, there is a penalty to pay with these. Cereal fibres are fundamentally different from vegetable and fruit fibre in that they also contain a material called phytate which binds with many nutrients, reduces their bioavailability and stops them from being digested.

Glucose is a simple sugar molecule. It is an important source of energy within the body. Glucose is the building block from which sugars and starches are composed. All sugar and starch carbohydrates are converted back to glucose by the process of digestion. Glucose is stored in the body's muscles in the form of glycogen. Any excess is converted and stored as fat.

Glycaemic Index (GI) is a measurement of the rate at which foods raise glucose and, thus, insulin levels in the blood. It is a simple scale based on glucose being given the number 100 and other foods measured in relation to glucose. The higher the number against a food, the quicker it raises insulin levels.

GI has provided new insights into the relationship between foods and chronic disease, but it should not be taken in isolation. While observational studies suggest that diets with a high **glycaemic load** – that is a food's GI as well as its carbohydrate content – is an important consideration, GI and carb content are both independently associated with increased risk of type-2 diabetes and cardiovascular disease.

Glycaemic Load (see Glycaemic Index)

Glycogen, a carbohydrate, is the principal form in which glucose is stored in the body: the counterpart of the starch that is stored in plants. It is stored in the liver and muscles but any excess is converted into and stored as fat. As glycogen it is readily broken down into glucose for use. After it has been converted into fat, however, the process is more difficult.

HDL. High density lipoprotein cholesterol (see Cholesterol).

Insulin resistance occurs when the normal amount of insulin secreted by the pancreas is not able to unlock the door to cells and tissues have a diminished ability to respond to the action of insulin. In an attempt to maintain a normal level of blood glucose, the pancreas secretes more insulin. Insulin-resistant persons, therefore, also have high blood insulin levels (*hyperinsulinaemia*). Many people who are insulin resistant produce large enough quantities of insulin to maintain near normal blood glucose levels. But in about one-third of the people with insulin resistance, when the body cells resist or do not respond even to high levels of insulin, glucose builds up in the blood to an abnormally high level. This is the definition of type-2 diabetes.

Intermittent claudication is a cramping pain induced by exercise and relieved by rest that is caused by an inadequate supply of blood to the affected area. It is most often seen in the calf and leg muscles as the result of partial or complete blockages of the leg arteries. The leg pulses are often absent and the feet cold. A complication of diabetes, claudication is the most common reason for leg amputation.

Intervention trials. Whenever a new drug, diet or other treatment is devised, it has to be tested to make sure that it is both effective and safe. In these circumstances the usual method is to select two groups of people who are matched for age, sex, lifestyle and so on. One, *the intervention* group, is then given the treatment while the other, the *control* group, is not. By comparing the responses of the two groups, it is then possible to assess the efficacy and/or safety of the treatment.

To ensure that there is no bias and to minimise the placebo effect, where a medicine is tested, such intervention trials are usually 'double blind'. This means that both the doctors administering the treatment and the subjects taking part have no idea who is receiving the active treatment and who is receiving an inactive placebo.

Ischaemic means lacking oxygen. It usually refers to an inadequate flow of blood to a part of the body caused by constriction or blockage of the arteries supplying it.

Ketones are a group of organic compounds related to acetone. They are normal products formed during the metabolism of fats and can be used by the body as a source of energy. Elevated levels arise when there is an imbalance in fat metabolism as may occur in diabetes or starvation.

LDL. Low density lipoprotein cholesterol (see Cholesterol, page 287).

Lipids are a group of compounds which occur naturally. They are soluble in solvents such as alcohol but not in water. The group includes fats and steroids that are important parts of a diet, not only because of their high energy value but because they are associated with certain vitamins and essential fatty acids.

Metabolic Syndrome (see Syndrome X)

Metabolism is the sum of all the chemical and physical processes which take place within the living body to enable its continued growth and function. It also means the process by which energy and heat are made available to the body.

The Basal Metabolic Rate (BMR) is the minimum amount of energy the body needs to expend to maintain vital processes such as breathing, circulation, hormone production and digestion.

Phytate (or phytic acid) is a compound found in certain foods which binds with minerals such as calcium, iron and zinc to form compounds which are indigestible. The body treats these as waste products. In this way, foods high in phytates inhibit the absorption of these minerals leading to deficiencies. Wholegrain cereals, soybeans and peanuts are the major sources of phytate.

Proteins are essential components in the body, being the materials from which the organs, muscles and tissues are made. They are organic compounds composed of hydrogen, carbon, oxygen and nitrogen. They are synthesised in the body from amino acids which in turn are absorbed from digested dietary proteins.

Protein is unstable. Body cells undergo a constant cycle of breakdown and rebuilding. Amino acids in the cells have to be replaced on a daily basis, and newly digested amino acids in food are used for this purpose. Your intake of proteins must be sufficient for this purpose every day. Less than this will lead to deficiency diseases. More than the body needs can be used to supply energy.

Retinopathy is damage to the retina of the eye resulting in loss of sight. It is usually due to a blockage in the blood vessels that supply the retina. The major causes are diabetes, and high blood pressure.

Syndrome X is a term used to describe a collection of symptoms – *hyper-triglyceridaemia* (high blood fats), low HDL-cholesterol, *hyperinsulinaemia* (high blood insulin), often *hyperglycaemia* (high blood glucose), and *hypertension* (high blood pressure), elevated uric acid, and small, dense LDL molecules – that collectively appear to be caused by disturbed insulin metabolism. These symptoms appear in turn to increase risk of heart disease, type-2 diabetes and many other conditions. Syndrome X may be responsible for a large percentage of the heart and artery disease that occurs throughout the world today. The term Syndrome X is often an expression interchangeable with insulin resistance.

Triglycerides are the form in which fat is stored in the body. They are lipids composed of glycerol combined with three fatty acids, and are synthesised in the body from the digestion of dietary fat. They are transported around the body with very low density (VLDL) cholesterol.

Appendix D

Reliable sources of information

There are several useful websites that will fill in any gaps and provide more information – reliable information that is. But beware, there are many more that publish misleading nonsense.

My own website at **www.second-opinions.co.uk** carries many papers and articles about the nutritional treatments and prevention of many diseases. You can also e-mail me via this website. My videos and DVDs are available through **www.theperfectweight.com**

On eating a natural low-carbohydrate diet

The Weston A. Price Foundation at **www.westonaprice.org** has a copious amount of information on eating a natural diet.

There are several low-carb sites in the UK. Here are two of the best.

Low Carb in the UK, a site dedicated to bringing to the UK the best in information about a Controlled Carbohydrate style of eating for weight loss is at **www.low-carb.org.uk**

www.lowcarbportal.com is very good for the latest news and opinions on a whole range of health conditions helped or prevented by a low-carb way of eating.

The full Glycaemic Index tables are at **www.mendosa.com/gi.htm**

If you are still worried about cholesterol and heart disease

Professor Uffe Ravnskov MD, PhD, author of *The Cholesterol Myths* has researched this myth and published many papers on the subject. See **www.ravnskov.nu/cholesterol.htm**

Another very useful site is that of The International Network of Cholesterol Skeptics at **www.thincs.org** This website carries discussions by internationally renowned experts in the medical world. Just look at the membership list.

Another good site about the benefits of cholesterol is at **www.cholesterol-and-health.com**

On dietary fats and oils

There are several papers about dietary fats and oils by Mary Enig, PhD and Sally Fallon at: **www.westonaprice.org/facts_about_fats/facts_about_fats.html**

Dr Mary Enig and associates also give valuable information refuting many myths about fat and its role in the human diet, and discuss one form of fat they do believe is dangerous: the *trans*-fatty acids in margarines and other hydrogenated and partially hydrogenated oils. See **www.enig.com/trans.html**

Uncovering the truth about soy

Soy is promoted as the miracle food that will feed the world while at the same time prevent and cure all manner of diseases. Now read about the dark side. **www.soyonlineservice.co.nz**

On fluoride

www.fluoridealert.org is an international site devoted to telling the truth about water fluoridation. But be careful: the pro-fluoride lobby has collared **www.fluoridealert.com** in an effort to mislead you.

The National Pure Water Association, the campaign for pure drinking water in the UK, is at **www.npwa.org.uk**

On BSE and CJD

Is BSE caused by feeding meat to cows? Not according to farmer turned scientist, Mark Purdey, whose researches into organophosphate pesticides and environmental factors suggest that we are not being told the truth. His site is at **www.purdeyenvironment.com**

Searching references

Lastly, I have included references, most of which can be accessed on the internet via one of the international medical databases such as Medline and PubMed. You will find the latter at:

http://www.ncbi.nlm.nih.gov/entrez/query.fcgi

Appendix E

Carbohydrate content and Glycaemic Loads of foods

This appendix contains three tables. The first gives the carbohydrate content of common foods in normal servings. This is for easy reference. The second table lists foods with their Glycaemic Index where it is known. This is more comprehensive and more informative when planning meal menus. The third lists the Glycaemic Load. This is most realistic as it is a measure of the Glycaemic Index multiplied by the amount eaten.

Carbohydrate contents of common foods

For easy reference, below is a list of the carbohydrate content (in grams) of common foods. As all foods from animals, fish and birds are low in carbohydrate and may be eaten freely, these are not included. Only foods of vegetable origin, and then only those which have a relatively concentrated carbohydrate content, need be avoided.

Food	Carbohydrate (g)
Fruit	
Apple, small	10
medium	13
large	21
Apricot, raw	2
dried	10

Food	Carbohydrate (g)
Banana, small, ripe	15
medium	16
Blackberries, raw, 1 oz (25 g)	2
Cherries, raw, 1 oz (25 g)	40
Clementine	5
Currants, dried, 1 oz (25 g)	18
Damsons, raw, 1 oz (25 g)	2
Dates, dried, 1 oz (25 g)	18
Fig, raw, one	4
Gooseberries, raw, 1 oz (25 g)	1
Grapefruit, raw, 7 oz (175 g)	5
juice, unsweetened, ½ pint	20
Grapes, 1 oz (25 g)	4
Melon, raw, 6 oz (150 g)	5
Nectarine, raw, 5 oz (125 g)	16
Orange, 3″ diam	9
Orange juice, ½ pint	24
Peach, 2″ diam	9
Pear, medium	14
Pineapple, raw, 1 oz (25 g)	3
Plums, raw, 4 oz (100 g)	
10 Prunes, dried, with stones	9
Raspberries, raw, 1 oz (25 g)	2
Rhubarb, stewed, no sugar, 5 oz (125 g)	1
Strawberries, raw, 1 oz (25 g)	2
Nuts	
Almonds, 1 oz (25 g)	1
Brazils, 1 oz (25 g)	1
Cashews, roast, 4 oz (100 g) packet	18
Chestnuts, shelled, 1 oz (25 g)	10
Cobs, 1 oz (25 g)	2
Coconut, raw, 1 oz (25 g)	1
Coconut, desiccated, 1 oz (25 g)	2
Hazelnuts, 1 oz (25 g)	2

Food	Carbohydrate (g)
Peanuts, roasted, 1 oz (25 g)	2
Pistachios	25
Walnuts, raw, 1 oz (25 g)	1
Cereals	
Breakfast cereals, see below	
Butter biscuit, (2)	15
Cream cracker (4)	19
Digestive (2)	19
Water biscuit (4)	21
Bread, slice, small	12
Croissant (1)	30
Crumpet (1)	16
Muffin (1)	28
Roll (1)	30
Flour, plain, 1 oz (25 g)	23
Oats, raw, 1 oz (25 g)	21
Pasta, (all types), dry, 1 oz (25 g)	7
Pasta verde, dry, 1 oz (25 g)	22
cooked, 1 oz (25 g)	6
Pastry, 1 oz (25 g)	10–14
Porridge, made with water, 4 oz (100 g)	9
Rice, white, raw, 1 oz (25 g)	25
boiled, 1 oz (25 g)	8
Sugar, 1 oz (25 g)	28
Honey, 1 oz (25 g)	22

The carbohydrate content of breakfast cereals is marked on their packets.

Vegetables

Most green vegetables are low in carbohydrate and are not listed. It is the root vegetables and seeds which tend to have a relatively high carbohydrate content. They are listed below. As a rough guide, restrict yourself to about a cup of vegetables (measured after cooking) per meal. Greens may be eaten in larger quantities.

Food	Carbohydrate (g)
Beans, baked, 2 tbs	4
broad, raw, 1 oz (25 g)	2
butter, dried, 1 oz (25 g)	14
french, raw, 1 oz (25 g)	0
haricot, dried, 1 oz (25 g)	13
runner, raw, 1 oz (25 g)	1
Beetroot, raw, medium	6
Carrots, raw, 4 oz (100 g)	5
Corn on the cob, raw, 5"	34
Lentils, dried, 1 oz (25 g)	15
Onion, medium	3
Parsnips, raw, 1 oz (25 g)	3
Peas, raw, 1 oz (25 g)	3
Potatoes, raw, 4 oz (100 g)	24
Sweetcorn, canned, 1 oz (25 g)	5
Turnips, raw, 1 oz (25 g)	1

The following two lists of fruit and vegetables list the amount of a food that gives either 10 g (fruit) or 5 g (vegetables) of commonly available products. Use these tables to determine how much of each you can eat.

I suggest that you photocopy them or print them out from www.hammersmithpress.co.uk and keep them handy.

The following quantities of fruit will give 10 g of carbohydrate (raw weights):

75 g/3 oz of:	100 g/4 oz of:	150 g/6 oz of:	200 g/8 oz of:
Apples	Apricots	Avocados	Rhubarb
Blackcurrants	Blackberries	Gooseberries	
Blueberries	Cherries	Grapefruit (white)	
Plums	Cranberries	Melon	
Elderberries	Guavas	Raspberries	
Kiwi fruit	Lemons (peeled)		
Kumquats	Limes		
Loganberries	Mulberries		
Mangoes	Nectarine		
Pears	Oranges		(cont'd)

75 g/3 oz of:	100 g/4 oz of:	150 g/6 oz of:	200 g/8 oz of:
Pineapple	Papaya		
	Peach		
	Red currants		
	Satsumas		
	Strawberries		
	Tangerines		

The following quantities of vegetables will provide 5 g of carbohydrate (raw weights):

50 g/2 oz of:	75 g/3 oz of:	100 g/4 oz of:	200 g/8 oz of:
Beetroot	Leeks	Asparagus	Broccoli
Carrots	Squash (winter)	Aubergine	Brussels sprouts
Celeriac		Bean sprouts	Cabbage
		Cauliflower	Celery
		Chicory leaves	Courgette
		Chives	Cucumber
		Fennel bulb	Endive
		Flax seed	Gherkins
		Green beans	Gourd (calabash)
		Kale	Lettuce
		Kohlrabi	Marrow
		Mangetout	Mustard greens
		Mung beans	Okra
		(sprouted)	Radishes
		Mushrooms	Spirulina
		Onions	Spinach
		Peppers (sweet)	Spring greens
		Pumpkin	Swiss chard
		Squash	Spring onions
		(summer)	Turnip greens
		Swede	
		Tomato (fresh	
		or canned)	
		Turnips	

Glycaemic Index

Carbohydrate content of foods in grams per 100 grams (3½ oz) and their Glycaemic Index (GI)

The Glycaemic Index (GI) is a numerical system of measuring how fast a carbohydrate triggers a rise in circulating blood sugar – the higher the number, the greater the blood sugar response. A low GI food will cause a small rise, while a high GI food will trigger a dramatic spike. A list of carbohydrates with their glycaemic values is shown below. A GI of 70 or more is classed as high and should be avoided, a GI of 56 to 69 inclusive is medium so go easy on it, and a GI of 55 or less is low and you can be more liberal. Where no Glycaemic Index is given, this is because it hasn't yet been determined. (Highest measured figures used.)

Food	Carb (g/100 g)	GI
Milk		
Cream – single	3	0
Milk, liquid, whole	5	21
Milk, liquid, skimmed	5	32
Yoghurt, low-fat, natural	10	36
Yoghurt, low-fat, fruit	18	47
Cheese		
Brie	0	0
Cheddar	0	0
Cheese spread	1	
Cottage	1	
Feta	0	0
Meat		
Bacon, rashers	0	0
Beef, mince, stewed	0	0
Stewing steak	0	0
Black pudding, fried	15	
Chicken, roast, meat and skin	0	0
Corned beef	0	0
Ham	0	0

Food	Carb (g/100 g)	GI
Kidney, pig's, fried	0	0
Lamb, roast	0	0
Liver, lamb's, fried	0	0
Luncheon meat	3	
Pâté, average	1	
Pork chop, cooked	0	0
Sausage, beef, cooked	15	28
Sausage, pork, cooked	11	28
Steak and kidney pie	2	
Turkey, roast, meat and skin	0	0
Fish		
White fish	0	0
Cod, fried	7	
Fish fingers	16	38
Herrings	0	0
Mackerel	0	0
Pilchards, canned in tomato sauce	1	
Prawns, boiled	0	0
Sardines, canned in oil, fish only	0	0
Tuna in oil	0	0
Eggs		
Eggs, served any way	0	0
Fats		
Lard, cooking fat, dripping	0	0
Margarine, average	0	0
Cooking and salad oil	0	0
Preserves, etc.		
Chocolate, milk	59	51
Honey	76	83
Jam	69	51
Marmalade	70	48
Sugar, white	105	110

Food	Carb (g/100 g)	GI
Syrup	79	
Peppermints	100	70
Vegetables		
Aubergines	3	
Baked beans	15	56
Beans, runner, boiled	3	
Beans, red kidney, raw	45	52
Beans, soya, boiled	9	25
Beetroot, boiled	10	64
Brussels sprouts, boiled	2	
Cabbage, raw	3	
boiled	2	
Carrots, (not new)	5	47
Cauliflower, cooked	1	
Celery, raw	1	
Courgettes, raw	5	
Cucumber	2	
Lentils, cooked	17	41
Lettuce	1	
Mushrooms	0	0
Onion	5	
Parsnips, cooked	14	97
Peas, frozen, boiled	11	51
Peas canned, processed	19	48
Peppers, green	2	
Potatoes, boiled	18	54
Potatoes, fried (chips)	34	75
Potatoes, instant	30	85
Potatoes, roast	26	85
Potato crisps	50	77
Spinach, boiled	1	
Sweetcorn, canned	17	53
Sweet potato	22	61
Tomatoes, fresh	3	36

Food	Carb (g/100 g)	GI
Turnips, cooked	2	
Watercress	1	
Yam, boiled	30	37
Nuts		
Almonds	4	
Brazils	4	
Cashews	27	22
Coconut, desiccated	6	
Hazelnuts	7	
Peanuts, roasted, salted	9	21
Peanut butter	13	
Walnuts	3	
Fruit		
Apples	12	38
Apricots,		
canned, in syrup	28	64
stewed, no sugar	5	57
dried	43	30
fresh, raw	11	57
Avocado	2	
Bananas, ripe	19	52
Blackberries, raw	7	
Blackcurrants	7	
Cherries	12	22
Clementine	8	
Cranberries, raw	4	
Currants, dried	59	
Dates, dried	64	103
Figs, dried	53	61
Gooseberries, raw	4	
Gooseberries, cooked, unsweetened	3	
Grapes	16	49
Grapefruit	5	25
Lemon juice	2	

Food	Carb (g/100 g)	GI
Mango	15	51
Melon, cantaloupe, raw	4	65
Mulberries, raw	7	
Nectarine, raw	10	
Oranges	9	42
Orange juice	9	50
Peaches, raw	9	56
Peaches, canned in syrup	23	58
Pears	11	42
Pineapple	12	59
Plums	8	39
Prunes, dried	40	29
Raisins	60	64
Raspberries	6	
Rhubarb, cooked, no sugar	1	
Strawberries	6	40
Sultanas	65	56
Cereals		
Biscuits, chocolate	67	
Biscuits, plain, digestive	69	84
Biscuits, semi-sweet	75	79
Bread, brown	44	
Bread, white	49	70
Bread, wholemeal	42	71
Chelsea bun, (1)	58	
Cream crackers	68	65
Crispbread, rye	71	69
Flour, white	77	71
Flour, wholemeal	63	69
Pearl barley	79	25
Popcorn	66	79
Rice, raw	86	
Rice, instant, boiled 6 min	30	69
Spaghetti, raw	74	68
Tapioca	90	70

Food	Carb (g/100 g)	GI
Breakfast cereals		
Cornflakes	85	81
Muesli	66	66
Oats, porridge	66	58
Weetabix	70	70
Cakes, pastries		
Chocolate cake with butter icing	53	38
Fruit cake, rich	51	
Jam tarts	63	
Plain cake, Madeira	58	46
Puddings		
Apple pie	57	
Bread and butter pudding	17	
Cheesecake, frozen, fruit topping	33	
Custard	17	43
Ice-cream, dairy	21	61
Rice pudding	20	69
Trifle	20	
Beverages		
Chocolate, drinking	77	51
Coca Cola	11	63
Fanta	7	58
Lucozade	18	95

Alcohol

There is some dispute over the effect of alcohol. One theory has it that alcohol reduces the combustion of fat in the body in a similar way to carbohydrate. On the other hand, there is a school of thought that suggests that by dilating the blood vessels in the skin, making it work harder, alcohol may step up the metabolism sufficiently to compensate for the added calories taken in the alcohol. There is also experimental evidence that such increased metabolism coupled with increased loss of water from the skin and in urine could result in weight loss. It is also known that alcohol does not raise blood sugar or insulin levels. So, while alcohol might stop weight loss, it doesn't put weight on.

Alcohol really is a case of try it and see. Dry wines and spirits will have the least affect. Drinks to avoid are those which contain sugar. These include beer, lager and sweet drinks.

Glycaemic Load

Although carbs are what put glucose in the bloodstream, not all foods with carbs raise glucose to the same height. This difference is thought to be important. The rate at which blood glucose is affected by foods is measured by the 'Glycaemic Index' (GI); the higher the number against a food, the faster it raises blood glucose levels.

However, there is still a problem because this increase in blood glucose levels is also dependent on the amount of the food you eat and what it is eaten with. And so another scale has been created which takes this into consideration. This scale is the Glycaemic Load.

In the tables that follow, foods are listed with their carb contents and with both their GI and Glycaemic Load values. As you will see, these can be quite complicated. Although I have included them to give you the whole picture, I think it is much easier just to take note of the carb content and keep the total for the day around 60 g, spread equally between meals.

When planning meals, try to keep your Glycaemic Load at no more than 15 per meal.

Food	Serving	GI	Carb (g)	Glycaemic Load
Breads				
Wholemeal (wheat flour)	1 slice, 35 g	69	14	**9.6**
White (wheat flour)	1 slice, 30 g	70	15	**10**
Gluten-free bread, multigrain	1 slice, 35 g	79	15	**12**
Melba toast	4 squares, 30 g	70	19	**13**
French baguette	30 g	95	15	**14**
Rye bread	1 slice, 50 g	65	23	**15**
Croissant	1, 50 g	67	27	**18**

Food	Serving	GI	Carb (g)	Glycaemic Load
Muffins, apple	1 muffin, 80 g	44	44	**19**
Muffins, bran	1 muffin, 80 g	60	34	**20**
Pita bread	1 piece, 65 g	57	38	**22**
Muffins, blueberry	1 muffin, 80 g	59	41	**24**
Bagel	1, 70 g	72	35	**25**
Breakfast cereals				
Oat bran, raw	1 tbsp, 10 g	55	7	**4**
Bran Buds	½ cup, 30 g	58	14	**8**
All-Bran	½ cup, 40 g	42	22	**9**
Porridge (cooked with water)	1 cup, 245 g	42	24	**10**
Special K	1 cup, 30 g	54	21	**11**
Shredded wheat	½ cup, 25 g	67	18	**12**
Weetabix	2 Biscuits, 30 g	69	19	**13**
Nutri-grain	1 cup, 30 g	66	20	**13**
Cheerios	30 g	74	20	**15**
Frosties	¾ cup, 30 g	55	27	**15**
Puffed wheat	1 cup, 30 g	80	22	**18**
Bran Flakes	¾ cup, 30 g	74	24	**18**
Muesli, non-toasted	½ cup, 60 g	56	32	**18**
Crunchy Nut Cornflakes	30 g	72	25	**18**
Coco Pops	¾ cup, 30 g	77	26	**20**
Corn Flakes	1 cup, 30 g	84	26	**22**
Rice Krispies	1 cup, 30 g	82	27	**22**
Sultana Bran	1 cup, 45 g	73	35	**26**
Grape Nuts	½ cup, 58 g	71	47	**33**
Cakes				
Sponge cake	1 slice, 60 g	46	32	**15**
Scones, made from packet mix	1 scone, 40 g	92	20	**18**
Pound cake	1 slice, 80 g	54	42	**23**
Cracker biscuits				
Ryvita	2 biscuits, 20 g	69	16	**11**
Soda crackers	3 biscuits, 25 g	74	17	**13**

Food	Serving	GI	Carb (g)	Glycaemic Load
Water biscuits	5 biscuits, 25 g	78	18	**14**
Rice cakes	2 pieces, 25 g	82	21	**17**
Fruit				
Grapefruit, raw	½ med, 100 g	25	5	**1**
Cherries	20 cherries, 80 g	22	10	**2**
Plums	3–4 small, 100 g	39	7	**3**
Peach, fresh,	1 large, 110 g	42	7	**3**
Apricots, fresh	3 medium, 100 g	57	7	**4**
Apricots, dried	5–6 pieces, 30 g	31	13	**4**
Kiwi fruit	1 raw, peeled, 80 g	52	8	**4**
Orange	1 medium, 130 g	44	10	**4**
Watermelon	1 cup, 150 g	72	8	**6**
Pineapple, fresh	2 slices, 125 g	66	10	**7**
Apple	1 medium, 150 g	38	18	**7**
Grapes, green	1 cup, 100 g	46	15	**7**
Prunes, pitted	6, 40 g	29	15	**7**
Pear, fresh	1 medium, 150 g	38	21	**8**
Fruit cocktail, canned, natural juice	½ cup, 125 g	55	15	**8**
Mango	1 small, 150 g	55	19	**10**
Lychee, canned and drained	7 lychees, 90 g	79	16	**13**
Sultanas	¼ cup, 40 g	56	30	**14**
Banana, raw	1 medium, 150 g	55	32	**18**
Raisins	¼ cup, 40 g	64	28	**18**
Dates, dried	5 dates, 40 g	103	27	**21**
Grains				
Barley, pearled, boiled	½ cup, 80 g	25	17	**4**
Millet, cooked	½ cup, 120 g	71	12	**8**
Bulgur, cooked	½ cup, 120 g	48	21	**10**
Couscous, cooked	½ cup, 120 g	65	28	**12**
Rice, Basmati, white, boiled	1 cup, 180 g	58	50	**30**
Bengal gram dahl	½ cup, 100 g	54	57	**31**
Buckwheat, cooked	½ cup, 80 g	54	57	**31**
Rice, instant, cooked	1 cup, 180 g	87	38	**33**

Food	Serving	GI	Carb (g)	Glycaemic Load
Rice, glutinous, white, steamed	1 cup, 174 g	98	37	**36**
Tapioca (steamed 1 hour)	100 g	70	54	**37**
Tapioca (boiled with milk)	1 cup, 265 g	81	51	**41**
Pasta				
Tortellini, cheese, cooked	1 cup, 180 g	50	21	**10**
Ravioli, meat-filled, cooked	1 cup, 220 g	39	30	**11**
Vermicelli, cooked	1 cup, 180 g	35	45	**16**
Rice noodles, fresh, boiled	1 cup, 176 g	40	44	**18**
Spaghetti, wholemeal, cooked	1 cup, 180 g	37	48	**18**
Fettucini, cooked	1 cup, 180 g	32	57	**18**
Spaghetti, gluten-free in tomato sauce	1 small tin, 220 g	68	27	**18**
Macaroni and cheese, packaged, cooked	220 g	64	30	**19**
Macaroni, cooked	1 cup, 180 g	45	56	**25**
Linguine thin, cooked	1 cup, 180 g	55	56	**31**
Rice vermicelli, cooked	1 cup, 180 g	58	58	**34**
Rice pasta, brown, cooked	1 cup, 180 g	92	57	**52**
Vegetables				
Carrots, peeled, boiled	½ cup, 70 g	49	3	**1.5**
Swede, peeled, boiled	60 g	72	3	**2**
Peas, green, fresh/frozen, boiled	½ cup, 80 g	48	5	**2**
Beetroot, canned, drained	2–3 slices, 60 g	64	5	**3**
Beans, haricot, boiled	½ cup, 90 g	38	11	**4**
Pumpkin, peeled, boiled	½ cup, 85 g	75	6	**5**
Peas, split, yellow, boiled	½ cup, 90 g	32	16	**5**
Lentils (average)	100 g	28	19	**5**
Peas, chick, canned, drained,	½ cup, 95 g	42	15	**6**
Beans, kidney, canned, drained	½ cup, 95 g	52	13	**7**
Beans, broad, frozen, boiled	½ cup, 80 g	79	9	**7**
Parsnips, boiled	½ cup, 75 g	97	8	**8**
Sweet potato, peeled, boiled	½ cup, 80 g	54	16	**9**
Sweet corn	½ cup, 80 g	55	18	**10**

Food	Serving	GI	Carb (g)	Glycaemic Load
Beans, baked, canned in tomato sauce	½ cup, 120 g	48	21	**10**
Potatoes, Desirée, peeled, boiled	1 medium, 120 g	101	13	**13**
Potatoes, new, canned, drained	5 small, 175 g	65	21	**14**
Potatoes, instant, prepared	½ cup	83	18	**15**
Potatoes, French fries, fine cut	small serving, 120 g	75	49	**37**

Don't forget that foods which do not contain carbs have a Glycaemic Index and a Glycaemic Load of zero. So meats, poultry, fish, eggs, cheese, fats, et cetera, can be eaten without limit.

Recipes, menus and food preparation

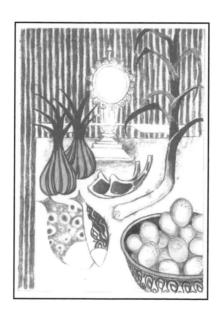

Recipes, menus and food preparation

No-one these days wants to spend hours slaving over a hot stove, but we do have to eat, and commercially-made, packaged meals are a nutritional nightmare. So, you have a choice: make your own meals or live an unhealthy life. It's up to you. But, I hear you say, I don't know how to cook.

Preparing good, wholesome meals really need not be time-consuming or difficult. While some of the more elaborate recipes are for the more adventurous, most are simple and quick to produce. As this way of eating is simply a matter of reducing the carbohydrate content of meals, you do not really need special menus. However, a few examples of daily menus are given in this section, in which the carbohydrate content has been calculated to give some idea of minimum daily amounts.

Margarine is not recommended (see Chapter 14). In the menus and recipes which follow, however, margarine may be substituted for butter if you wish. Do not use low-fat spreads.

Drinks with each meal: water, or coffee, tea or cocoa with milk – or preferably cream – as desired, sweetened with artificial sweetener if necessary, but cut down on this until you don't need it.

Miscellaneous ideas

Frying

It is important to choose the right fat for frying as it must be able to stand a temperature of up to 200°C without burning or oxidising. It should also be free of water as this will make it spit. Clarified butter is by far the best fat for frying, but it is prohibitively expensive. The best all-round alternative is probably lard. Beef dripping or other animal fats are suitable for frying but, as they tend to flavour the food being cooked, they should only be used to fry savoury dishes. Vegetable margarines usually contain a high proportion of water, thus they spit. There are white vegetable-oil based cooking fats which can be used for frying, and pure oils such as sunflower, and blended cooking oils which are suitable for frying. However, when heated, vegetable oils that are high in polyunsaturated fats oxidise readily, can cause free radicals to form and increase the risk of some cancers. It may be unwise to use vegetable-based cooking oils, such as sunflower oil, for cooking at high temperature, namely, frying, grilling or roasting. Olive oil is not suitable for the high temperatures of frying. It also has a distinctive taste that may not go with the food being cooked.

If you use different oils and fats, do not mix them.

How to clean saved fat

The use of fat is an essential element of this way of eating. You will (I hope) buy the fattest meat you can get. When roasting this, you will collect quantities of dripping in the oven pan. Don't throw this away, it is valuable, but it may need cleaning.

Most of the fat will be clear and can be poured through a sieve into a suitable bowl. Cleaning accumulated fat, dripping, et cetera, which has been left to set is also quite easy. Put it in a large heatproof bowl and pour boiling water over it. Stir it until it has all melted and then leave it to set hard. The fat will set in a layer on top of the water and all the impurities and bits will be mostly in the water and can be thrown away. Skim off the fat and keep it in the fridge. It will last for a very long time.

7-Days' menus

In the recipes and menus that follow, the total carbohydrate content for the days is less than the recommended 60 grams. This will allow you to add other foods you like to make the totals up to the required amount. If you include bread, reckon its carbohydrate content at 12 grams per slice. We suggest that you aim for equal amounts at each meal.

The figure given for carbohydrate content is calculated per person.

Day 1

Breakfast

MIXED GRILL

2 slices lamb's liver	Salt and black pepper to taste
2 lamb's kidneys	2 tomatoes, halved
40 g (1½ oz) lard	4 large mushrooms

Skin and core the kidneys and halve them lengthways.

Line a grill pan with foil and melt the lard and spread in it. Put the liver in the middle of the pan surrounded with the kidneys. Brush with lard.

Grill under a medium heat until the liver and kidneys change colour (approx 3 min), and turn them over. Sprinkle with salt and pepper to taste.

Arrange the tomatoes and mushrooms around the kidneys, with the cut sides of tomatoes and caps of mushrooms uppermost. Sprinkle them with salt and pepper and brush with fat.

Grill for a further 5 minutes and serve hot.

Serves 2

Carbohydrate: 3 grams per portion
Follow with a piece of fruit.
Tea, coffee or cocoa with cream.

Lunch

PORK WITH CHEESE SAUCE

240 g (8 oz) minced pork
2 onions, chopped
4 cloves garlic, crushed
Cinnamon
2 large tomatoes

2 handfuls fresh parsley
Salt and pepper to taste
25 g (1 oz) butter
4 tbsp grated cheddar cheese
2 tbsp single cream

Fry minced pork with an onion, garlic and a sprinkle of cinnamon. Stir in chopped tomato.

Simmer. Add a large handful of chopped flat leaf parsley. Season if necessary. Tip the minced pork mixture onto a flat-bottomed ovenproof dish. Make a cheese sauce (basic roux: butter, cheese and cream). Pour on top of pork.

Bake in moderate oven until top is crispy.

It's just as good hot as it is cold.

Serve with salad or cooked leafy vegetables.

Serves 2

Carbohydrate: just the veges
Tea, coffee or cocoa with cream.

Evening meal

After all that, you shouldn't need to eat much in the evening. So try:

120 g (4 oz) Brie or other full-fat cheese that you like
Medium apple each.
Tea, coffee or cocoa with cream.

Carbohydrate: 12–15 g

Day's total carbohydrate: 30–50 g depending on veges

Day 2

Breakfast

HERBED SCRAMBLED EGGS

6 eggs	50 g butter
4 tbsp single cream	2 tsp chopped chives
Salt	2 tsp chopped parsley
White pepper	

Break the eggs into a bowl, add the cream and season to taste. Whisk with a fork until mixed.

Melt the butter in a small saucepan. Add the egg mixture and cook gently, stirring constantly, until the eggs begin to set, but are not fully set. Use a low heat or lift the pan occasionally.

While the eggs are setting but still creamy, stir in the chives and parsley.
Follow with a piece of fruit.
Tea, coffee or cocoa with cream.

Serves 2

Carbohydrate: 15–20 g

Lunch

FISH, CHEESE AND EGG SALAD

2, 120 g smoked mackerel	2 large eggs, hard-boiled
Vinegar	Salad veges: onion, lettuce,
Salt and pepper	cucumber, radish, etc.
100 g (4 oz) cheese	

Take olive oil into a large bowl, add a similar amount of vinegar and season to taste to make French dressing.

Arrange fish, cheese and egg on a plate. Chop or tear salad ingredients and put in the olive oil/vinegar mixture to coat. Remove to the plate of fish, egg and cheese.
Tea, coffee or cocoa with cream.

Serves 2

Carbohydrate: 10 g

Evening meal

A plate of cold meat and cheese with unsweetened pickles, red cabbage, etc.
Follow with a bowl of chopped fruit or berries and single cream.
Tea, coffee or cocoa with cream.

Carbohydrate: 20 g

Day's total carbohydrate: 50 g

Day 3

Breakfast

REAL CONTINENTAL BREAKFAST

4 hard-boiled eggs
50 g (2 oz) cold meat, salami
   or continental sausage

50 g (2 oz) cheese (any full-fat)
Tomatoes

This real continental breakfast takes no time in the morning, as it can be prepared the previous evening.
   Follow with a piece of fruit.
   Tea, coffee or cocoa with cream.

Serves 2

Carbohydrate: about 15–20 g

Lunch

KIDNEYS À L'ORANGE

4 sheep's kidneys	1 tsp flour
25 g (1 oz) butter	½ pint stock
1 shallot	Orange peel, grated
2 mushrooms	2 slices of toast
Salt and pepper	Butter

Cut the kidneys in half, lengthways, skin them and remove the white parts (if using ox kidneys, cut into pieces). Melt the butter in a deep frying pan or a saucepan, put in the kidneys and fry brown. Chop the shallot and mushrooms small and add to the kidneys, season with salt and pepper. When these have fried brown, stir in the flour and brown this. Pour in the stock and simmer for about 20 minutes, with the lid off to reduce the stock. Flavour with grated orange peel and serve hot on a buttered almond and parmesan pancake or slice of buttered toast.

Tea, coffee or cocoa with cream.

Serves 2

Carbohydrate: 15 g with the toast

Evening meal

Make one breakfast pancake per person (see Basic recipes, page 328). Top with grated cheese and grill until cheese is lightly brown.

Follow with a piece of fruit.

Tea, coffee or cocoa with cream.

Carbohydrate: 15 g

Day's total carbohydrate: 50 g

Day 4

Breakfast

CREAMED EGGS

25 g (1 oz) butter
50 g (2 oz) cream cheese
3 tbsp double cream

½ tsp onion powder (or to taste)
Salt and pepper to taste
5 eggs

In a small saucepan, melt butter over medium heat. Add cream cheese, a small piece at a time, stirring until cheese and butter are well blended. Add cream and seasonings; mix well. Continue to heat, stirring frequently, until mixture is heated through. Add eggs while stirring and cook gently until set stirring continually.

Follow with a piece of fruit.

Tea, coffee or cocoa with cream.

Serves 2

Carbohydrate: 4 g + fruit = 15–20 g

Lunch

MEAT, CHEESE AND EGG SALAD

As for Day 2, except the fish is replaced with cold meat. Dress salad with mayonnaise or pesto (see page 330–331).

Tea, coffee or cocoa with cream.

Carbohydrate: 15–20 g

Evening meal

CHICKEN LIVERS WITH ONION

220 g (8 oz) organic chicken livers,
    chopped
Lard

1 medium onion
1 hard boiled egg, chopped

In a frying pan, heat the lard until it is hot but not smoking and sauté the chicken livers and onion over a moderately high heat until the liver is cooked right through. Transfer the mixture to a food processor, add the egg and salt and pepper to taste, and blend until the mixture is smooth. Serve on a bed of lettuce or a breakfast pancake (see Basic recipes, page 328).

Follow with fruit alone or with cream.

Tea, coffee or cocoa with cream.

Serves 2

Carbohydrate: about 20 g

Day's total carbohydrate: 50–60 g

Day 5

Breakfast

Breakfast pancake

Breakfast pancake (see Basic recipes) per person topped with: scrambled egg or bacon pieces or cold meat or grated cheese and spring onions, with fried tomato and/or mushrooms, and so on.

Follow with a piece of fruit.

Tea, coffee or cocoa with cream.

Carbohydrate: 15 g

Lunch

Packed lunches other than sandwiches can be taken to work in covered plastic boxes and eaten with either your fingers or a knife and fork. These can reduce the necessity for bread and, thus, the carbohydrate content.

Finger salads

If the constituents of a salad are dry, they may be eaten with the fingers.

100 g (4 oz) full-fat cheese, (Cheddar, Brie, Gouda, Maarsdam, et cetera) or
100 g (4 oz) cooked sliced ham rolled around a soft cheese such as Philadelphia or
chicken legs or
hard-boiled eggs or
any mixture of the above
with a salad composed of, say, a stick of celery, 1 tomato, 2 green pepper and 1 raw
    carrot.

Carbohydrate content: approx 10 grams

A similar meal, replacing the cheese with an individual pork pie, or egg and bacon
flan, would have a carbohydrate content of about 20 grams.
Tea, coffee or cocoa with cream.

Evening meal

SMOKED SALMON AND SCRAMBLED EGGS

4 eggs scrambled in butter   100 g (3½ oz) smoked salmon

Fresh fruit salad with cream
    Tea, coffee or cocoa with cream.

Serves 2

Carbohydrate: 15 g

Day's total carbohydrate: 40–50 g

Day 6

Breakfast

SCRAMBLED EGGS

This is easier than fried eggs and bacon.

50 g lard or butter   4 tbs single cream
6 large eggs   salt and pepper

Heat the lard or butter in a saucepan or frying pan. Mix the other ingredients. Pour into the pan and cook gently, stirring constantly, until set.

To make it even quicker, break the eggs directly into the frying pan and stir. Follow with a piece of fruit.

Tea, coffee or cocoa with cream.

Serves 2

Carbohydrate: 15 g

Lunch

HERBED SEAFOOD SALAD

This salad is ideal where a small meal is required: lunch for example. Or it may be divided among more people as a starter to a dinner. It is quick and easy to prepare.

2 tbsp olive oil	2 tbsp fresh basil, chopped
2 tbsp chilli oil, basil oil or other	85 g (3 oz) mixed salad leaves
flavoured oil	55 g (2 oz) sugar peas, chopped
Rind of 1 small lemon, grated finely	200 g (7 oz) packet of frozen seafood
1 tbsp lemon juice	mix defrosted and drained
1 clove of garlic, crushed	Salt and ground black pepper

Put 1 tbsp of the olive oil, the flavoured oil, grated lemon rind, lemon juice, garlic and basil into a small bowl or jug. Season with salt and pepper to taste and whisk until thoroughly mixed.

In another bowl, toss together the salad leaves and snap peas.

Heat the remaining olive oil in a large frying pan or wok, add the seafood and stir-fry over a medium heat until cooked (approx 5 minutes).

Scatter the cooked seafood over the salad mixture, toss together to mix and serve.

Tea, coffee or cocoa with cream.

Serves 2

Carbohydrate: 4 g

Evening meal

2 Egg omelette with diced kidney and basil

4 eggs	Salt and pepper to taste
Butter or lard for frying	10 basil leaves, chopped finely
4 lamb's kidneys, diced	

Beat and season the two eggs. Fry the kidneys and mix with the eggs. Pour the mixture back into the frying pan and cook through. Sprinkle with basil when almost cooked. Serve on a bed of lettuce.

Follow with fruit alone or with cream.

Tea, coffee or cocoa with cream.

Serves 2

Carbohydrate: 15 g

Day's total carbohydrate: 35 g

Day 7

Breakfast

Fish omelette

This dish is a useful way of using up leftovers of a fish dish from the previous day. Any white fish may be used.

Remains of cold boiled white fish	40 g (1½ oz) butter
1 tbsp milk or cream	A little white sauce
4 eggs	Salt and cayenne pepper

Remove any skin and bones from the fish and break it into small flakes. Melt a little butter in a frying pan, add the fish, seasonings and enough white sauce to moisten the fish. Keep it hot.

Lightly beat the eggs in a basin, add the milk and season to taste. Melt a full 30 grams (ounce) of butter in an omelette pan or small frying pan, pour in the eggs and stir over a high heat until the mixture begins to set. Then release from the bottom of the pan, put the prepared fish in the middle, fold the omelette over, allow it to colour, then serve immediately.

Follow with a piece of fruit.

Tea, coffee or cocoa with cream.

Serves 2

Carbohydrate: 15 g

Lunch

BRAISED TROUT

2 trout   1 tbsp cider vinegar
2 cups white wine   ¼ tsp ginger

Fry the fish until brown and then simmer in a dish with the other ingredients until the fish flakes easily. Simultaneously, cook 150 g (5 oz) vegetables of your choice until tender.

Place fish on a warm serving dish, reduce the cooking liquid by half, pour over the fish and serve with the veges.

Tea, coffee or cocoa with cream.

Serves 2

Carbohydrate: 15 g

Evening meal

DARK CHOCOLATE MOUSSE WITH FRUIT

225 g (8 oz) continental dark chocolate (70% or more cocoa solids)
4 large eggs, separated
2 tbsp orange liqueur (or juice from mandarin oranges)
6 tbsp double cream
Sliced fruit of your choice

Line a shallow 200 mm (8-inch) round cake tin with cling film.
Break up and melt the chocolate in a bowl over a pan of hot water.

Beat the egg yolks and orange liqueur into the chocolate then fold in the cream, mixing well.

In a separate bowl whisk the egg whites until stiff, then gently fold them into the chocolate mixture.

Pour the mixture into the prepared cake tin, level the surface and chill in a refrigerator for several hours until set.

Turn out the mousse onto a plate and serve with the fruit.

Tea, coffee or cocoa with cream.

Serves up to 4

Carbohydrate: 17 g

Day's total carbohydrate: 47 g

Basic recipes

ALMOND AND PARMESAN PANCAKES

This is a sort of thick pancake that is useful as it can be used for many things and is easy and quick to make. Parmesan is expensive, but supermarkets sell similar, but much cheaper cheeses.

1 large egg
1 tbsp ground almonds
1 tbsp grated Italian cheese (Parmesan type)

Mix all together and fry in lard or butter.

Each pancake serves 1.

Carbohydrate content: negligible.

This basic recipe has many uses: as a pizza base, breakfast pancake, bread substitute, sweet dessert base, and so on so why not experiment? By varying the ratio of ground almonds to cheese, a variety of textures and tastes are possible.

For a few ideas to start you off, you could use it like toast with lashings of butter, or top with savoury toppings: cheese, anchovies, tinned fish or meat, fried egg; you could even embed a little soft fruit in it while cooking for a dessert. For this last one, it is better to increase the ground almonds while reducing the amount of cheese, and fry on one side only, finishing off the top, if necessary, under a grill.

For a pizza base, place the mixture in a baking tin lined with non-stick baking parchment. Bake in a moderate oven until just set (approx 10 min). Add pizza topping of your choice and bake for a further 10 minutes or until topping is cooked and cheese melted.

Several of the meal recipes in this book use these pancakes as bases. They freeze well, so why not make a lot in one go and freeze them until required?

LOW-CARB PANCAKES

Here is a recipe which makes great low-carb pancakes. These are 10% carb, 20% protein and 70% fat by weight so you won't want more than one or two at a meal. This recipe makes about 30. They will keep in the freezer for use as required.

250 g (9 oz) curd cheese
500 g (1 lb 1 oz) eggs (about 8 large)
100 g (4 oz) potato flour
100 g (4 oz) lard for frying

Mix eggs and cheese together, add flour and mix well. Melt lard in pan and fry small pancakes (about 5 inches diameter) until light brown on both sides. Makes about 30.

These pancakes can be used as the base for breakfast meals, lunches or dinners.

COCONUT BISCUITS

3 egg whites
28 g (1 oz) grated (desiccated) coconut
Butter to fry in

Beat egg whites and mix with coconut. Place mix in hot frying pan and fry on both sides. Eat hot or cold.

Notes: do not beat egg whites too stiff.
These are also nice with grated cheese on top and popped under the grill.

Salad dressings

Many commercial mayos are not only high in carbs but their major ingredient is sunflower oil or a similar polyunsaturated vegetable oil. These are not at all healthy, so why not make your own? The easiest, by far, is the traditional French dressing.

FRENCH DRESSING

6 tbsp (90 ml) extra virgin olive oil
2 tbsp (30 ml) wine or cider vinegar
Salt and pepper to taste.

Put all ingredients in a bottle, shake vigorously to mix and drizzle over salads.

Variations on this can be made by adding herbs and/or spices to the basic mixture.

MAYONNAISE

1 egg
1 tbsp lemon juice
1 tsp mustard
Pepper and salt
2 tbsp vinegar or lemon juice
1 tsp crushed garlic or half that if using powder
1 cup olive oil

Put all ingredients except the oil into blender, whiz for a couple of seconds, then add oil in a steady slow drizzle. (If it curdles, pour it out, wash blender, put another egg in and trickle the curdled mix back in – problem solved.)

Notes: Any flavouring can be added, depending on your taste. Add 1 tbsp chilli sauce, 1 dstsp pimento and ½ tsp minced onion to the egg and oil basic mayonnaise for a Russian dressing. Or 1 tbsp horseradish and ¼ cup of very finely chopped celery leaves and parsley, plus 1 small spring onion to make a herb mayonnaise.

Because it is uncooked, this mayo will not keep for long – a few days in the fridge.

PESTO

Pesto is another salad dressing that is very popular in our house.

280 mL (½ pt) olive oil
2 generous handfuls of fresh basil leaves
2 cloves garlic, peeled
2 tbsp pine nuts
Freshly ground peppercorns to taste
Salt
2 tbsp grated Italian cheese (Parmesan type)

Whiz at fast speed olive oil, basil and garlic in a blender until the basil leaves are pulped.

Add pine nuts and season with peppercorns and salt to taste. Whiz at slower speed until pine nuts have blended into the sauce.

Add the Italian cheese and whiz slowly until it is absorbed. Taste and adjust seasoning, stirring in any added ingredients.

We use pesto mainly as a salad dressing, but it can be used to flavour soups and stews. It can be stored in a glass container in the fridge for use later.

Tip: Pesto tends to stick around the sides of the blender. To avoid wasting this, make pesto on a day when you will be having salad. You can then tear salad leaves and wipe them around the blender to coat them in the pesto and clean the blender at the same time.

Breakfast

The breakfast recipes that follow are designed to fill and satisfy, and to get you off to a good start. This is all important if you are to function at your best.

The ideas for lunches are aimed at the working man or woman who needs to carry a packed lunch to eat at the workplace.

As you only need to reduce your intake of carbohydrates to lose weight, dinners can probably consist of the foods you eat now with, perhaps, more meat and less potato. Therefore, the dinner recipes included here give ideas for you to adapt and for gourmet meals for dinner parties or special occasions.

The easy breakfast

If you are short of time, there is nothing easier than scrambled eggs for a cooked breakfast.

QUICK SCRAMBLED EGGS – THE QUICKEST BREAKFAST

Three large eggs   Salt and pepper seasoning
25 g (1 oz) butter or lard for frying

Put butter or lard in frying pan and begin to heat. As the fat melts, quickly break the eggs into the pan, add seasoning and mix until set. The eggs will soak up the butter or lard.

Serves 1

Carbohydrate: Negligible

Notes: This will probably only take about three minutes, so if you want a hot drink with your breakfast, it might be an idea to put the kettle on first.

To vary this meal, you can chop up meat or cheese and add as it cooks, or add chopped vegetables such as mushrooms, peas or anything else you fancy. It is also nice with smoked salmon or other fish and peas.

POACHED EGGS ON TOAST

300 mL (½ pint) of water   Butter
2 slices white bread   4 eggs
Pinch of salt   1 tsp yeast extract

Put the water and salt in an egg poacher and bring to the boil. Break the eggs into the poacher and simmer for three minutes until the eggs are set. Toast the bread lightly on both sides, then spread with butter and yeast extract. Remove the eggs and place on top of the toast.

Serves 2

Carbohydrate: 12 g

SCRAMBLED EGGS (2)

4 eggs	Salt
Butter	2 tsp chopped chives
4 tbsp single cream	White pepper
2 slices white bread	2 tsp chopped parsley

Break the eggs into a bowl, add the cream and salt and pepper to taste. Whisk with a fork until mixed.

Melt some butter in a small saucepan. Add the egg mixture and cook gently, stirring constantly, until the eggs begin to set, but are not fully set. Use a low light or lift the pan occasionally.

At the same time, toast the bread lightly and spread with butter. While the eggs are setting but still creamy, stir in the chives and parsley. Pile onto the toast and serve immediately.

Serves 2

Carbohydrate: 13 g

BREAKFAST OMELETTES

These are basic omelettes with a variety of toppings. You could use the toppings listed below one at a time or combine them for variety.

Basic ingredients

2 eggs per person	Salt and black pepper
1 tbsp milk or cream	Lard or butter

Toppings: Streaky bacon; cooked ham; mushrooms; Cheddar cheese; chopped lamb's kidney; anchovies; prawns mixed with cream; tomatoes; fried onions with grated cheese; herbs; flaked smoked haddock; cream cheese.

Break the eggs into a small bowl, add the cream or milk and salt and pepper to taste, and beat until frothy.

Melt the lard or butter into a frying pan and pour in the egg mixture. Cook over a moderate heat until it becomes firm.

When the omelette starts to set, spread the topping onto it and continue cooking until the omelette is set. Fold in half and serve.

Adding the toppings. The cooked ham should be cut small before adding and the Cheddar cheese grated before adding. If cream cheese is used, spread on the firm mixture and allow to melt. The bacon should be cut into small pieces and fried first, the omelette mixture being poured over it.

Carbohydrate: negligible

STACKED OMELETTES

If making breakfast for four or more people, you might try stacking omelettes. First make up three or four toppings which complement each other. Make an omelette and slide it onto a plate standing over hot water to keep it warm. Cover with one topping. Make a second omelette and place on top, followed by another topping, and so on. Make as many omelettes as there are people. Serve by cutting the stack of omelettes into wedge shaped portions.

Carbohydrate: negligible

AVOCADO AND CREAM CHEESE OMELETTE

4 eggs	20 g butter
2 tbsp single cream	50 g (2 oz) cream cheese
Salt and white pepper to taste	1 avocado, sliced
½ tsp paprika	Chives or spring onions, chopped

Beat eggs, cream, salt, pepper and paprika together.

Melt butter in a large frying pan over medium heat. Tilt pan to coat all sides evenly.

Pour egg mixture into pan, tilt to permit uncooked egg to run to sides and bottom. Prick egg with a fork to let heat through. Lower heat and cook 2 to 3 minutes or until egg is slightly firm through.

Spoon or drop cream cheese across the centre of eggs. Top with avocado slices and roll the edges of egg over filling.

Remove from heat and cover for 2 to 3 minutes or until cheese is melted.

Sprinkle with chopped chives. Serve hot.

Serves 2

Carbohydrate: 4 g

BAKED HAM, EGG AND TOMATO

4 tomatoes large enough to hold an egg	100 g (4 oz) cooked ham
	Salt and pepper
4 eggs	1 tsp chopped parsley

Cut the tops off the tomatoes and scoop out the seeds and pulp. Remove the seeds from the pulp with a sieve. Mix the ham, parsley and pulp in a bowl with added salt and pepper to taste.

Divide the mixture and put into the tomatoes, pressing it well down. With the tomatoes in a baking dish, break an egg into each and sprinkle with salt and pepper to taste.

Bake in a preheated oven at moderate heat (190°C/375°F/Gas Mark 5) until the eggs are set (about 15 minutes). Serve immediately.

Serves 4

Carbohydrate: 3 g

POACHED HADDOCK WITH EGG

450 g (1 lb) smoked haddock fillets	25 g (1 oz) butter
Black pepper	4 eggs
600 mL (1 pint) water	

In a frying pan, cover the fish with water. Bring slowly to the boil and simmer until the fish is tender but not breaking up (about 10–15 minutes). Transfer to warm plates and keep hot.

Break an egg into a cup.

Stir the cooking water, still in the frying pan, briskly to create a whirlpool and carefully slide the egg into it. Simmer until the egg is set (about 3 minutes) Repeat for the other eggs.

Cut the fish into 4 portions, sprinkle with pepper to taste and melt the butter on to it. Place one egg on each piece and serve immediately.

Serves 4

Carbohydrate: negligible

KIPPERS (SMOKED HERRING) AND SCRAMBLED EGGS

2 kipper fillets	Butter
Salt and pepper	Milk or cream
4 eggs	

Prepare the kippers: wash them well, cut off the head and just cover with boiling water. Cook gently for 2–3 minutes, drain and serve with a knob of butter.

Alternatively, brush with butter and grill for 5–6 minutes.

The kippers may also be fried in lard for 5–7 minutes.

Mix the eggs with a little milk or cream, and salt and pepper to taste. While the kippers are cooking scramble the eggs in butter. Serve together immediately.

Serves 2

Carbohydrate: 0

EGG CROQUETTES

4 hard-boiled eggs	30 g (1 oz) butter
Salt and pepper	2 eggs
30 g (1 oz) onion	30 g (1 oz) flour
1 tsp chopped parsley	55 g (2 oz) dry breadcrumbs
55 g (2 oz) mushrooms	150 mL (¼ pint) milk
Pinch of grated nutmeg	Oil for deep frying

Chop the hard-boiled eggs and reserve. Prepare, chop finely and mix together the onion and mushrooms. In a pan large enough to hold all the ingredients, melt the butter and fry the onion/mushroom mixture until the onion is soft. Stir in the flour and cook for 1 minute. Pour in the milk gradually while stirring and bring to a simmer, while continuing to stir. Still stirring, simmer until the sauce thickens (about 3 minutes). Mix in the hard-boiled eggs, seasoning parsley and nutmeg. Stir over a low heat for 1 minute.

Turn the mixture onto a plate, flatten the top and cover with a second plate. Allow to cool. When cold, divide into 6 or 8 portions.

On a floured board, form into rounds. Beat the 2 eggs in a bowl. Dip the croquettes into the egg ensuring that each one is covered all over and, on a sheet of greaseproof paper, roll each one in the breadcrumbs.

Heat the fat and fry the croquettes a few at a time until crisp and brown. Drain and serve.

Serves 2

Carbohydrate: negligible

More breakfast ideas

Chives, cheese and eggs – Add chives and grated hard cheese to beaten eggs and cook slowly in a buttered frying pan.

Eggs and anchovies – Add anchovy paste and cayenne to creamed hard boiled eggs.

Eggs and orange juice – Add a little orange juice to scrambled eggs.

Eggs in black butter – Brown the butter in a pan but don't burn it. Fry eggs in this, slowly, until the white over the yolk clouds over. Remove the eggs, add a little vinegar to the pan and bring to a bubble. Pour sauce over the eggs.

Tomato and eggs – Bake hollowed tomato halves seasoned with garlic butter in a hot oven. Top them with eggs scrambled with cream, to which a bit of grated cheese and parsley has been added.

Scrambled with cream cheese – Halfway through a batch of scrambled eggs, stir in small chunks of cream cheese and continue until the cheese melts. Top with minced chives.

Devilled eggs – Mix softened cream cheese with hardboiled egg yolks and season.

Easy recipes for lunch

If lunches are eaten at home, their preparation and serving should present few problems. These days, however, many people are away from home at lunchtime. This can make meal preparation more difficult. If you take your lunch in a restaurant or works' canteen, it is safest to choose meat, fish or cheese salads. Eat the lettuce, tomatoes, coleslaw, et cetera, but go easy on the potato or pasta salad. You could also have a hot meal of, say, roast beef, green vegetables and a little mashed potato, but decline the Yorkshire pudding and go easy on the puddings: finish with cheese rather than a sweet. At the 'Little Chef' type of restaurant, the All-day breakfasts are good. Just have a salad in place of the beans, chips, etc. If you eat in a pub, and normally have a drink, bear in mind the carbohydrate content of the alcohol. Have, say, a glass of dry wine – and restrict yourself to just the one.

If you normally take a packed lunch of sandwiches, however, it is not so easy. The ideas for lunches below, therefore, concentrate on meals to be eaten in an office or building site.

Sandwiches

Sandwiches should be used as sparingly as possible, and then be restricted to two slices of bread (carbohydrate content: 24 grams) at any one meal, spread liberally with butter. The secret is to ensure that what fills the sandwich is enough to fill you. The bread may be fresh or toasted.

FILLINGS

Cold beef, cut thickly with mustard and a slice of cheese.
Minced lamb or mutton and mint sauce.
Fried bacon and unsweetened pickles.
Cheddar cheese and sliced onions.
Cooked white fish with pickled walnuts.
Grilled cheese on bacon.
Cheese, ham and chicken slices.
2 egg omelette with diced kidney and basil.
Scrambled egg with anchovy paste and chopped watercress.
Smoked cods' roes with tomato, lettuce and lemon juice.
White fish with tomato sauce.

Packed lunches other than sandwiches can be taken to work in covered plastic boxes and eaten either with your fingers or a knife and fork. These can reduce the necessity for bread and, thus, the carbohydrate content.

Finger salads

If the constituents of a salad are dry, they may be eaten with your fingers.

100 g (4 oz) full-fat cheese (Cheddar, Brie, Gouda, Edam, Maarsdam, et cetera), or
100 g (4 oz) cooked sliced ham rolled around a soft cheese such as Philadelphia or chicken legs or
hard-boiled eggs or
any mixture of the above
with a salad composed of, say, a stick of celery, 1 tomato, 2 green pepper and 1 raw
    carrot.

Carbohydrate: about 10 g

A similar meal, replacing the cheese with an individual pork pie, or egg and bacon flan, would have a carbohydrate content of about 20 grams.

Knife and fork meals

Salads to be eaten with a knife and fork can be more adventurous. The basis may be any cold meat such as lamb cutlets, boiled bacon, chicken legs; fish such as sardines, salmon or tuna; hard-boiled eggs and/or cheese, together with a dressed salad. Carbohydrate content will be approximately 13 grams.

Easy dinners and main meals

SWISS SHEPHERD'S PIE

A shepherd's pie is a lamb mixture under a mashed potato topping. This recipe reduces the carb content by replacing the mashed potato with a Swiss cheese, hence the name. The recipe is really easy to make, and is a very tasty and filling dish. You can use any meat, although leftover cold meat from a lamb roast gives the best taste. You can also use pretty much any green leafy vegetable or tomatoes, instead of the spinach. Although Raclette cheese is best, other 'rubbery' cheeses, such as Maarsdam or Edam are also suitable.

1 medium onion, chopped into
    small pieces
450 g (1 lb) minced lamb, or beef
50 g lard or dripping for frying

100 g (4 oz) mushrooms, sliced
100 g (4 oz) spinach or broccoli
150 g (6 oz) Raclette cheese sliced
    6 mm thick

Fry chopped onion and meat in the lard. Add sliced mushrooms and fry until cooked. Mix well together.

In a saucepan, bring spinach, with very little water, to the boil and switch off. This will cook it sufficiently. If using broccoli, cook until tender.

Take the meat mixture out of the frying pan and place in an ovenproof dish. Cover with the spinach and then place slices of Raclette cheese over the spinach to form a 'crust'.

Place the dish under the grill until the cheese is golden.

Serve alone or with a salad

Serves 2–4

Carbohydrate: negligible

PORK CHOPS WITH TARRAGON AND MUSTARD

4 pork chops   30 g lard or butter for frying

Sauce
300 mL chicken stock   2 tsp grainy mustard
1 tsp English mustard   30 mL double cream
1 tsp Dijon mustard   2 tbsp tarragon, chopped

Melt 30 g fat in frying pan. Fry pork chops until liquid runs out clear when pricked.

Sauce
Add chicken stock and simmer for 10 minutes. Add mustards and cream and simmer for a further 5 minutes. Stir in tarragon.

Pour over pork chops and serve with green vegetables.

Serves 4

Carbohydrate: negligible plus veges

ROAST LAMB WITH CHILLI

1 kg (2¼ lb) lamb leg or shoulder   3 onions, peeled and halved
   joint, boned and rolled   2 red chilli peppers, halved

Sauce

2 tbsp sweet chilli sauce   2 tbsp olive or coconut oil
1 tbsp balsamic vinegar

Preheat oven to 180°C, 350°F, Gas mark 4.

Put joint on rack in roasting tin and roast for requisite time.

About 45 minutes before lamb is finished roasting, arrange onion halves and peppers on a baking tray and roast.

Mix the rest of the ingredients together to make the sauce. About 10 minutes before the end of the cooking time, drizzle the sauce over both the roast and the vegetables. Allow all to finish cooking.

Serve with any green vegetables or a salad.

Serves 4

Carbohydrate: negligible plus veges

LAMB IN RED WINE

Neck cutlets of lamb   28 g (1 oz) butter
1 tbsp olive oil   280 mL (½ pt) red wine
1 tbsp green peppercorns in brine 150 mL (¼ pt) chicken stock
1 tbsp fresh rosemary

Mix the lamb, oil, peppercorns and rosemary together in a bowl. Season with salt.

Heat the butter in a large frying pan, add the lamb and cook over a moderate to high heat for 2–3 minutes each side. The lamb should be lightly browned but still pink inside.

Remove the lamb from the frying pan and keep warm.

Add the wine and stock to the frying pan and bring to the boil, stirring and mixing in the residue from the pan. Reduce the heat and allow to simmer until the sauce has begun to thicken slightly (about 5–10 minutes). Pour over the lamb and serve with green vegetables.

Serves 4

Carbohydrate: negligible plus veges

SMOKED SALMON PARCELS

This recipe makes a small, light meal for an evening or as a starter. No cooking is required.

110 g (4 oz) cream or curd cheese
2 tbsp crème frâiche
2 tbsp dill, chopped
2 tbsp chives, chopped, plus eight complete chives for tying the parcels

140 g (5 oz) 4-slice smoked salmon pack
1 packet of salad leaves, or lambs leaves and rocket (to serve 4)
2 tbsp olive oil and vinegar, French dressing
Lemon juice

Mix together the cheese, crème frâiche, dill and chives. Season with pepper.

Line four deep bun tins with oversize cling film, then line with the salmon slices. Fill these with the cheese mixture and fold the salmon over the top, pressing to seal and firm.

Cover with the excess cling film.

Chill in a freezer for 15 minutes then refrigerate for 45 minutes or until ready to serve.

To serve, remove cling film, tie chives crosswise around the parcels, place on a bed of salad, and drizzle with dressing and lemon juice.

Serves 4

Carbohydrate : 1 gram

CHEESE AND BROCCOLI PIZZA

Makes enough for 8 people if part of a larger meal. You could also make larger pizzas, to serve as a main meal for 4 people.

Almond and parmesan pancake mixture (see first Basic recipe page 328)
50 g (2 oz) butter
1 medium onion, peeled and chopped
150 g (6 oz) broccoli florets

4 large eggs
280 mL (½ pt) milk
110 g (4 oz) mature cheese (Stilton or similar)
Ready made red pepper or tomato sauce

Preheat oven to 220°C, 425°F, Gas mark 7.

Mix the almond Parmesan pancake dough.

Grease eight 10 cm (4 inch) flan tins and spread the pancake mix over the bottoms of each tin. Put in the oven for 2–3 minutes to seal, then remove.

In a saucepan, melt the butter and cook the onion gently until softened.

Cook broccoli in boiling water for 2–3 minutes, pour into a sieve and rinse under cold water. Drain on kitchen paper.

Whisk the eggs with the milk and season with salt and black pepper to taste. Mix the onion in and the cheese and broccoli.

Spoon the mixture into the tins and bake until set and golden (about 25–30 minutes).

Remove from oven and allow to cool a little.

Serve with your choice of ready-made sauce.

Serves 4 or 8

Carbohydrate: negligible

CHICKEN TIKKA MASALA

Lard for frying
4 chicken fillets, cubed
2 tbsp tikka paste

295 g condensed cream of tomato soup
200 mL (7 fl oz) milk

Heat the lard in a large frying pan, add the chicken and fry for 5 minutes.

Add the other ingredients and simmer for 20 minutes, stirring regularly.

Serve on Almond Parmesan pancakes (see first Basic recipe page 328).

Serves 2

Carbohydrate: 5 g plus soup

BAKED COD

4 cod portions, 8 oz (250 g) each
295 g condensed cream of mushroom soup

50 g ground almonds
50 g Cheddar cheese, grated

Preheat oven to 190°C, 375°F, Gas mark 5.

Place the cod portions in a 1.2 litre (2 pint) ovenproof dish and pour the soup over them. Sprinkle top with ground almond and grated cheese and bake in the oven for 20 minutes.

Serve with buttered green vegetables.

Serves 4

Carbohydrate: see soup can

POTTED PRAWNS

200 g (7 oz) prawns, frozen or fresh
2 tbsp Greek yoghurt, full-fat
1 tsp lemon juice
Tabasco sauce

3 tbsp dill, fresh
Coarsely ground pepper to taste
80 g (3 oz) butter, melted

Whiz all the ingredients except the butter briefly in a food processor to form a coarse-textured paste.

Spoon into four ramekins and smooth the tops. Pour a thin layer of melted butter over the prawn mixture and chill for 2 or 3 hours before serving.

This dish would normally be served with toast or French bread. However, the almond, parmesan pancake is also ideal.

Serves 4

Carbohydrate: negligible

LIVER AND ONIONS

Marinate 1 lb liver in lemon juice overnight.

Slow-fry 1–2 onions in olive oil and butter until caramelised (you can do this bit quickly, but they are tastier if you make them cook on low for 20 minutes or so).

Remove onions from pan. Turn heat up to medium high.

Rinse liver and pat dry. Season with salt and pepper. Fry quickly on each side until browned. Leave in the pan.

To the pan add about 2 tbsp of balsamic vinegar, plus approx 250 mL of beef stock. Bring to boil and serve.

Liver should be pink in the middle.

I can't imagine this with the artificial taste of stock cubes. Use home-made beef stock, and it is just delicious.

Serves 4–6

Carbohydrate: negligible

Desserts

Many existing dessert recipes can be adapted merely by halving their sugar content. In my experience this makes very little difference to the taste, but a big difference to the carb content. Where you would normally serve with custard, use cream instead.

RICH CHOCOLATE PUDDING

There can't be many people who don't like chocolate, but normally it has far too high a carb count. This pudding isn't bad.

150 g (6 oz) Dark continental chocolate (at least 70% cocoa solids)	284 mL double cream
	250 g Marscapone cheese
	3 tbsp brandy (optional)

Melt chocolate in a bowl over a pan of simmering water. Take the bowl off the heat and add the cream, Marscapone and brandy. Mix together. The hot chocolate will melt the Marscapone and cream.

Divide into six individual dishes and chill for 20 minutes.

Decorate with whipped cream, or serve with pouring cream.

Note: This pudding is very rich and not to be eaten every day, but it is delicious. (Can be frozen.)

Serves 6

Carbohydrate: 12 g

BANANA SOUFFLÉ

Remove the skin and chop five firm bananas very fine. Stir five well beaten eggs into a pint of whipped cream, then quickly stir in the banana pulp.

Turn into a soufflé dish, bake in a quick oven until brown and light. Serve immediately with cream.

Serves 5

Carbohydrate: 30–40 g

Real ice-cream recipes

Most people love ice-cream, but the commercial products are suspect as far as their carbohydrate content – and chemical content – is concerned. Fortunately, *real* ice-cream is not only nicer, it is also healthier and less fattening.

REAL VANILLA ICE-CREAM

4 large eggs
400 mL (¾ pint) whipping or
    double cream

100 g (4 oz) caster sugar
Vanilla essence

Separate the eggs. In a bowl, whisk the egg whites until they are stiff. Add the yolks and sugar.

In another bowl, whip the cream until it is stiff. Combine the cream and the egg mixture and add the vanilla essence, then freeze.

Serves 4

Carbohydrate: 25 g

Some very nice ice-creams can be made quickly and easily using just cream and a sweetened flavour. For example: using whipping cream, whip the cream until it is stiff and combine with lemon curd, or black cherry jam, any other smooth jam or honey.

Note: if lemon curd is used, it must be one made with butter, not margarine.

STRAWBERRIES AND CREAM

Fresh strawberries and cream are delicious, and strawberries are low in carbohydrate. However, normally they are sugared, which increases the carbohydrate content considerably. If you think that you have to add sugar, try this: after washing the fruit, place for about 30 minutes in a pint of water, in which a teaspoon of salt has been mixed, then drain and serve. You will be surprised how much sweeter they taste. The same can be done with raspberries, melon and apple.

Children's recipes

RED FRUIT COMPÔTE

Choose a variety of mainly red, soft fruit: strawberries, raspberries, cherries, papaya, mango, melon, passion fruit, banana, pears, peach, and nectarines. Cut the large fruit into cubes or slices and mix all the fruit in a small amount of fresh orange juice. Marinate for an hour. Serve with unsweetened whipped cream.

FRUIT JELLY

300 mL (½ pt) orange juice
20 g (¾ oz) powdered gelatine
½ a Canteloupe melon, sliced thinly
3 oranges, segmented

3 kiwi fruit, peeled sliced thinly
A few raspberries or strawberries
100 g (4 oz) washed strawberries,
   sliced in halves

Heat half the orange juice in a small saucepan. Off the heat sprinkle in the gelatine and stir well to dissolve. Reheat gently if any grains do not dissolve. Do not allow to boil. Add the rest of the juice, mix and set aside.

Using an empty butter wrapper, lightly grease a large loaf tin. Put the fruit into the tin in neat layers, kiwi fruit first. Scatter the raspberries throughout as you go.

When all the fruit is in, pour in the juice. Put in the fridge to set.

To turn out, run a blunt knife around the sides and warm the bottom. Place a serving plate on top and invert.

Serve with whipped or double cream.

FRESH FRUIT TRIFLE

This is a trifle based on the fruit jelly above.

Any light sponge cake
140 mL (½ pt) double cream

Fruit jelly (see above)
140 mL (½ pt) Greek yogurt

Slice the sponge in half, lengthways and place in the bottom of a serving bowl. Pour over the jelly and place in the fridge to set.

Whisk the cream until it is just firm and fold in the yogurt. Spread this mixture over the jelly.

Decorate the top with the raspberries, or any other fruit except pineapple, but leave this until just before serving to avoid staining the cream.

Surviving Christmas

A low-carb, or at least lower-carb, Christmas need not be as difficult as you might think.

Give turkey a miss at Christmas. Turkey is a much overrated bird – it's dry and fatless. A goose or duck, in that order of preference, are much moister, tastier and more satisfying. These, particularly the goose, will also provide lots of lovely fat to use for frying later, although that will reduce the weight of the bird somewhat. (Goose fat is not only tasty, it is mainly mono-unsaturated, like olive oil.)

The rest of the meal is usually vegetables, which hardly count unless they are root veges, and if you do have the odd roast spud or parsnip – never mind, it's Christmas.

You might think that Christmas cake is a no-no, but it need not be. Use ground almonds in place of flour. As Christmas cake contains lots of fruit, why add sugar? You shouldn't ice it, of course, but icing is so sickly sweet, that it tastes better without anyway.

There is a recipe for Christmas cake below. Make Christmas pudding the same as you would normally, but leave the sugar out. It probably won't taste any less sweet, but you've lowered the carb count by an enormous amount. Eat it with cream instead of custard.

SAGE AND ONION 'STUFFING' TO GO WITH POULTRY

Boil and chop up an onion; add sage, either a few fresh leaves chopped up or a teaspoon of dried leaves. Pour off most of the liquid into a bowl and reserve. Add ground almonds to the onion to make a thick paste, adjusting the consistency with the reserved cooking water as necessary. Season with salt and pepper.

Grease an ovenproof pan, put in the stuffing paste and cook in the oven until brown on top (about 15–20 minutes). Serve with the poultry.

Use the reserved onion water for gravy or use in soups, etc. You could also cook the other Christmas veges in it.

Low(er)-carb Christmas cake

This is the Christmas cake Monica makes. It contains no cereal flour, sugar or treacle, but it is delicious. There is one caveat. This cake will not keep for long so must be frozen if you want to keep it for several weeks. If made within about three weeks of Christmas it may be kept in the fridge.

225 g (8 oz) raisins
140 g (5 oz sultanas
140 g (5 oz) currants
80 g (3 oz) mixed peel
80 g (3 oz) glace cherries

6 large eggs
250 g (9 oz) ground almonds plus a
   little more for coating cake tin
1 tsp baking powder
1 tbsp brandy

Mince all the dried fruit.

Beat eggs in a large bowl, add all the other ingredients and mix thoroughly.

Grease a large round cake tin (Springform is best) and coat with almond flour. Pour in the cake mixture and cover top with foil to stop it browning too soon and drying out. Cook at 180°C, 350°F, Gas mark 4 for 30 minutes, turn down to 160°C, 320°F, Gas mark 3 for approx 1 hour or until skewer comes out clean.

Let the cake cool in the tin before turning out.

Enjoy.

Because it isn't iced, we tend to eat it in a bowl with cream.

Serves 12

Carbohydrate content: Who's counting, it's Christmas

Advanced suggestions

Make your own sausage meat

I call it sausage meat, but as I don't use sausage skins it is probably more accurate to call this a burger mixture. Buy minced pork or beef meat and ask the butcher to make it up into 500 g bags. Freeze all but that which you want immediately.

In a bowl, put 500 g of minced meat and open up with a fork. Sprinkle with a little dried mixed herbs and salt to taste, and mix. Do this several times until you have sufficient herbs and salt and these are well mixed with the meat. This amount will make about 6–8 good-sized burgers. We use them with eggs for breakfast. Try also curry powder, garlic powder, turmeric, cumin, Worcestershire sauce, et cetera for other flavours.

To cook, heat fat in a frying pan, cut out a lump about the size of a large egg, place in the frying pan and spread to a flat about 12 mm (½ inch) thick. (I find this easier than making burgers.) Fry for about 4 minutes each side.

The rest, if it will be used within three days, can be kept in a sealed bowl in the fridge.

Cure your own bacon

You have probably already found that supermarket bacon is terrible – all slimy and wet, and when you fry it, it spits and exudes a load of gunge that sticks to the pan. This is because bacon is not cured these days, it is 'pumped'. Bacon is sold by weight: the more it weighs, the more it costs you. So, to increase the weight cheaply, it's filled with water – and other things, but you don't have to buy it. Farmers' markets are usually a good source of 'dry-cured' bacon and, if you have the right equipment, curing your own bacon need not be difficult.

You will need space in a fridge with a temperature between 2.5° and 6.0°C (35° to 41°F). Too warm and the meat may spoil, too cold and it won't cure properly. You also need something to put the bacon in. I use a plastic washing up bowl, but a shallower tray may be easier.

Buy as much belly of pork as you can handle and as fatty as you can get it. I would suggest a side of about 12 lb. Gloucester Old Spot is a good bacon pig in the UK. Ask the butcher to bone it out.

Mix 2 parts sea salt with 1 part caster sugar. This is the cure (the salt and sugar will not be eaten). Sea salt is too coarse to use as it is, so use a blender's coffee grinder attachment to grind the salt to a fine powder and mix it with the sugar.

Cut off as much pork as will fit in the bowl. Rub the cure mixture all over it, paying attention to the ends and inside where the bones have been removed. It doesn't have to be put on thickly. When it is covered, place in the bowl, put the bowl in the fridge and tilt it so that liquid from the bacon runs to one end, or place the meat on a wire tray. The aim when curing bacon is to remove the moisture from it by osmosis. This mixture will do that.

Each day for a week pour away the water that has run out from the bowl and recoat the meat with cure.

After about seven to ten days, depending on thickness, the bacon should be ready to eat. Rinse the outside of the bacon to remove the cure, pat dry, and slice. Keep in the fridge or freeze what cannot be used within a week.

I find that I can do 12 lb at a time this way by stacking one piece on top of another. They last me about a month.

The sugar is not essential but if salt alone is used it is a bit sharp to the taste. The sugar takes this away. You will note that I do not use nitrates or nitrites; these are not necessary.

You could also buy a commercially produced cure; there are several available via the Internet. The method of curing is similar, however.

Index

Index

About the author

Barry Groves, who lives with his wife, Monica, in the Oxfordshire Cotswolds, can rightfully claim to be Britain's leading exponent of the low-carb way of life as he has lived on, researched, lectured and written about it for well over 40 years.

He and Monica were overweight from 1957 to 1962, when he discovered the low-carb regime for weight loss. It worked: they haven't been overweight since. This started his questioning of conventional diets. As a consequence he took up full-time research into the relationship between diet and 'diseases of civilisation' such as obesity, diabetes, heart disease and cancer.

As a result of his researches, he realised that the perceived wisdoms, both of low-calorie dieting for weight loss and 'healthy eating' for the control of heart disease, were seriously flawed.

Now an award winning international author with a doctorate in nutritional science, Barry has written both popular and more technical books which have been published in countries as far apart as Argentina and Russia, as well as all English-speaking countries.

He currently divides his time between researching and writing books, and lecturing to medical professionals and to the food industry about the management and prevention of obesity, diabetes and associated conditions. He also gives less technical talks to Rotary, Women's Institute, Probus, and similar groups.

Barry Groves is a director of the Foundation for Thymic Cancer Research, (www.thymic.org), an honorary board member of the Weston A. Price Foundation, (www.westonaprice.org), a founder member of The International Network of Cholesterol Sceptics (www.thincs.org), and a founder member of the Fluoride Action Network (www.fluoridealert.org). He also maintains an internationally respected health information website at www.second-opinions.co.uk.

Barry Groves does not confine himself to medical and dietary research. With a long-term interest in energy conservation, he and his wife, Monica, designed and built their own solar-heated house over three years from 1977 to 1980.

For relaxation, in 1982, Barry took up archery. He has been a British Champion every year since 1987 taking over 20 British records. He is also a six times World Champion with five World Records.